AORTIC VALVE

Edited by **Ying-Fu Chen** and **Chwan-Yau Luo**

Aortic Valve
Edited by Ying-Fu Chen and Chwan-Yau Luo

Published by InTech
Janeza Trdine 9, 51000 Rijeka, Croatia

Publishing Process Manager Alenka Urbancic

Technical Editor Teodora Smiljanic

Cover Designer InTech Design Team

Additional hard copies can be obtained from orders@intechopen.com

Aortic Valve, Edited by Ying-Fu Chen and Chwan-Yau Luo
p. cm.
ISBN 978-953-307-561-7

For EU product safety concerns:
IN TECH d.o.o., Prolaz Marije Krucifikse Kozulić 3, 51000 Rijeka, Croatia, info@intechopen.com or visit our website at intechopen.com.

Meet the editors

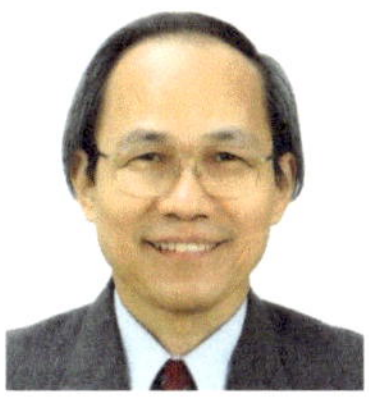

Dr. Ying-Fu Chen was born in Changhua, Taiwan, in 1946. He received an MD degree from Kaohsiung Medical College, Kaohsiung, Taiwan, in 1973, and a PhD degree from Graduate Institute of Medicine, Kaohsiung Medical University, in 1992.

In 1983, Dr. Chen was a clinical fellow at the Heart Institute of Japan, Tokyo Women Medical University in 1983, before moving to Durham, North Carolina in 1985, where he worked as a research fellow at the Duke University Medical Center. He was appointed Professor of Surgery at the Kaohsiung Medical University in 1992, and is currently appointed Professor of Graduate Institute of Medicine as well, also at the Kaohsiung Medical University. His main research interests include stem cells and inflammation in basic studies, and thoracic aorta aneurysms/dissections in clinical fields. He has served as an editor of 2 books and is also an editorial member of several national and international journals. Currently, he also serves as a managing editor of Frontiers of Bioscience.

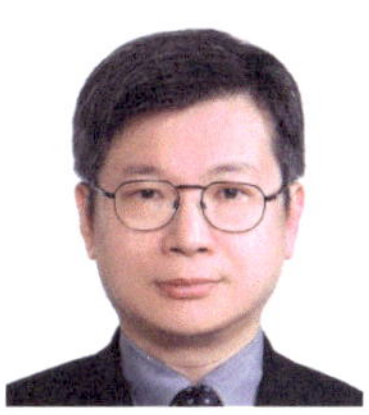

Dr. Chwan-Yau Luo received his MD degree from Kaohsiung Medical University, Kaohsiung, Taiwan, in 1986, and his Master of Science in Experimental Surgery, under the supervision of Prof. Ray C-J Chiu, from McGill University, Montreal, Canada, in 2004. He was trained in thoracic organ transplantation at Papworth Hospital at Cambridge University, England, in 1999. Currently, he is the Chief of the Cardiovascular Surgery Department, Director of the Heart Transplantation and Mechanical Circulatory Assisted Device Programs, and an active cardiovascular surgeon at National Cheng Kung University Hospital in Tainan, Taiwan. Moreover, he is also an Associate Professor and a Fellow of the Cardiovascular Research Center at National Cheng Kung University. His current clinical research interest is focused on the surgical treatment of heart failure, including heart transplantation, mechanically assisted support and post-transplantation therapeutic immunosuppressive drug monitoring. In addition, his basic research interest is concentrated on angiogenesis therapies for peripheral artery occlusive disease.

Contents

Preface

The book "**Aortic Valve**" is comprised of 18 chapters and is further organized into seven sections. **Section I** (Basic Science) includes two chapters. In Chapter 1 titled "Rapid quantitation of aortic valve flow using spiral Fourier velocity encoded MRI" by Joao LA Carvalho and Krishna S Nayak, the authors introduced spiral Fourier velocity encoding, a new method for rapid and non-invasive measurement of cardiovascular blood flow using magnetic resonance imaging (MRI), which is capable of accurately capturing peak velocities in flow jets due to stenosis or regurgitation. In Chapter 2, titled "State-of-the-art methods for the numerical simulation of aortic BMHVs" by Annerel Sebastiaan et al., the authors say that modern bileaflet mechanical heart valves (BMHVs) are still far from perfect and still face major design challenges. Authors introduce that numerical simulation techniques can provide valuable information and are considered as crucial in order to gain insights into the blood flow, and assess the performance of future valve prototypes. **Section II** (General Consideration of Aortic Valve Disease) includes chapter 3 with the title "Aortic valve disease from etiology to bedside" by Shahab Shahrzad and Samira Taban. The authors provide basic information that is essential to understanding aortic root anatomy and the general knowledge of aortic valve diseases, including management. **Section III** (Infective Endocarditis) includes two chapters covering infective endocarditis. Chapter 4, "Aortic valve endocarditis" by Lazar Velicki and Chapter titled "Native and prosthetic aortic valve endocarditis" by Ioan Tilea et al. These chapters describe various aspects of native and prosthetic aortic valve endocarditis, including epidemiology, pathogenesis, clinical presentation, microbiology, diagnosis, complications and updated medical and surgical treatments, and it will be informative to readers. **Section IV** (Aortic Sclerosis / Aortic Stenosis) includes two chapters. In Chapter 6, "The progression of aortic sclerosis to aortic stenosis" by Uzma Jalal et al., the authors propose some thoughts that early, aggressive medical intervention be undertaken before the irrevocable process of calcification occurs. Chapter 7, titled "Calcific aortic valve disease" by Jesper Hjortnaes and Elena Aikawa, attempts to characterize the studies that have identified the molecular biology of calcific aortic valve disease, to understand the cellular mechanisms of the disease, and potentially preventing this disease procession. **Section V** (Bioprosthetic Valve) includes two chapters on cardiac valvular prosthesis. Chapter 8 which is titled "Clinical and hemodynamic performance of the Sorin Mitroflow pericardial bioprothesis" by Jamieson et al., and Chapter 9, "Influence of prosthesis-patient mismatch on survival with aortic valve replacement" by Jamieson et al. These chapters describe the various issues of cardiac prostheses including the newly developed bioprosthesis with excellent hemodynamic performance and a comprehensive review of prosthesis-patient mismatch after aortic valve replacement. **Section VI** (Transcatheter Aortic Valve Implantation) is comprised of four chapters. Chapter 10, "Current indications for transcatheter aortic valve implantation" by Ibrahim Akin et al. Chapter 11, "Transcatheter aortic valve implantation: State of the art" by Alice Le Huu et al., Chapter 12, "Transcatheter aortic valve implantation" by Hunaid A Vohra et al. These chapters provide the most recent evidence of transcatheter aortic valve implantation that has recently emerged as an effective therapeutic alternative to conventional aortic valve replacement for high-risk patients with severe aortic valvular stenosis. In Chapter 13, titled "Image-guided transcatheter aortic valve implantation assistance system" by Mohamed Esmail Karar et al. the authors have developed a novel system to overcome the current technical difficulties with the TAVI under 2D fluoroscopy guidance. It would be a promising design for helping the physician more accurately to put the aortic valve prosthesis in the exact position. **The Last Section** (Congenital Anomalies of the Aortic Valve) includes 5 chapters. Chapters 14, "Unicuspid aortic valve" by Venkata Thota and Farouk Mookadam, and 15, "Bicuspid aortic valve" by Blerim Berisha et al. clearly describe the anomalies of the congenital aortic valve diseases from the perspective of embryology, epidemiology, clinical presentation, diagnosis, and treatment. In Chapter 16, which is titled "A case-control investigation of the relation between bicuspid aortic valve disease and coronary heart disease", by Mehmet Necded Akkus, the author conducts a prospective case-control study to search for a relationship between bicuspid aortic valve disease and coronary artery disease. Chapter 17, "Novel phenotypes in bicuspid aortic valve disease" by Evaldas Girdauskas et al. addresses the recent updated phenotype studies of bicuspid aortic valve disease. It is a novel concept and comprehensive to the readers. The final chapter is titled "Surgical treatment of bicuspid aortic valve disease", written by Ying-Fu Chen and Shou-Tsan Lee. The authors describe the updated information regarding surgical treatment for patients with bicuspid aortic valve disease, including balloon valvuloplasty, valve replacement, Ross procedure, repair of regurgitant valve, valve-sparing aortic root replacement, and ascending aortic replacement.

In assuming the editorship of this book, we felt it was important to publish it as soon as possible to maximize the effect of the most up-to-date knowledge in the field of aortic valve for the reader. While we hope this book will be particularly useful to cardiologists and cardiovascular surgeons and trainees, we also believe that this book will be a valuable resource for radiologists, cardiovascular anesthesiologist, and other healthcare professionals who have a special interest in treating or caring for patients with aortic valve disease.

We wish to express our gratitude to many people whose efforts made completion of this book possible. We are especially indebted to our esteemed contributing authors, who generously shared their extraordinary expertise and timely contribution. We sincerely appreciate the efforts of the team at InTech Open Access Publisher, especially publishing process managers, including Alenka Urbacic, and Zeljko Spalj, who patiently, with the editorial process, led to the production process, and editorial consultant, Viktorija Zgela, who invited us to carry out this very important book. We are indebted to our English editor, Bill Franke, at National Cheng Kung University in Tainan. His help has been incredibly important, and his experience is invaluable. We are also very grateful to Man-Lin Chen and Shan-Tsu Kuo, the administrative assistants in the Division of Cardiovascular Surgery and Graduate Institute of Medicine at Kaohsiung Medical University, who were extremely helpful and have made important contributions to this book.

Finally, we wish to acknowledge the support of our families and the many sacrifices they have made to make this book possible. Our wives, Jane-Jane Wang and Ruey-Ling Huang, were our greatest support and encouragement, whose love and support make it all worthwhile.

Ying-Fu Chen, MD, PhD
Professor
Division of Cardiovascular Surgery,
Kaohsiung Medical University Hospital
Graduate Institute of Medicine,
Kaohsiung Medical University
Kaohsiung,
Taiwan

Chwan-Yau Luo, MD, MSc
Associate Professor
Division of Cardiovascular Surgery,
National Cheng Kung University Hospital
School of Medicine,
National Cheng Kung University
Tainan,
Taiwan

Part 1

Basic Science

1

Rapid Quantitation of Aortic Valve Flow Using Spiral Fourier Velocity Encoded MRI

Joao L. A. Carvalho[1] and Krishna S. Nayak[2]
[1]*Universidade de Brasília*
[2]*University of Southern California*
[1]*Brazil*
[2]*USA*

1. Introduction

Aortic stenosis consists in a narrowing or incomplete opening of the aortic valve. This typically alters the blood flow, causing turbulent and/or complex flow jets. Such jets display peak velocities considerably higher than those of normal flow, and a much broader range of flow velocities. Another form of aortic valve disease is aortic insufficiency, or regurgitation. This condition occurs when the aortic valve fails to close completely. This is also known as "leaky valve", as flow jets in the reverse direction are observed when no flow should occur. The visualization and quantitation of cardiovascular blood flow is an important component of the assessment of aortic valve disease. For example, peak velocity measurements in flow jets are used to estimate pressure drop, which is an indicator of the hemodynamic load of a stenosis (Tsai et al., 1999).

1.1 Doppler ultrasound

The current non-invasive gold standard for flow quantitation is Doppler ultrasound. The ultrasound equipment is relatively inexpensive, small, and portable. Measurements are typically obtained in real-time, with excellent temporal resolution. The most popular techniques for ultrasound flow assessment are color Doppler and spectral Doppler.
Evaluation by ultrasound is impossible when there is air, bone, or surgical scar in the ultrasound path. Examination by ultrasound in obese patients is difficult, as the overlying adipose tissue (fat) scatters the sound waves. Doppler flow measurements may be inaccurate when the ultrasound beam cannot be properly aligned with the vessel axis, requiring measured velocities to be "angle-corrected" by the operator. Peak-velocity overestimation on the order of 18–40% have been reported in the literature (Hoskins, 1996; Winkler & Wu, 1995), usually due to spectral broadening at large insonation angles, and to Doppler gain settings.

1.2 Magnetic resonance imaging

Magnetic resonance imaging (MRI) is potentially the most appropriate technique for addressing all aspects of cardiovascular disease examination, which includes assessing myocardial function and perfusion, as well as visualizing and measuring blood flow. MRI overcomes the acoustical window limitations of ultrasound, potentially allowing flow measurements to be obtained along any direction, and for any vessel in the cardiovascular system. Magnetic resonance (MR) measurements are also less operator-dependent than those of Doppler ultrasound, and the true direction of flow can generally be precisely measured. The main MR techniques for measuring flow are phase contrast and Fourier velocity encoding. These techniques are introduced below, and will be discussed in further detail in section 2.

1.2.1 Phase contrast

Phase contrast (O'Donnell, 1985) is a technique in which a bipolar gradient (see section 2) aligned with the axis of flow is used to obtain a velocity measurement associated with each pixel (or "voxel") of the image. In practice, two acquisitions are used, and the first moment of the bipolar gradient is varied between measurements. The velocity estimate is obtained from the phase difference between the images obtained in each acquisition.

Phase contrast can be combined with dynamic (cine) MRI (Glover & Pelc, 1988), in which short acquisitions and some form of cardiac synchronization are used to produce images throughout the cardiac cycle. The combined technique (cine phase contrast) can depict motion and flow throughout the cardiac cycle (Nayler et al., 1986). Alternatively, phase contrast can be combined with real-time MRI (Holsinger et al., 1990; Riederer et al., 1988), in which the encodings are applied sequentially, periodically, and continuously. In real-time MRI, images are formed by sliding a window along the acquired data and reconstructing an image for each position of the window. The display of real-time phase contrast data is typically implemented as color overlay of flow information (phase difference) over the anatomical (magnitude) image, which is called real-time color flow (Nayak et al., 2000; Riederer et al., 1991).

In phase contrast, data inconsistency, partial volume effects, and intravoxel phase dispersion can lead to peak velocity underestimation (Clarke et al., 1996; Tang et al., 1993). Partial voluming is particularly problematic when flow is highly localized and/or turbulent. When a large voxel size is adopted to measure the flow rate, not only may moving spins and stationary spins coexist in a voxel, but also the velocity distribution of spins within a voxel may spread over a wide range of velocities. This results in signal loss, distortion and erroneous velocity estimates. As a result, phase contrast imaging can not provide accurate peak velocity measurements in turbulent and/or complex flow jets. Such jets are commonly observed in narrowed vessels, and in valves presenting stenotis and/or regurgitation.

1.2.2 Fourier velocity encoding

The limitations mentioned above can be overcome using Fourier velocity encoding (FVE) (Moran, 1982). FVE can be considered the MR equivalent to spectral Doppler. In this technique, the full spectrum of velocities within each voxel is measured by phase-encoding the velocity information in Fourier domain. Therefore, FVE is robust to partial voluming, and flow measurements from low spatial resolution images are still accurate (Tsai et al., 1999). FVE shows satisfactory agreement with Doppler ultrasound (Mohiaddin et al., 1997). However, it is typically not used clinically, because the acquisition time required by this technique is in principle considerably longer than that of phase contrast.

Different approaches to accelerating FVE have been proposed. One example is the use of two-dimensional cylindrical excitation to restrict the field-of-view to a beam that can be imaged without phase encoding (Dumoulin et al., 1991). This approach makes it possible to perform spatial encoding and velocity encoding simultaneously, and in a single pulse repetition time (TR) (DiCarlo et al., 2005; Hu et al., 1993; Irarrazabal et al., 1993; Macgowan et al., 2005). This allows FVE measurements to be obtained in real-time. However, real-time FVE has problems related to the precise placement of the imaging beam, especially when the

region of interest (e.g., mitral valve) moves during the cardiac cycle. Other problems include the large voxel size and low temporal resolution.
FVE has also been accelerated by simply neglecting spatial encoding along one of the spatial dimensions (Feinberg et al., 1985; Hennig et al., 1988), or by acquiring velocity images with no spatial encoding other than slice selection (Galea et al., 2002). In these techniques, the velocity measurement is a projection of all signal along a line or a plane in 3D space, respectively. As a consequence, both methods have dynamic range issues, as the signal of flowing blood has to be distinguished from all the background signal from static tissue observed along the projection. Furthermore, these approaches are unable to resolve different sources of flow that may co-exist in the projected line or plane.

1.3 Chapter outline

This chapter introduces spiral FVE, a novel method for MR flow quantitation that addresses the limitations discussed above. The proposed method provides fully-localized time-velocity distribution measurements, in a single acquisition, that is one short breath-hold long (approximately 10 seconds). Spiral FVE uses conventional slice-selective excitation (Bernstein et al., 2004; Nishimura, 2010), which excites (selects) a thin slice of the body to be imaged. The two-dimensional plane defined by this slice is imaged using spiral acquisitions (Ahn et al., 1986; Meyer et al., 1992), which encode both spatial dimensions simultaneously. Therefore, no spatial encoding is neglected, and measurements are fully localized in 3D space. 2D-resolved spatial encoding allows for easy localization of the region of interest, and the ability to resolve multiple sources of through-plane flow in the imaged field-of-view, without requiring static tissue suppression. Scan-plane prescription is performed using classic protocols, which is considerably less laborious than the beam-placing process used in real-time FVE.
Without acceleration, spiral FVE presents some limitations: (1) insufficient velocity field-of-view (the maximum range of velocities allowed without aliasing); (2) low in-plane spatial resolution, which limits the ability of spatially localizing the flow; (3) long readouts, which causes spatial blurring at 3 T, due to off-resonance effects (Noll, Meyer, Pauly, Nishimura & Macovski, 1991); and (4) moderate temporal resolution, which may blur certain features of the flow waveform. We address these limitations using the following acceleration techniques: variable-density spirals (Tsai & Nishimura, 2000), partial Fourier reconstruction (Noll, Nishimura & Macovski, 1991), and temporal acceleration (Madore et al., 1999; Tsao, 2002). By combining these techniques, we achieve a total 18-fold acceleration in spiral FVE.

2. MR flow imaging

2.1 Basic principles of MRI

MRI is a modality uniquely capable of imaging all aspects of heart disease, and is a potential "one-stop shop" for cardiovascular health assessment. MRI can generate cross-sectional images in any plane (including oblique planes), and can also measure blood flow. The image acquisition is based on using strong magnetic fields and non-ionizing radiation in the radio frequency range, which are harmless to the patient.
The main component of a MRI scanner is a strong magnetic field, called the B_0 field. This magnetic field is always on, even when the scanner is not being used. Typically, MR is used to image hydrogen nuclei, because of its abundance in the human body. Spinning charged particles (or "spins"), such as hydrogen nuclei, act like a tiny bar magnet, presenting a very small magnetic field, emanating from the south pole to the north pole. In normal conditions,

each nucleus points to a random direction, resulting in a null net magnetization. However, in the presence of an external magnetic field (such as the B_0 field), they will line up with that field. However, they will not all line up in the same direction. Approximately half will point north, and half will point south. Slightly more than half of these spins (about one in a million) will point north, creating a small net magnetization M_0, which is strong enough to be detected. The net magnetization is proportional to the strength of the B_0 field, so MRI scanners with stronger magnetic fields (e.g., 3 Tesla) provide higher signal-to-noise ratio (SNR).

Another important component of the scanner are the gradient coils. There are typically three gradient coils (G_x, G_y, and G_z), that produce an intentional perturbation in the B_0 field when turned on ("played"). This perturbation varies linearly along each spatial direction (x, y and z), such that no perturbation is perceived at the iso-center of the magnet when these gradients are used. In the presence of an external magnetic field, the spins rotate about the axis of that field. B_0 is (approximately) spatially uniform, so all spins initially rotate at the same frequency (the Larmor frequency), $\omega = \gamma B_0$, where γ is the gyromagnetic ratio (γ = 42.6 MHz/Tesla for hydrogen protons). However, when any of the gradients is played, the magnetic field becomes spatially varying, and so does the rotation frequency of the spins. Therefore, G_x, G_y, and G_z are used to frequency-encode (or phase-encode) spatial position along the x, y and z directions, respectively.

The final major component of the MR scanner is the radio-frequency (RF) coil. This is used to transmit a RF "excitation" pulse to the body, and also to receive the frequency-encoded signal from the "excited" portion of the body. In practice, independent coils may be used for transmission and reception. The RF pulse is typically modulated to the Larmor frequency. While B_0 is aligned with the z-axis (by definition), B_1, which is a very weak magnetic field associated with the RF pulse, is aligned with the x-axis (also by definition). When the RF pulse is played, some of the spins which are in resonance with the RF pulse (i.e., rotating at the RF pulse's frequency) will now begin to rotate around the x-axis (thus the name magnetic resonance). This tilts the net magnetization towards the x-y plane, and the net magnetization will now have a component in the x-y plane (M_{xy}).

The RF pulse is typically designed to have a somewhat rectangular profile in Fourier domain, centered at the modulation frequency (e.g., a modulated windowed sinc). This implies that the RF pulse in fact contains a certain range of frequencies, thus all spins rotating within that range become "excited", or tilted towards the x-axis. So, by playing gradient(s) of an appropriate amplitude, and designing the RF pulse accordingly, one can excite only a thin slice of the body, which correspond to the region containing all spins that are in resonance with the RF pulse's range of frequencies. Excitation profiles other than "slices" may also be obtained (e.g., a pencil beam, or cylindrical excitation (Hu et al., 1993)), by designing an appropriate gradient/pulse combination.

When the RF pulse is turned off, M_{xy} begins to rotate (at the Larmor frequency) around the z-axis, as the net magnetization begins to realign with B_0. This rotating magnetization generates an oscillating signal, which can be detected by the receive coil. The frequency content of the received signal can be used to obtain spatial information about the excited portion of the body. In order to frequency-encode spatial information, gradients are also played during signal acquisition. These are called readout gradients. For imaging a slice perpendicular to the z-axis (an axial image) , G_z is played during excitation (for slice-selection), and G_x and G_y are played during acquisition. These can be switched, for acquiring sagittal or coronal images, or all three gradients may be used during both excitation and acquisition to image oblique planes.

When the readout gradients are played, the acquired signal at a particular time instant corresponds to the sum of different sinusoidal signals generated by spins located at different regions of the body, each rotating at different frequencies corresponding to their spatial locations. If an axial slice is being acquired, for example, the demodulated signal value is equivalent to a sample of the Fourier transform $M(k_x, k_y)$ of the cross-sectional image $m(x, y)$. In this case, by changing the amplitudes of G_x and G_y during acquisition, one may acquire different samples of $M(k_x, k_y)$. In fact, by playing G_x and/or G_y, one can move along the k_x-k_y plane (which is known in MRI as k-space), collecting samples of $M(k_x, k_y)$. When enough samples of $M(k_x, k_y)$ have been collected, an inverse Fourier transform produces $m(x, y)$.
The required coverage of k-space, and the number of samples, depend on the specified spatial resolution and field-of-view. For low spatial resolution imaging, only the central portion of k_x-k_y needs to be sampled. For higher spatial resolution, the periphery of k-space must also be covered. The field of view is associated with the spacing between samples. For a larger field-of-view, k-space needs to be more densely sampled, requiring an increased number of samples. If k-space is not sufficiently sampled, and the resulting field-of-view is not large enough to cover the entire object, overlap in spatial domain is observed (aliasing).
Because signal amplitude is lost as the net magnetization realigns with B_0 (this is called relaxation), multiple acquisitions (excitation + readout) may be needed in order to cover the entire k-space. Different trajectories are more efficient in covering k-space than others. For example, spiral imaging, which uses oscillating gradients to achieve spiral k-space trajectories (Figure 1b), are generally faster than 2DFT imaging, i.e., require fewer acquisitions. In 2DFT imaging, each acquisition readout acquires a single line of k-space, sampling k_x-k_y in a Cartesian fashion (Figure 1a). This is generally slower, but may be advantageous in some applications with respect to the nature of associated image artifacts. The fashion in which RF pulses and gradients are played is called pulse sequence. The time between acquisitions is called pulse repetition time, or TR.

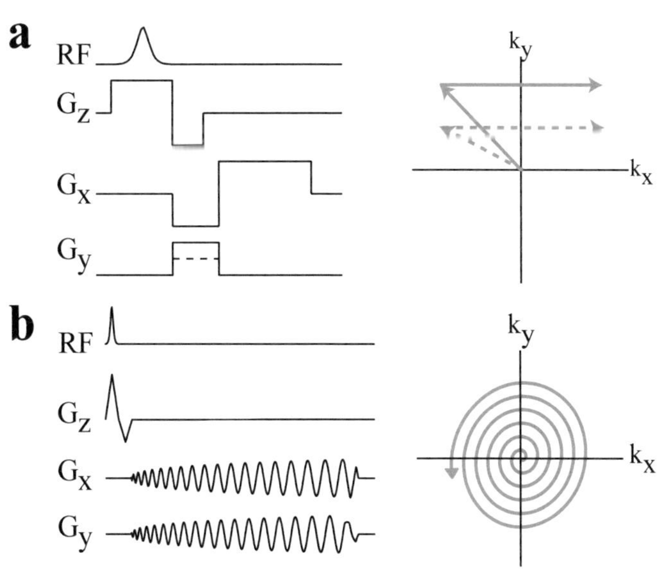

Fig. 1. Timing diagram (left) and corresponding k-space trajectories (right) for (a) 2DFT, and (b) spiral acquisitions.

2.2 Mathematical formalism

As discussed on section 2.1, the acquired MR signal $s(t)$ at a particular time instant corresponds to a sample of the Fourier transform $M(k_x, k_y)$ of the cross-sectional image $m(x,y)$:

$$M(k_x, k_y) = \int_x \int_y m(x,y)\, e^{-j2\pi(k_x x + k_y y)}\, dx\, dy. \quad (1)$$

The Fourier coordinates k_x and k_y vary with time, according to the zeroth moment of the readout gradients G_x and G_y:

$$k_x(t) = \frac{\gamma}{2\pi} \int_0^t G_x(\tau)\, d\tau \quad (2)$$

$$k_y(t) = \frac{\gamma}{2\pi} \int_0^t G_y(\tau)\, d\tau. \quad (3)$$

These equations explain how the gradients can be used to "move" along k-space, as discussed on section 2.1. This formalism can be generalized for any combination of the gradients G_x, G_y and G_z as:

$$M(\vec{k}_r) = \int_{\vec{r}} m(\vec{r}) \cdot e^{-j2\pi \vec{k}_r \cdot \vec{r}}\, d\vec{r} \quad (4)$$

$$\vec{k}_r(t) = \frac{\gamma}{2\pi} \int_0^t \vec{G}_r(\tau)\, d\tau, \quad (5)$$

where $\vec{G}_r$ is the oblique gradient resulting from the combination of the G_x, G_y and G_z gradients, and $\vec{r}$ is its corresponding axis, along which the linear variation in magnetic field intensity is perceived.

Given a spatial position function $\vec{r}(t)$ and a magnetic field gradient $\vec{G}_r(t)$, the magnetization phase is:

$$\phi(\vec{r}, t) = \gamma \int_0^t \vec{G}_r(\tau) \cdot \vec{r}(\tau)\, d\tau, \quad (6)$$

For static spins, $\vec{r}(t)$ is constant ($\vec{r}$), and this becomes:

$$\phi = \gamma \vec{r} \cdot \int_0^t \vec{G}_r(\tau)\, d\tau \quad (7)$$

$$= 2\pi \vec{k}_r \cdot \vec{r}, \quad (8)$$

as in the exponential in equation 4.

2.3 Principles of MR flow imaging

The basic principles of quantitative flow measurement using magnetic resonance were first proposed by Singer (1959) and Hahn (1960) in the late 1950's. However, clinical applications of MR flow quantitation weren't reported until the early 1980's (Moran et al., 1985; Nayler et al., 1986; Singer & Crooks, 1983; van Dijk, 1984). Current MR flow imaging methods are based on the fact that spins moving at a constant velocity accrue a phase proportional to the

velocity times the first moment of the gradient waveform along the direction in which they are moving.
For spins moving along the $\vec{r}$-axis with a constant velocity $\vec{v}$, and initial position $\vec{r}_0$, we can write $\vec{r}(t) = \vec{r_0} + \vec{v}t$. Rewriting equation 6, for $t = t_0$:

$$\phi = \gamma \int_0^{t_0} \vec{G}_r(t) \cdot (\vec{r}_0 + \vec{v}t)\, dt \tag{9}$$

$$= \gamma \vec{r}_0 \cdot \int_0^{t_0} \vec{G}_r(t)\, dt + \gamma \vec{v} \cdot \int_0^{t_0} \vec{G}_r(t)\, t\, dt \tag{10}$$

$$= \gamma \vec{r}_0 \cdot \vec{M}_0 + \gamma \vec{v} \cdot \vec{M}_1, \tag{11}$$

where $\vec{M}_0$ and $\vec{M}_1$ are the zeroth and first moments of the $\vec{r}$-gradient waveform at echo time, respectively. Thus, if a gradient with null zeroth moment is used (e.g., a bipolar gradient, aligned with $\vec{v}$), the phase accrued for a constant velocity spin is $\phi = \gamma \vec{v} \cdot \vec{M}_1$.
Therefore, if a bipolar gradient waveform is played between the excitation and the readout, the phase measured in a pixel of the acquired image is directly proportional to the velocity of the spins contained within its corresponding voxel. However, factors other than flow (such as inhomogeneities of the magnetic field) may cause additional phase shifts that would cause erroneous interpretation of the local velocity (Rebergen et al., 1993).

2.3.1 Phase contrast

The phase contrast method addresses the problem mentioned above by using two gradient-echo data acquisitions in which the first moment of the bipolar gradient waveform is varied between measurements (O'Donnell, 1985). The velocity in each voxel is measured as:

$$v(x,y) = \frac{\phi_a(x,y) - \phi_b(x,y)}{\gamma(M_1^a - M_1^b)}, \tag{12}$$

where $\phi_a(x,y)$ and $\phi_b(x,y)$ are the phase images acquired in each acquisition, and M_1^a and M_1^b are the first moment of the bipolar gradients used in each acquisition.

2.3.2 Fourier velocity encoding

While phase contrast provides a single velocity measurement associated with each voxel, Fourier velocity encoding (FVE) (Moran, 1982) provides a velocity histogram for each spatial location, which is a measurement of the velocity distribution within each voxel.
FVE involves phase-encoding along a velocity dimension. Instead of only two acquisitions, as in phase contrast, multiple acquisitions are performed, and a bipolar gradient with a different amplitude (and first moment) is used in each acquisition. Equation 10 can be rewritten as:

$$\phi(\vec{r}, \vec{v}, t) = 2\pi(\vec{k}_r \cdot \vec{r} + \vec{k}_v \cdot \vec{v}), \tag{13}$$

where $\vec{k}_v$ is the velocity frequency variable associated with $\vec{v}$, and is proportional to the first moment of $\vec{G}_r(t)$:

$$\vec{k}_v = \frac{\gamma}{2\pi} \vec{M}_1. \tag{14}$$

Each voxel of the two-dimensional image is associated with a distribution of velocities. This three-dimensional function, $m(x, y, v)$, is associated with a three-dimensional Fourier space, $M(k_x, k_y, k_v)$. Thus, an extra dimension is added to k-space, and multiple acquisitions are required to cover the entire k_x-k_y-k_v space. In order to move along k_v, a bipolar gradient with the appropriate amplitude (and first moment) is played before the k_x-k_y readout gradients, in each acquisition. Placing the bipolar gradient along the z-axis will encode through-plane velocities. Placing the bipolar gradient along x or y will encode in-plane velocities. Oblique flow can be encoded using a combination of bipolar gradients along the x, y and z axes.
Each acquisition along k_v is called a velocity encode. The number of required velocity encodes depends on the desired velocity resolution and velocity field-of-view (the maximum range of velocities measured without aliasing). For example, to obtain a 25 cm/s resolution over a 600 cm/s field-of-view, 24 velocity encodes are needed. The velocity distributions along the cross-sectional image $m(x, y, v)$ is obtained by inverse Fourier transforming the acquired data $M(k_x, k_y, k_v)$. If cine imaging (Glover & Pelc, 1988) is used, measurements are also time resolved, resulting in a four-dimensional dataset: $m(x, y, v, t)$.
The main drawback of FVE is scan time, as k_x-k_y should be fully sampled for each value of k_v. As discussed in section 1.2.2, different approaches to accelerating FVE have been proposed. Those techniques are typically inefficient in spatially separating flowing blood from nearby static tissue. Furthermore, they are not capable of resolving multiple flows in a single acquisition. The spiral FVE method, proposed in section 4, addresses these limitations.

3. Experimental setup

Most experiments were performed on a Signa 3 T EXCITE HD system (GE Healthcare), with gradients capable of 40 mT/m amplitude and 150 T/m/s slew rate, and a receiver with sampling interval of 4 μs. Sequence designs were optimized for this scanner configuration. The body coil was used for RF transmission in all studies. An 8-channel phase array cardiac coil was used in the healthy volunteer studies, but data from only 1 or 2 elements were used in reconstruction. In phantom studies, a single channel 5-inch surface coil was used. In the patient experiments presented in section 4, a Signa 1.5 T LX system (GE Healthcare) with the same gradient and receiver configuration was used, and acquisition was performed using a 5-inch surface coil.
The institutional review boards of the University of Southern California and Stanford University approved the imaging protocols. Subjects were screened for magnetic resonance imaging risk factors and provided informed consent in accordance with institutional policy.

4. Slice-selective FVE with spiral readouts (spiral FVE)

In order to address the limitations of existing flow imaging methods, we propose the use of slice-selective FVE MRI with spiral acquisitions. The proposed spiral FVE method is capable of acquiring fully localized, time-resolved velocity distributions in a short breath-hold. Scan-plane prescription is performed using classic protocols.
We present practical implementations for measuring blood flow through the aortic valve, and comparisons with Doppler ultrasound and high-resolution 2DFT phase contrast MRI. The proposed method is demonstrated in healthy volunteers and in a patient.

4.1 Pulse sequence

The spiral FVE imaging pulse sequence (Figure 2) consists of a slice-selective excitation, a velocity-encoding bipolar gradient, a spiral readout, and refocusing and spoiling gradients. The dataset corresponding to each temporal frame is a stack-of-spirals in k_x-k_y-k_v space (Figure 3). The bipolar gradient effectively phase-encodes in k_v, while each spiral readout acquires one "disc" in k_x-k_y.

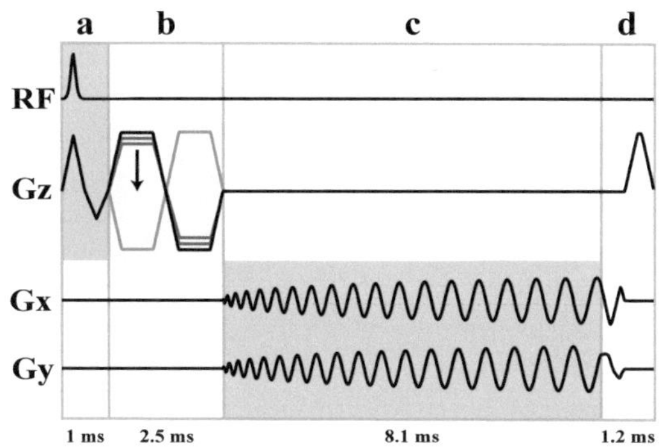

Fig. 2. Spiral FVE pulse sequence. It consists of (a) slice selective excitation, (b) velocity encoding bipolar gradient, (c) spiral readout, and (d) refocusing and spoiling gradients. This timing corresponds to the studies shown in Figures 5 and 6.

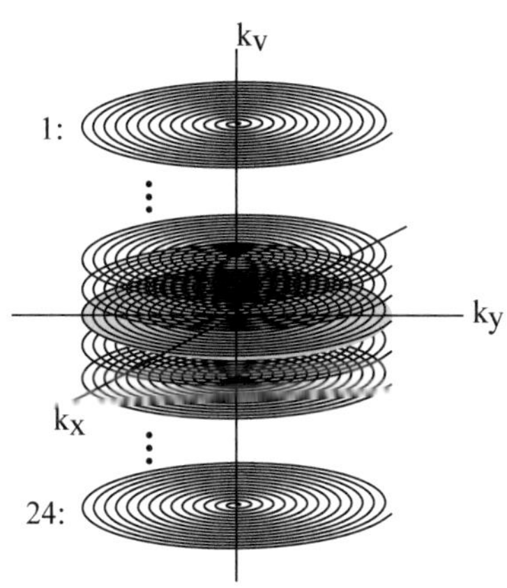

Fig. 3. Spiral FVE k-space sampling scheme. The dataset corresponding to each temporal frame is a stack-of-spirals in k_x-k_y-k_v space. Each spiral acquisition corresponds to a different k_v encode level.

4.2 Signal model

2DFT phase contrast provides two two-dimensional functions, $m(x,y)$ and $v_o(x,y)$, the magnitude and velocity maps, respectively. If these maps are measured with sufficiently high spatial resolution, and flow is laminar, one can assume that each voxel contains only one velocity, and therefore the spatial-velocity distribution associated with the object is approximately:

$$s(x,y,v) = m(x,y) \times \delta(\ v - v_o(x,y)\ ), \tag{15}$$

where $\delta(v)$ is the Dirac delta function.
As spiral FVE acquisitions follow a stack-of-spirals pattern in k_x-k_y-k_v space (Figure 3), k-space data is truncated to a cylinder, i.e., a circle along k_x-k_y (with diameter $1/\Delta r$), and a rectangle along k_v (with width $1/\Delta v$), where Δr and Δv are the prescribed spatial and velocity resolutions, respectively. The associated object domain spatial-velocity blurring can be modeled as a convolution of the true object distribution, $s(x, y, v)$, with $\text{jinc}(\sqrt{x^2+y^2}/\Delta r)$ and $\text{sinc}(v/\Delta v)$, resulting in:

$$\hat{s}(x,y,v) = [m(x,y) \times \delta(\, v - v_o(x,y)\,)] * \text{sinc}\left(\frac{v}{\Delta v}\right) * \text{jinc}\left(\frac{\sqrt{x^2+y^2}}{\Delta r}\right)$$
$$= \left[m(x,y) \times \text{sinc}\left(\frac{v - v_o(x,y)}{\Delta v}\right)\right] * \text{jinc}\left(\frac{\sqrt{x^2+y^2}}{\Delta r}\right), \qquad (16)$$

where $\hat{s}(x, y, v)$ is the measured object distribution, and $*$ denotes convolution.

4.3 Data acquisition

The excitation achieved a 5 mm slice thickness and 30° flip angle, with a 0.5 ms RF pulse and a 1 ms gradient. Through-plane velocity encoding was implemented using a large bipolar pulse along the z direction that was scaled to achieve different k_v encodes. The velocity resolution is determined by the first moment of the largest bipolar gradient, and the velocity field-of-view is determined by the increment in gradient first moment for different velocity encodes. A bipolar duration of 2.5 ms achieves a velocity resolution of 25 cm/s. Gradient duration increases if velocity resolution is improved.
An 8.1 ms optimized uniform-density single-shot spiral acquisition (Hargreaves, 2001) acquires k_x-k_y at each velocity encode, and zeroth and first moments are refocused in 0.5 ms. The readout and refocusing gradients were designed using public domain software[1]. A 0.65 ms spoiling gradient (Zur et al., 1991) achieves a 6π phase-wrap over the slice thickness. The spoiling gradient was not overlapped with the refocusing gradients, but this could be done to further shorten the TR. The minimum TR (approximately 13 ms) was used in all studies. Other scan dependent pulse sequence parameters are listed in Table 1.
Prospective ECG gating was used to synchronize acquisitions with the cardiac cycle. Two k_v levels were repeatedly acquired during each heartbeat in order to resolve 25 to 35 cardiac phases and produce a cine dataset (Figure 5, discussed later). The true temporal resolution was 26 ms (2 TRs). Sliding window reconstruction (Riederer et al., 1988) was used to produce a new image every 13 ms.

4.4 Data reconstruction

Reconstruction was performed in Matlab (The MathWorks, Inc., Natick, MA, USA). Each spiral interleaf is first gridded (Jackson et al., 1991) and inverse Fourier transformed to form an image, $m(x, y)$, for each temporal frame. This step converts the acquired data $S_{k_x,k_y}(k_v, t)$ to $S_{x,y}(k_v, t)$. The operator manually defines a region of interest (ROI) in the x-y plane using the image corresponding to $k_v = 0$ and $t = 0$. Pixel intensities within the ROI are averaged at each temporal frame, resulting in a 2D dataset: $S_{\text{ROI}}(k_v, t) = \sum_{x,y}^{\text{ROI}} S_{x,y}(k_v, t)$. View sharing is

[1] http://www-mrsrl.stanford.edu/~brian/vdspiral/

	healthy volunteer	patient
field-of-view	25 cm	20 cm
spatial resolution	7 mm	6.5 mm
k_v **encodes**	24	64
velocity field-of-view	600 or 800 cm/s	1200 cm/s
velocity resolution	25 or 33 cm/s	19 cms/s
k_v **encodes/heartbeat**	2	4
TR	12.8 or 12.5 ms	12.8 ms
temporal resolution	25.6 or 25 ms	51.2 ms
scan time	12 heartbeats	16 heartbeats

Table 1. Scan parameters used in the different spiral FVE studies.

then applied to $S_{\text{ROI}}(k_v, t)$ to increase the number of temporal frames (Riederer et al., 1988). Saturation effects (Gao et al., 1988) are compensated by normalizing the ℓ_2-norm of $S_{\text{ROI}}(k_v)$ independently for each temporal frame, which effectively normalizes each cardiac phase. $S_{\text{ROI}}(k_v, t)$ is then zero-padded along the k_v axis, and an inverse Fourier transform produces $s_{\text{ROI}}(v, t)$. The time-velocity histogram for the ROI is $|s_{\text{ROI}}(v, t)|$, and for display purposes, smoother histograms are obtained by cubic spline interpolation along t (Bartels et al., 1987). The reconstruction process can be repeated for each voxel, or for multiple regions of interest, using the same data (see Figure 8, discussed later).

4.5 Accuracy of spiral FVE measurements

An *in vitro* comparison of velocity distributions measured with spiral FVE with those derived from high-resolution 2DFT phase contrast — the current MR gold standard — was performed. The signal model presented on section 4.2 was used to generate simulated FVE data based on high-resolution 2DFT phase contrast data.

The validation experiments were performed using a pulsatile carotid flow phantom (Phantoms by Design, Inc., Bothell, WA). A slice perpendicular to the phantom's carotid bifurcation was prescribed, and through-plane velocities were measured. A cine gradient-echo 2DFT phase contrast sequence with high spatial resolution and high SNR (0.33 mm resolution, 10 averages, 80 cm/s Venc) was used as a reference. Cine spiral FVE data with $\Delta r = 3$ mm and $\Delta v = 10$ cm/s was obtained from the same scan plane. Both acquisitions were prospectively gated, and used the same TR (11.6 ms), flip angle (30°), slice profile (3 mm), temporal resolution (23.2 ms), and pre-scan settings. The total scan time was 40 minutes for phase contrast, and 12 seconds for FVE.

A simulated spiral FVE dataset was computed from the PC magnitude and velocity maps, using the convolution model described in Eq. 16. The PC-derived and FVE-measured data were registered by taking one magnitude image $m(x, y)$ from each dataset, and then using the phase difference between their Fourier transforms $M(k_x, k_y)$ to estimate the spatial shift between the images. Amplitude scaling was performed by normalizing the ℓ_2-norm of each FVE dataset. The difference between PC-derived and FVE-measured time-velocity distributions was calculated for select voxels, and the associated signal-to-error ratios were computed. This was used as a quantitative assessment of spiral FVE's accuracy.

Figure 4 shows measured and PC-derived time-velocity FVE distributions from nine representative voxels, selected around the circumference of the vessel wall of the pulsatile carotid flow phantom's bifurcation. The signal-to-error ratio between measured and PC-derived time-velocity distributions was measured to be within 9.3–11.7 dB. Imperfect registration between the datasets, combined with spatial blurring due to off-resonance in the measured spiral FVE data, may have contributed to this moderate signal-to-error ratio. Nevertheless, the two datasets show good visual agreement, and no significant spatial variation was observed in terms of accuracy. These results show that velocity distributions measured with spiral FVE agree well with those obtained with 2DFT phase contrast, the current MRI gold standard. This approach for deriving FVE data from high-resolution velocity maps (Eq. 16) can be used for many simulation purposes (Carvalho et al., 2010).

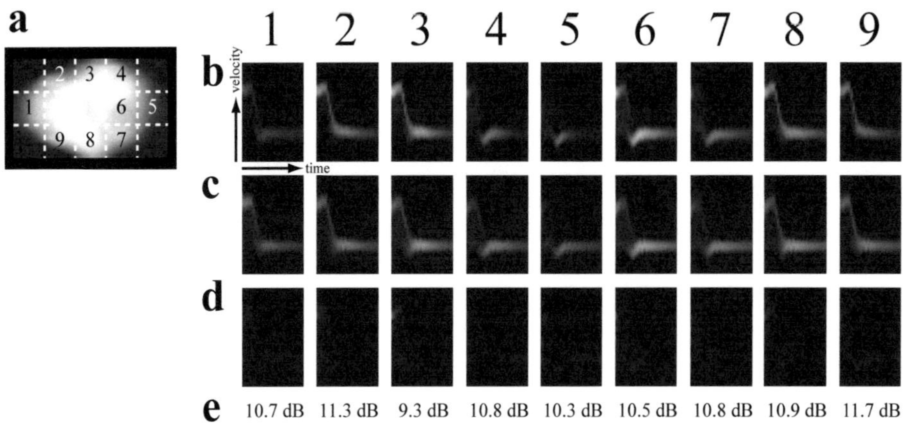

Fig. 4. *In vitro* evaluation of the accuracy of spiral FVE velocity histograms. Results are shown for nine representative voxels, selected around the circumference of the vessel wall of the pulsatile carotid flow phantom's bifurcation (a). For each voxel, it is shown: (b) time-velocity distribution derived from high-resolution 2DFT phase contrast; (c) time-velocity distribution measured with spiral FVE; (d) absolute difference between spiral FVE and 2DFT PC-derived histograms; (e) signal-to-error ratio.

4.6 Aortic valve flow assessment using spiral FVE

The proposed method was evaluated *in vivo*, aiming at quantifying flow through the aortic valve. Scan-plane prescription was performed using a real-time imaging sequence.

For a severely stenosed heart valve, peak velocities can reach up to 600 cm/s (Galea et al., 2002). As regurgitant jets don't overlap in time with forward flow, we used a 600 cm/s velocity field-of-view ($\pm$300 cm/s). This value could be increased by extending the scan time, or by sacrificing temporal, velocity and/or spatial resolutions (see Figure 9, discussed later). Scan parameters were summarized in Table 1.

4.6.1 Order of velocity encode acquisitions

When the k_v levels are acquired in a sequential fashion, ghosting artifacts due to data inconsistency appear shifted by one half of the velocity field-of-view (Figure 5). Using this sampling scheme and an appropriate velocity field-of-view, the artifacts will not overlap with the flow profile and may be easily identified and masked out.

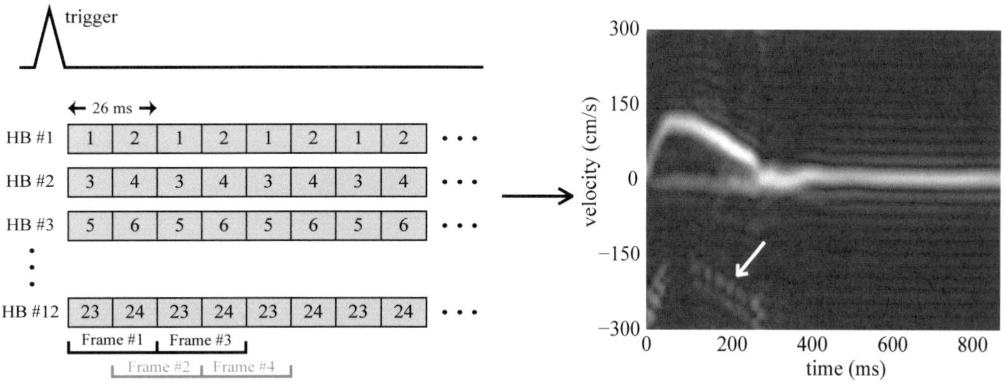

Fig. 5. Artifacts with sequential view-ordering scheme. Each box represents the acquisition of one k_v level, during one imaging TR. A sliding window is used to produce a new image every TR. Ghosting artifacts appear shifted by 1/2 of the velocity field-of-view when the k_v levels are acquired in this sequential fashion (see white arrow).

Artifacts and loss of temporal resolution due to view sharing can be avoided or corrected using different approaches. Acquiring multiple k_v levels per heartbeat reduces scan time, but causes blurring along the time axis and ghosting along the velocity axis. Blurring is caused by the reduction in temporal resolution, and ghosting artifacts arise when the velocity distribution changes between the acquisition of consecutive velocity encodes. Both ghosting and blurring can be overcome by acquiring only one view per heartbeat, but this would require increase in scan time or reduction in velocity resolution. As an alternative, these artifacts may be corrected using techniques that exploit efficient use of *k-t* space, such as the approach proposed in section 5.

4.6.2 Spiral FVE vs. doppler ultrasound

A representative *in vivo* result is compared with Doppler ultrasound in Figure 6. The MRI measured time-velocity histogram show good agreement with the ultrasound measurement, as the peak velocity and the shape of the flow waveform were comparable to those observed in the ultrasound study.

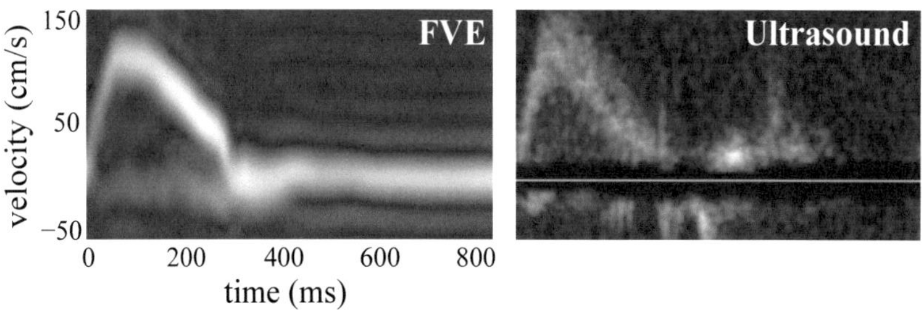

Fig. 6. Comparison of the spiral FVE method with Doppler ultrasound, in a healthy volunteer aortic valve study.

4.6.3 Patient evaluation

Figure 7 shows the time-velocity distribution measured through the aortic valve of a patient with aortic stenosis. This result demonstrate that spiral FVE can accurately detect complex flow, as a high-speed jet with a wide distribution of velocities is clearly visible.

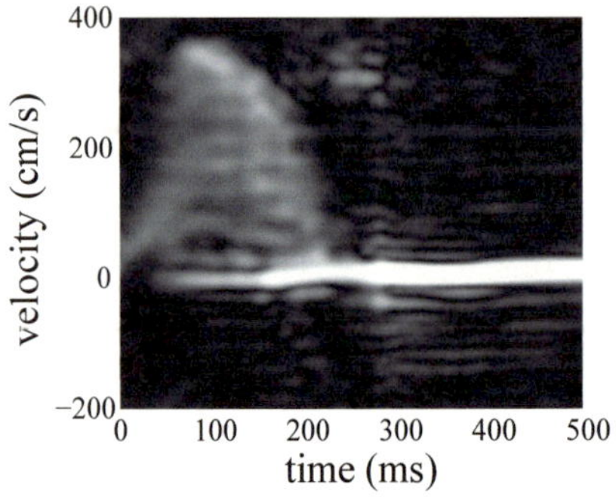

Fig. 7. Evaluation of spiral FVE in a patient with aortic stenosis. Note the high-speed jet with a wide distribution of velocities.

4.6.4 Measurement of multiple flows

Figure 8 illustrates spiral FVE's ability of resolving different flows from a single dataset. A different flow distribution was calculated for each voxel, and the distributions from single voxels from different ROIs are displayed. Red and blue dots indicate voxels where ascending and descending blood flows were detected, respectively, and the color intensity of each dot indicates the highest velocity detected in that voxel in a particular temporal frame.

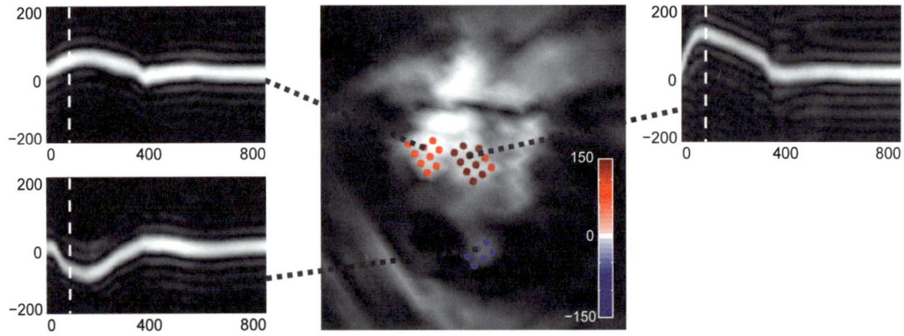

Fig. 8. Multiple flow distributions obtained from a single spiral FVE dataset. For each voxel in the image, a flow distribution was calculated, and the red and blue dots indicate voxels where ascending and descending blood flows were detected, respectively. The color intensity of each dot indicates the highest velocity detected in that voxel in a particular temporal frame (indicated by the white dashed lines).

4.7 Resolution trade-offs

In spiral FVE, there is an important trade-off between velocity resolution, temporal resolution, and scan time (Figure 9). This trade-off also involves other scan parameters, such as velocity field-of-view, number of spiral interleaves, spiral readout duration, spatial resolution, and spatial field-of-view. Velocity resolution can be improved in many ways, such as increasing the breath-hold duration to acquire more k_v levels, or by reducing the velocity field-of-view. Temporal resolution can be made as high as one TR duration (13 ms) by segmenting the k_v encodes across additional heartbeats (longer breath-holds), or by compromising velocity resolution or field-of-view. Spatial resolution can be improved by reducing the spatial field-of-view, or by increasing the number of spiral interleaves, which would require compromising other scan parameters such as scan time, temporal resolution and/or velocity resolution.

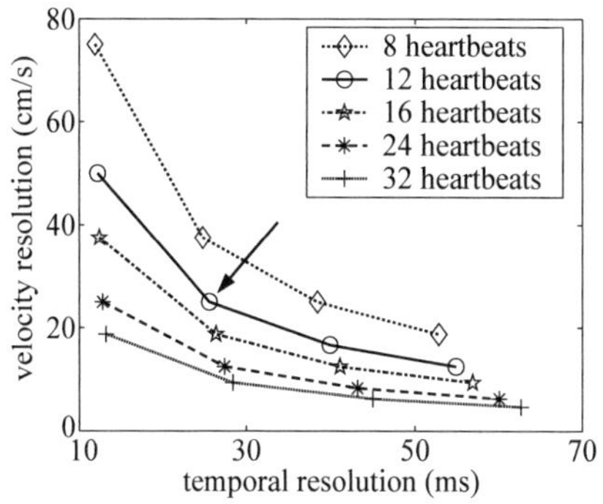

Fig. 9. Spiral FVE trade-offs between temporal resolution, velocity resolution, and breath-hold duration. Velocity resolution corresponds to a 600 cm/s field-of-view, temporal resolution corresponds to a 8.1 ms spiral readout, and scan time corresponds to a single-shot spiral acquisition. The arrow indicates the configuration used in the study in Figure 6 (2·TR temporal resolution, 24 velocity encodes).

4.8 Issues with spiral FVE

As the spiral readouts are considerably long, a potential issue in spiral FVE imaging is blurring in image domain, due to off-resonance. Because SNR was not a limiting issue for the applications we have presented, spiral FVE may perform better at lower field strengths where there is reduced off-resonance. At 3 T, localized shimming and off-resonance correction techniques can be used to reduce blurring. Furthermore, readout duration can be reduced by decreasing the spatial resolution or field-of-view, or by using variable-density spirals (Tsai & Nishimura, 2000). Another alternative is to use multiple short spiral interleaves, which would require longer scan times, but parallel imaging techniques (Pruessmann et al., 2001; Samsonov et al., 2006) can potentially accelerate acquisition if multi-channel receiver coils are used. This approach also has the benefit of allowing increase in the frame rate, as the number of imaged cardiac phases is limited by the minimum TR. Another possible solution to the off-resonance problem is the use of echo-planar imaging trajectories, which produce different off-resonance effects (geometric warping) (Feinberg & Oshio, 1992), but are also more sensitive to artifacts from in-plane flow or motion.

A noticeable artifact in spiral FVE is Gibbs ringing along the velocity dimension. These artifacts can be less noticeable if velocity resolution is increased, which would also improve the ability to visualize features in the flow waveform and the precision to resolve the peak velocity, but would require longer breath-holds. Alternatively, the velocity resolution can be improved by using variable-density sampling along k_v (Carvalho et al., 2007; DiCarlo et al., 2005), or partial Fourier techniques (Noll, Nishimura & Macovski, 1991). Another approach to reducing ringing artifacts is to window the k_v samples before applying the inverse

Fourier transform (Bernstein et al., 2001). However, windows with lower sidelobes generally have wider mainlobes, which would cause blurring along the velocity axis and consequent reduction in velocity resolution.

One drawback of the proposed method is the requirement of cardiac gating and breath-holding. Cardiac gating does not work well in patients with arrhythmias, and breath-holding may cause hemodynamic changes and is not possible for some patients (Macgowan et al., 2005). However, arrhythmia rejection (Chia et al., 2000) and respiratory gating schemes may overcome these problems, at the cost of increased scan time.

5. Accelerated spiral FVE

As introduced in section 4, spiral FVE presents limitations such as insufficient velocity field-of-view (FOV), low spatial resolution, and moderate temporal resolution. In particular, the use of view sharing (Riederer et al., 1988) causes blurring along the temporal dimension (t) and ghosting along the velocity dimension (v) (Figure 5), and the use of long spiral readouts makes the technique sensitive to off-resonance, resulting in blurring along the in-plane spatial axes (x and y). The approach proposed in this section aims to address these limitations.

Spiral FVE datasets are four-dimensional, which makes this method particularly suitable for accelerated acquisition (Hansen et al., 2004). In this section, we achieve 18-fold acceleration using a combination of three techniques: variable-density spiral sampling along k_x-k_y (Tsai & Nishimura, 2000); partial Fourier (Noll, Nishimura & Macovski, 1991) along k_v; and temporal acceleration through a novel implementation of the UNFOLD method (Madore et al., 1999; Tsao, 2002). The improved acquisition is performed without increase in scan time compared with the original implementation, and is demonstrated *in vivo* in a healthy volunteer.

5.1 Accelerated data acquisition

5.1.1 Acceleration via variable-density sampling

Variable-density spirals have been shown to increase spatiotemporal resolution and improve accuracy in flow quantitation (Liu et al., 2008). The spatial aliasing resulting from variable-density spiral sampling is incoherent, and, in the regions-of-interest (e.g., cardiac chambers, valves, great vessels), it typically originates from static or slow moving material located at the periphery of the spatial FOV (e.g., chest wall). FVE resolves the distribution of velocities within the voxel, thus moderate low-velocity aliasing artifacts generally do not affect one's ability to calculate diagnostically important parameters — such as peak velocity and acceleration — from the time-velocity distribution. Spiral FVE's single-shot uniform-density spiral readout was replaced with a multi-shot variable-density spiral acquisition (Tsai & Nishimura, 2000). The use of multi-shot acquisitions provides the possibility of multi-dimensional temporal acceleration, and allows reduction of readout duration and TR, which reduce off-resonance artifacts and temporal aliasing, respectively. The use of a shorter TR also allows improving the temporal resolution. Gradient waveforms were designed using public domain software[2], based on the hardware limits of our scanner. The spatial FOV was varied linearly from 25 cm at the center of k-space to 6.25 cm at the periphery.

[2] http://www-mrsrl.stanford.edu/~brian/vdspiral/

5.1.2 Acceleration via UNFOLD

Scan time in FVE imaging can be significantly reduced using multi-dimensional temporal acceleration (Gamper et al., 2008; Hansen et al., 2004). An implementation of the UNFOLD method (Madore et al., 1999; Tsao, 2002) was specially designed for spiral FVE. A view-ordering scheme that reduces overlap in v-f space (f denotes temporal frequency) was designed. It consists in alternating spiral interleaves and k_v encodings for each cardiac phase, according to Figure 10a. The associated point spread function is such that aliasing replicas, caused by temporal undersampling, are separated from the main lobe both in velocity (by half of the velocity FOV) and in temporal frequency (by 1/2TR) (Figure 10b) (Hansen et al., 2004; Tsao, 2002). Aliasing components caused by the sidelobes at ±20 and ±40 Hz are expected to correspond to static or slow moving spins, and hence will have a small footprint in v-f space. This is because these sidelobes spread around the periphery of the spatial FOV, but are null at the center, where high-velocity pulsatile flow is located. The aliasing signal is filtered using the two-dimensional filter shown in Figure 11. This filter has a bandwidth of 107 Hz for velocities below ±150 cm/s. For higher velocities, the bandwidth varies from 69 to 30 Hz. This results in effective temporal resolutions of 9.3 ms and 14.5–33.3 ms, respectively. The temporal resolution is lower for higher velocities, but this may prove unnoticeable, as the velocity distribution of high-velocity flow jets within large voxels is typically temporally smooth. For comparison, the temporal resolution with the conventional approach — view sharing (Riederer et al., 1988) — would be 50 ms for all v. The remaining narrow-bandwidth aliasing components at ±20 and ±40 Hz are filtered using a tight zero-phase one-dimensional notch filter along t.

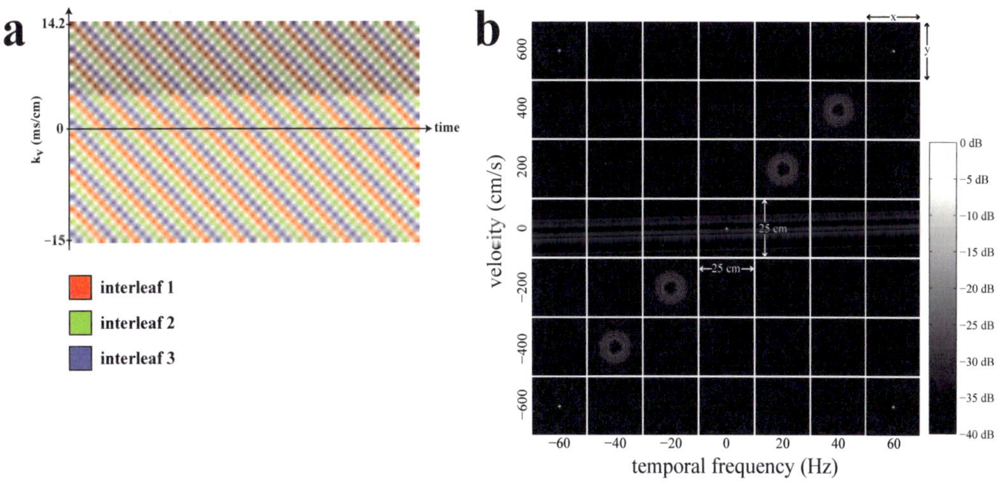

Fig. 10. Proposed view-ordering scheme for accelerated spiral FVE (a) and its corresponding point spread function (b). In (a), each color represents a different spiral interleaf, and darker tones indicate "views" that are discarded in the partial Fourier experiments. Views aligned in k_v are acquired sequentially throughout the cardiac cycle. Views aligned in time (same cardiac phase) are acquired in different heartbeats. In (b), each square shows the point spread function in x-y for a particular v-f coordinate. Aliasing replicas are separated from the main lobe by half of the velocity FOV, and half of the temporal frequency bandwidth, which reduces overlaps and facilitates filtering.

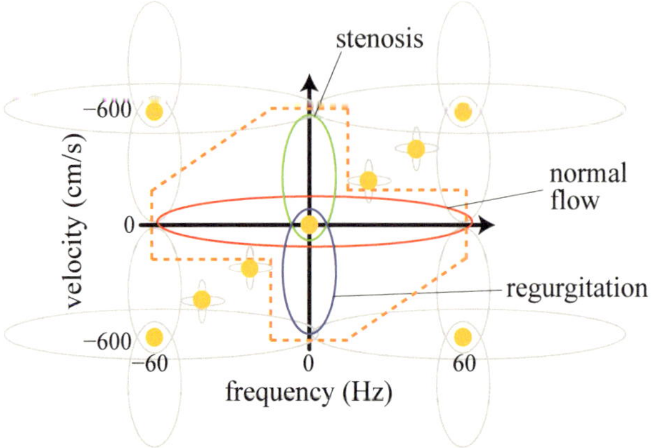

Fig. 11. Aliasing in v-f space as a result of temporal undersampling. The red, green and blue ellipses illustrate the expected footprints for aortic valve flow for normal, stenotic, and regurgitant flows, respectively. Yellow dots represent peaks in the point spread function for the proposed undersampling scheme (see Figure 10). Grey ellipses represent potential aliasing components. Replicas at ±60 Hz are exact copies of the true signal. The potential aliasing at ±20 and ±40 Hz have a small footprint, because they are composed of signal from the periphery of the spatial FOV, i.e. static tissue or slow moving flow. A 2D filter (dashed lines) is capable of avoiding aliasing while preserving all signal content.

5.1.3 Acceleration via partial Fourier

Partial Fourier along the velocity dimension has been successfully used in FVE for scan time reduction, without significant loss of velocity resolution. This approach has been previously demonstrated in studies with healthy volunteers (Carvalho & Nayak, 2007; Macgowan et al., 2005) and patients (Carvalho & Nayak, 2007; Santos et al., 2007), and in phantom experiments (DiCarlo et al., 2005). Data was acquired with full coverage of k_v space, and 33% of the data was retrospectively discarded before reconstruction (dark-colored squares in Figure 10a). The missing data was synthesized using homodyne reconstruction (Noll, Nishimura & Macovski, 1991).

5.2 Data reconstruction

Reconstruction was performed in Matlab (The MathWorks, Inc., Natick, MA, USA). The acquired data, $S(k_x, k_y, k_v, t)$, is first re-sampled onto a Cartesian grid (Jackson et al., 1991) using a Kaiser-Bessel kernel designed for the largest FOV (25 cm). Each spiral interleaf is gridded separately, and inverse Fourier transformed to form a spatial image for its corresponding k_v-t coordinate, resulting in $S(x, y, k_v, t)$. The data corresponding to the two central k_v values ($k_v = 0$ and $k_v = \frac{1}{\text{FOV}_v}$) are separately filtered using a 6-tap moving average temporal filter that effectively implements view sharing (Riederer et al., 1988). A color-flow video (Riederer et al., 1991) is obtained from the filtered data. The operator draws one or multiple ROIs over the video. Pixel values within each ROI are averaged, resulting in multiple 2D datasets: $S_{\text{ROI}_i}(k_v, t) = \sum_{x,y}^{\text{ROI}_i} S(x, y, k_v, t)$. Each of these 2D datasets is filtered using the 2D filter and the notch filter described in section 5.1.2. Saturation effects (Gao et al., 1988) are compensated by normalizing the data in each cardiac phase. The data is then zero-padded along the k_v axis, and homodyne reconstruction (Noll, Nishimura & Macovski, 1991) is used to produce each $s_{\text{ROI}_i}(v, t)$ distribution. The time-velocity histogram for each

ROI is $\left|s_{\text{ROI}_i}(v,t)\right|$, and smoother histograms are generated by one-dimensional cubic spline interpolation (Bartels et al., 1987) along t.

5.3 Acceleration experiments

The use of variable-density sampling in spiral FVE for improving spatial resolution and reducing off-resonance artifacts was evaluated in the following experiment. Three acquisitions were performed, measuring flow at the aortic valve plane of a healthy volunteer. A different spiral design was used in each acquisition (Table 2). A reduced velocity FOV (200 cm/s) was used, in order to limit each acquisition to a single feasible breath-hold. The FOV was adjusted to either the -50 to 150 cm/s range or the -150 to 50 cm/s range, depending on the flow of interest. Six k_v encoding steps were acquired, resulting in a velocity resolution of 33 cm/s. No temporal undersampling was performed, and the acquisition was segmented across multiple heartbeats. The temporal resolution was one TR. The results were qualitatively compared in spatial and time-velocity domains.

	original design	**proposed design**	**ground truth reference**
interleaves	1	3	6
sampling	UD	VD	UD
readout	8 ms	4 ms	4 ms
field-of-view	25 cm	6–25 cm	25 cm
resolution	7.2 mm	3.6 mm	3.6 mm
heartbeats†	6	18	36
TR‡	12.4 ms	8.4 ms	8.4 ms

UD=uniform-density; VD=variable-density; †scan time with 6 k_v encodes; ‡TR for 33 cm/s velocity resolution.

Table 2. Design parameters used to evaluate the use of variable-density sampling in spiral FVE.

The proposed temporal acceleration scheme was then evaluated in a second experiment. Aortic valve flow was measured using the proposed variable-density spiral design (Table 2), and the proposed view-ordering scheme (Figure 10a). The velocity resolution and FOV were set to 33 and 1200 cm/s, respectively. The data was acquired in an 18-heartbeat breath-hold, and was reconstructed using view sharing, the proposed 2D filter, and the proposed notch filter after 2D-filtering. The reduced velocity FOV results from the previous experiment were used as ground truth reference for a qualitative comparison.

Partial Fourier acceleration was evaluated by discarding, before reconstruction, 12 of the 36 k_v encodes from the temporally-undersampled data from the previous experiment, as indicated in Figure 10a. The reconstructed time-velocity distribution was qualitatively compared with the fully sampled reference.

5.4 Acceleration results

Figure 12 contains results from the experiment using different spiral designs from Table 2. The data in Figure 12a was obtained using the 8 ms readout uniform-density spiral design used in section 4. The proposed variable-density design provided higher spatial resolution and reduced off-resonance artifacts, and thus better spatial localization of flow (Figure 12b). Some aliasing artifacts were observed in spatial domain (see asterisk), but these were not observed in the time-velocity distributions. A fully sampled reference is shown in Figure 12c, for comparison.

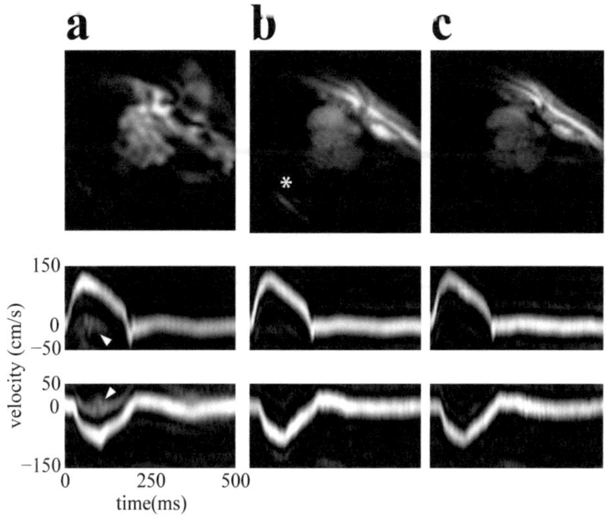

Fig. 12. Effect of variable-density sampling on image quality and spatial localization of flow: (a) original design; (b) new design; (c) ground truth reference. Top row: spatial images from the first cardiac phase; center row: time-velocity distributions measured at the aortic valve; bottom row: time-velocity distributions measured in the descending aorta. The use of higher spatial resolution and shorter readout duration improves the spatial localization of flow, which is identified by the reduced signal from static material in the time-velocity histograms (see arrows). Some aliasing artifacts were observed in spatial domain (see asterisk), but these were not observed in the time-velocity distributions.

Figure 13 contains results from the temporal acceleration experiment. Figure 13a shows the undersampled data in both v-f and v-t domains (compare this with Figure 11). Aliasing components were significantly reduced using the proposed 2D filter (dashed lines), while all of the signal energy was preserved (Figure 13b). The notch filter (dotted line) removed the majority of the remaining aliasing at ± 20 and ± 40 Hz (solid arrows) (Figure 13c). These results show that the proposed temporal acceleration scheme is capable of achieving 6-fold acceleration in multi-interleaf spiral FVE, without noticeable loss of temporal resolution, and without introducing significant artifacts. A result using view sharing is shown in Figure 13d, for comparison. This approach is equivalent to a moving-average low-pass filter, which reduces the temporal frequency bandwidth (dashed arrows), and causes loss of temporal resolution, perceived as blurring along t (circled).
Figure 14 shows a comparison between the accelerated results and the fully sampled reference. Two-fold acceleration was achieved using variable-density sampling (Figure 14b), with no noticeable artifacts in the time-velocity histogram when compared with the fully sampled reference (Figure 14a). Additional 6-fold acceleration was achieved using the proposed temporal acceleration scheme (Figure 14c). Those results were achieved in a single 18-heartbeat acquisition, while a fully sampled acquisition with the same scan parameters would require 216 heartbeats. Partial Fourier was then used to reduce the acquisition time to 12 heartbeats (i.e., by 1.5-fold), which represents a combined 18-fold acceleration (Figure 14d).

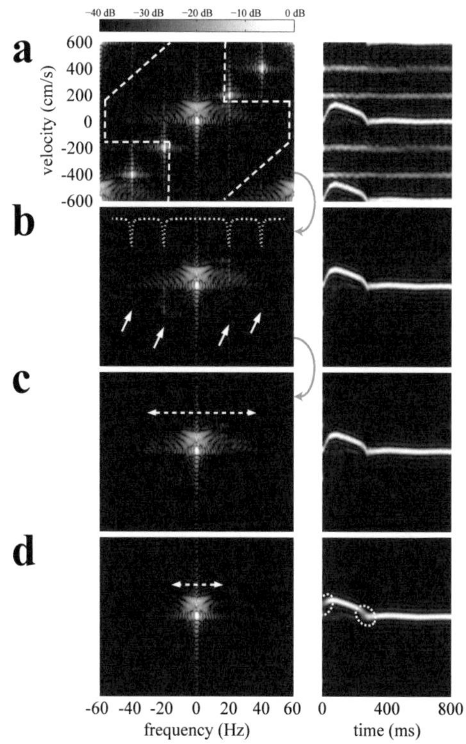

Fig. 13. Temporal acceleration compared with view sharing in (left) v-f space and (right) v-t space: (a) undersampled data; (b) with 2D filtering; (c) with 2D and notch filtering (proposed approach); and (d) with view sharing (conventional approach). The 2D filter (dashed lines) removes a majority of the aliasing, and the notch filter (dotted line) removes the remaining aliasing signal (solid arrows). The proposed method removes aliasing components without noticeable loss of temporal resolution. View sharing reduces the temporal frequency bandwidth (dashed arrows), which causes temporal blurring (circles). Compare the v-f representation in (a) with Figure 11.

No significant artifacts were observed when comparing the reference dataset with the 18-fold accelerated result.

Figure 15 presents time-velocity distributions from multiple ROIs. These distributions were reconstructed from the 18-fold undersampled dataset used in Figure 14d. Very few artifacts were observed in time-velocity histograms measured in voxels from different locations in the heart. Artifacts could be further reduced by designing different 2D filters for each ROI, based on typical characteristics of the targeted flow. For example, the artifacts observed in the descending aorta (see arrow), could be reduced by more aggressively filtering high positive-velocity components, as no ascending flow is expected in that vessel. These results, when compared with those in Figure 8, also illustrate the different improvements achieved with this approach. The spatial resolution was improved from 7 mm to 3.6 mm, and off-resonance effects were reduced. The velocity FOV was increased from $\pm$400 to $\pm$600 cm/s, without loss of velocity resolution (33 cm/s). The effective temporal resolution was improved from 26 ms to 9 ms, and ghosting artifacts due to view sharing were eliminated. Both acquisitions were performed in 12-heartbeat breath-holds.

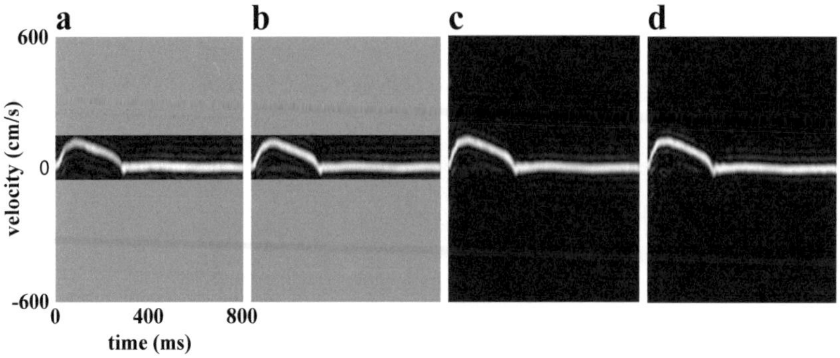

Fig. 14. Accelerated spiral FVE results: (a) fully sampled reference (36 heartbeats); (b) 2-fold acceleration, using variable-density sampling (18 heartbeats); (c) 12-fold acceleration, using variable-density sampling and temporal acceleration (18 heartbeats); and (d) 18-fold acceleration, using variable-density sampling, temporal acceleration, and partial Fourier (12 heartbeats). A reduced velocity FOV (200 cm/s) was used in (a) and (b) to limit the acquisition to a single feasible breath-hold. If acquiring a full 1200 cm/s velocity FOV, as in (c) and (d), the total acquisition time for (a) and (b) would have been 216 and 108 heartbeats, respectively. All other scan parameters were identical for the four acquisitions. No significant differences were observed when comparing the 18-fold accelerated result with the fully sampled reference.

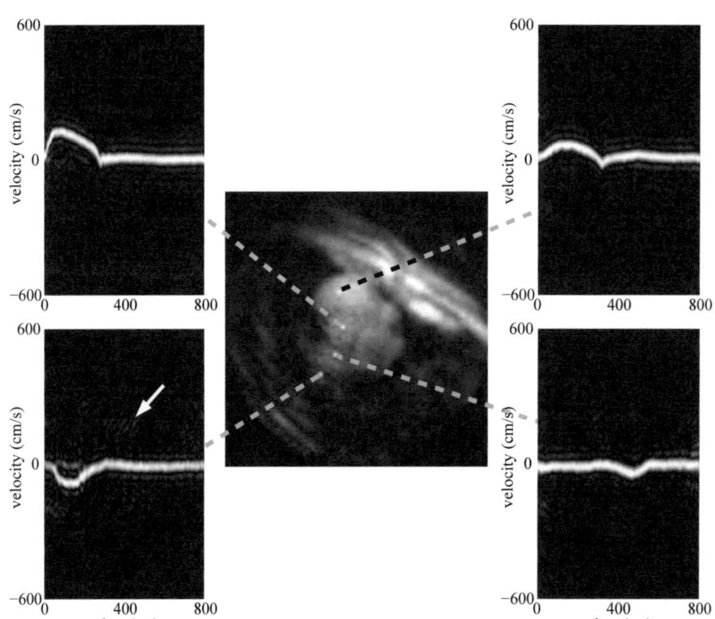

Fig. 15. Flow in multiple ROIs measured in a single 12-heartbeat spiral FVE acquisition using 18-fold acceleration. Voxels of interest are highlighted. Time-velocity histograms reveal only minimal artifacts (see arrow). The data illustrates significant improvements in spatial resolution, velocity field-of-view, and temporal resolution (compare with Figure 8).

Signal-to-noise ratio was not a limiting issue for the presented application. This is in part due to the large voxel sizes and the multi-dimensional characteristics of spiral FVE. The proposed acceleration scheme reduced scan time and improved spatiotemporal resolution, and did not compromise the quality of the time-velocity histograms. Aliasing artifacts in spatial domain due to variable-density sampling are negligible in time-velocity domain (Figure 12b). The proposed *k-t* filters remove a majority of the temporal aliasing artifacts, and also filter high-frequency noise for high velocities (Figure 13c). Partial Fourier acceleration may cause some artifacts due to the use of a low-resolution phase estimate, thus a low acceleration factor was used (Figure 14d). Further acceleration could be achieved using parallel imaging techniques (Pruessmann et al., 2001; Samsonov et al., 2006), and further reduction in off-resonance effects could be achieved by imaging at lower field strengths.

6. Conclusion

In this chapter, we have addressed the issue of non-invasive aortic valve flow quantitation through magnetic resonance imaging. We addressed both imaging and reconstruction aspects, including accelerated acquisitions and reconstruction from undersampled data. We introduced spiral FVE, a new method for MR flow quantitation, which is capable of accurately capturing peak velocities in flow jets due to stenosis or regurgitation. Spiral FVE compared well against Doppler ultrasound, the current gold standard for cardiovascular flow imaging, and against high-resolution 2DFT phase contrast, the current MRI gold standard. Our method was demonstrated in both healthy volunteers and in a patient.

Using a combination of three different techniques (variable-density spirals, temporal acceleration, and partial Fourier reconstruction), we are able to improve the spiral FVE method by 18-fold. Improvements consisted of increased velocity field-of-view, higher spatial resolution, reduced off-resonance effects, and higher temporal resolution. The improved acquisition was performed in only 12 heartbeats, whereas 216 heartbeats would be necessary to achieve such improvements without acceleration. No significant artifacts were observed.

Magnetic resonance imaging is potentially the most appropriate technique for addressing all aspects of cardiovascular disease examination. The evaluation of valvular disease and intracardiac flow will be a necessary capability in a comprehensive cardiac MR examination. The imaging and reconstruction techniques proposed in this chapter can be an important contribution towards making such exam feasible.

7. References

Ahn, C. B., Park, J. H. & Cho, Z. H. (1986). High-speed spiral-scan echo planar NMR imaging, *IEEE Trans Med Imaging* 5(1): 2–7.

Bartels, R. H., Beatty, J. C. & Barsky, B. A. (1987). *An introduction to splines for use in computer graphics and geometric modelling*, Morgan Kaufmann, San Francisco, California.

Bernstein, M. A., Fain, S. B. & Riederer, S. J. (2001). Effect of windowing and zero-filled reconstruction of MRI data on spatial resolution and acquisition strategy, *J Magn Reson Imaging* 14(3): 270–280.

Bernstein, M. A., King, K. F. & Zhou, X. J. (2004). *Handbook of MRI Pulse Sequences*, Academic Press.

Carvalho, J. L. A., DiCarlo, J. C., Kerr, A. B. & Nayak, K. S. (2007). Reconstruction of variable-density data in Fourier velocity encoding, *Proc, ISMRM, 15th Annual Meeting*, Berlin, p. 2514.

Carvalho, J. L. A. & Nayak, K. S. (2007). Rapid quantitation of cardiovascular flow using slice-selective Fourier velocity encoding with spiral readouts, *Magn Reson Med* 57(4): 639–646.

Carvalho, J. L. A., Nielsen, J. F. & Nayak, K. S. (2010). Feasibility of in vivo measurement of carotid wall shear rate using spiral Fourier velocity encoded MRI, *Magn Reson Med* 63(6): 1537–1547.

Chia, J. M., Fischer, S. E., Wickline, S. A. & Lorenz, C. H. (2000). Arrhythmia rejection using a VCG-based triggering algorithm, *Proc, ISMRM, 8th Annual Meeting*, Denver, p. 201.

Clarke, G. D., Hundley, W. G., McColl, R. W., Eckels, R., Smith, D., Chaney, C., Li, H. F. & Peshock, R. M. (1996). Velocity-encoded, phase-difference cine MRI measurements of coronary artery flow: dependence of flow accuracy on the number of cine frames, *J Magn Reson Imaging* 6(5): 733–742.

DiCarlo, J. C., Hargreaves, B. A., Nayak, K. S., Hu, B. S., Pauly, J. M. & Nishimura, D. G. (2005). Variable-density one-shot Fourier velocity encoding, *Magn Reson Med* 54(3): 645–655.

Dumoulin, C. L., Souza, S. P., Hardy, C. J. & Ash, S. A. (1991). Quantitative measurement of blood flow using cylindrically localized Fourier velocity encoding, *Magn Reson Med* 21(2): 242–250.

Feinberg, D. A., Crooks, L. E., Sheldon, P., Hoenninger III, J., Watts, J. & Arakawa, M. (1985). Magnetic resonance imaging the velocity vector components of fluid flow, *Magn Reson Med* 2(6): 555–566.

Feinberg, D. A. & Oshio, K. (1992). Gradient-echo shifting in fast MRI techniques (GRASE imaging) for correction of field inhomogeneity errors and chemical shift, *J Magn Reson* 97: 177–183.

Galea, D., Lauzon, M. L. & Drangova, M. (2002). Peak velocity determination using fast Fourier velocity encoding with minimal spatial encoding, *Med Phys* 29(8): 1719–1728.

Gamper, U., Boesiger, P. & Kozerke, S. (2008). Compressed sensing in dynamic MRI, *Magn Reson Med* 59(2): 365–373.

Gao, J. H., Holland, S. K. & Gore, J. C. (1988). Nuclear magnetic resonance signal from flowing nuclei in rapid imaging using gradient echoes, *Med Phys* 15(6): 809–814.

Glover, G. H. & Pelc, N. J. (1988). A rapid-gated cine MRI technique, *Magn Reson Annu* pp. 299–333.

Hahn, E. L. (1960). Detection of sea-water motion by nuclear precession, *J Geophys Res* 65(2): 776–777.

Hansen, M. S., Baltes, C., Tsao, J., Kozerke, S., Pruessmann, K. P., Boesiger, P. & Pedersen, E. M. (2004). Accelerated dynamic Fourier velocity encoding by exploiting velocity-spatio-temporal correlations, *MAGMA* 17(2): 86–94.

Hargreaves, B. A. (2001). *Spin-Manipulation Methods for Efficient Magnetic Resonance Imaging*, PhD thesis, Stanford University.

Hennig, J., Mueri, M., Brunner, P. & Friedburg, H. (1988). Fast and exact flow measurements with the fast Fourier flow technique, *Magn Reson Med* 6(4): 369–372.

Holsinger, A. E., Wright, R. C., Riederer, S. J., Farzaneh, F., Grimm, R. C. & Maier, J. K. (1990). Real-time interactive magnetic resonance imaging, *Magn Reson Med* 14(3): 547–553.

Hoskins, P. R. (1996). Accuracy of maximum velocity estimates made using Doppler ultrasound systems, *Br J Radiol* 69(818): 172–177.

Hu, B. S., Pauly, J. M. & Macovski, A. (1993). Localized real-time velocity spectra determination, *Magn Reson Med* 30(3): 393–398.

Irarrazabal, P., Hu, B. S., Pauly, J. M. & Nishimura, D. G. (1993). Spatially resolved and localized real-time velocity distribution, *Magn Reson Med* 30(2): 207–212.

Jackson, J. I., Meyer, C. H., Nishimura, D. G. & Macovski, A. (1991). Selection of a convolution function for Fourier inversion using gridding, *IEEE Trans Med Imaging* 10(3): 473–478.

Liu, C.-Y., Varadarajan, P., Pohost, G. M. & Nayak, K. S. (2008). Real-time color-flow MRI at 3 T using variable-density spiral phase contrast, *Magn Reson Imaging* 26(5): 661–666.

Macgowan, C. K., Kellenberger, C. J., Detsky, J. S., Roman, K. & Yoo, S. J. (2005). Real-time Fourier velocity encoding: an in vivo evaluation, *J Magn Reson Imaging* 21(3): 297–304.

Madore, B., Glover, G. H. & Pelc, N. J. (1999). Unaliasing by Fourier-encoding the overlaps using the temporal dimension (UNFOLD), applied to cardiac imaging and fMRI, *Magn Reson Med* 42(5): 813–828.

Meyer, C. H., Hu, B. S., Nishimura, D. G. & Macovski, A. (1992). Fast spiral coronary artery imaging, *Magn Reson Med* 28(2): 202–213.

Mohiaddin, R. H., Gatehouse, P. D., Henien, M. & Firmin, D. N. (1997). Cine MR Fourier velocimetry of blood flow through cardiac valves: comparison with Doppler echocardiography., *J Magn Reson Imaging* 7(4): 657–663.

Moran, P. R. (1982). A flow velocity zeugmatographic interlace for NMR imaging in humans, *Magn Reson Imaging* 1(4): 197–203.

Moran, P. R., Moran, R. A. & Karstaedt, N. (1985). Verification and evaluation of internal flow and motion. true magnetic resonance imaging by the phase gradient modulation method, *Radiology* 154(2): 433–441.

Nayak, K. S., Pauly, J. M., Kerr, A. B., Hu, B. S. & Nishimura, D. G. (2000). Real-time color flow MRI, *Magn Reson Med* 43: 251–258.

Nayler, G. L., Firmin, D. N. & Longmore, D. B. (1986). Blood flow imaging by cine magnetic resonance, *J Comput Assist Tomogr* 10: 715–722.

Nishimura, D. G. (2010). *Principles of Magnetic Resonance Imaging*, Stanford University, Palo Alto, California.

Noll, D. C., Meyer, C. H., Pauly, J. M., Nishimura, D. G. & Macovski, A. (1991). A homogeneity correction method for magnetic resonance imaging with time-varying gradients, *IEEE Trans Med Imaging* 10(4): 629–637.

Noll, D. C., Nishimura, D. G. & Macovski, A. (1991). Homodyne detection in magnetic resonance imaging, *IEEE Trans Med Imaging* 10(2): 154–163.

O'Donnell, M. (1985). NMR blood flow imaging using multiecho, phase contrast sequences, *Med Phys* 12(1): 59–64.

Pruessmann, K. P., Weiger, M., Bornert, P. & Boesiger, P. (2001). Advances in sensitivity encoding with arbitrary k-space trajectories, *Magn Reson Med* 46(4): 638–651.

Rebergen, S. A., van der Wall, E. E., Doornbos, J. & de Roos, A. (1993). Magnetic resonance measurement of velocity and flow: technique, validation, and cardiovascular applications, *Am Heart J* 126(6): 1439–1456.

Riederer, S. J., Tasciyan, T., Farzaneh, F., Lee, J. N., Wright, R. C. & Herfkens, R. J. (1988). MR fluoroscopy: technical feasibility, *Magn Reson Med* 8(1): 1–15.

Riederer, S. J., Wright, R. C., Ehman, R. L., Rossman, P. J., Holsinger-Bampton, A. E., Hangiangdreu, N. J. & Grimm, R. C. (1991). Real-time interactive color flow MR imaging, *Radiology* 181: 33–39.

Samsonov, A. A., Block, W. F., Arunachalam, A. & Field, A. S. (2006). Advances in locally constrained k-space-based parallel MRI, *Magn Reson Med* 55(2): 431–438.

Santos, J. M., Kerr, A. B., Lee, D., McConnell, M. V., Yang, P. C., Hu, B. S. & Pauly, J. M. (2007). Comprehensive valve evaluation system, *Proc, ISMRM, 15th Annual Meeting*, Berlin, p. 2551.

Singer, J. R. (1959). Blood flow rates by nuclear magnetic resonance measurements, *Science* 130(3389): 1652–1653.

Singer, J. R. & Crooks, L. E. (1983). Nuclear magnetic resonance blood flow measurements in the human brain, *Science* 221(4611): 654–656.

Tang, C., Blatter, D. D. & Parker, D. L. (1993). Accuracy of phase-contrast flow measurements in the presence of partial-volume effects, *J Magn Reson Imaging* 3(3): 377–385.

Tsai, C.-M. & Nishimura, D. G. (2000). Reduced aliasing artifacts using variable-density k-space sampling trajectories, *Magn Reson Med* 43: 452–458.

Tsai, C.-M., Olcott, E. W. & Nishimura, D. G. (1999). Flow quantification using low-spatial-resolution and low-velocity-resolution velocity images, *Magn Reson Med* 42(4): 682–690.

Tsao, J. (2002). On the UNFOLD method, *Magn Reson Med* 47(1): 202–207.

van Dijk, P. (1984). Direct cardiac NMR imaging of heart wall and blood flow velocity, *J Comput Assist Tomogr* 8(3): 429–436.

Winkler, A. J. & Wu, J. (1995). Correction of intrinsic spectral broadening errors in Doppler peak velocity measurements made with phased sector and linear array transducers, *Ultrasound Med Biol* 21(8): 1029–1035.

Zur, Y., Wood, M. L. & Neuringer, L. J. (1991). Spoiling of transverse magnetization in steady-state sequences, *Magn Reson Med* 21(2): 251–263.

2

State-Of-The-Art Methods for the Numerical Simulation of Aortic BMHVs

Sebastiaan Annerel[1], Tom Claessens[2], Peter Van Ransbeeck[2], Patrick Segers[3], Pascal Verdonck[3] and Jan Vierendeels[1]
[1]*Department of Flow, Heat and Combustion Mechanics, Ghent University,*
[2]*Department of Mechanics, University College Ghent,*
[3]*IBiTech-bioMMeda, Ghent University,*
Belgium

1. Introduction

Since the first clinical implantation of an artificial aortic valve by Dr. Charles A. Hufnagel in 1952 (Hufnagel et al., 1954), the use of such prostheses has gained strong interest and has become a routine treatment for severe heart valve failure. During the past 60 years, various mechanical heart valve designs have been developed for use in both aortic and mitral positions (Butany et al., 2003; Aslam et al., 2007). Nowadays, bileaflet mechanical heart valves (BMHVs) are widely preferred for aortic valve replacement because of their long lifespan. However, current BMHVs still induce pannus and thromboembolism, among other undesired side effects, which are believed to be due to non-physiological flow and turbulence generated by the valve leaflets (Sotiropoulous & Borazjani, 2009).

One way to gain insight into the dynamics of a BMHV in order to improve its design is by experimental testing (Grigioni et al., 2004). Usually, *in vitro* testing is used, in which the functioning of the valve is assessed, for example, by using Doppler echocardiography (Dumont et al., 2002; Verdonck et al., 2002) or by visualizing the temporal and spatial flow field through velocimetry, like the laser Doppler anemometry (LDA) technique (Browne et al., 2000; Akutsu et al., 2001) or the particle image velocimetry (PIV) technique (Browne et al., 2000; Kaminsky et al., 2007). Also, the spectrum of the valve noise can be analyzed, as is done, for example, in Masson & Rieu (1998). Experimental *in vivo* testing is another option, using echocardiography and Doppler ultrasound to investigate the behavior of the valve after implantation in human patients (Bech-Hanssen, 2001; Aslam et al., 2007; Aljassim et al., 2008; Zogbi et al., 2009) or in animals (Yin et al., 2006).

Numerical (*"in silico"*) methods can provide an alternative way to obtain relevant and detailed information for valve design optimization, since they are capable of solving the valve dynamics with a high degree of resolution in time and space (Kelly et al., 1999; Grigioni et al., 2004; Yoganathan et al., 2005; Dasi et al., 2009; Sotiropoulous & Borazjani, 2009). Moreover, they are considerably less time-consuming and less expensive during the research and development phase compared with experimental testing (Dasi et al., 2009) and are, therefore, particularly efficient for sensitivity studies (Verdonck, 2002). Unfortunately, the numerical simulation of a BMHV is a complex fluid-structure interaction (FSI) problem

because the movement of the leaflets strongly interacts with the surrounding fluid motion; therefore, the equilibrium at the fluid-structure interface needs to be taken into account.
In this chapter, a review of numerical FSI methods for BMHVs is given. Subsequently, the general dynamics and flow fields of BMHVs are discussed and illustrated by numerical simulations. This flow field typically consists of three jets. Furthermore, the design optimization challenges are described. High-flow-velocity gradients give rise to high shear stresses that can induce blood damage (Yoganathan et al., 2004). Therefore, the blood damage is discussed. The flow through the hinge region is of special interest. Finally, the cavitation phenomenon in BMHVs is discussed, because it can induce blood damage as well as structural failure (due to pitting and erosion).

2. A review of FSI methods to simulate the dynamics of a BMHV

When numerically simulating a BMHV, three problems need to be solved, namely the structural problem, the flow problem, and the interaction of the fluid and the structure at the fluid-structure interface. In the following, each of these three problems is discussed in detail.
Since the leaflets of a BMHV have a small moment of inertia and are very stiff, they are usually assumed to be rigid. A BMHV can thus be modeled as a rigid casing in which two separate rigid leaflets rotate around their hinge axes (see Fig. 1). Because the position of each rigid leaflet is solely determined by its opening angle, the bileaflet valve has two degrees of freedom.

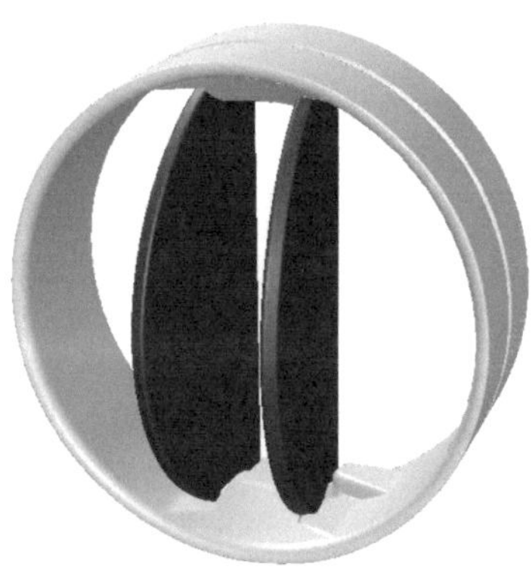

Fig. 1. View on the ATS Open Pivot™ Standard Heart Valve with leaflets (marked in black) in the open position. The casing is visible (in white) with the blocking mechanism at the hinges

The movement of a rigid leaflet i is governed by Newton's Second Law, which states that the (structural) moment $M_{s,i}$ about its rotation axis must be in equilibrium with the product of its moment of inertia I_i and its angular acceleration $\ddot{\theta}_{s,i}$. For two leaflets, this results in the following two equations:

$$\begin{cases} M_{s,1} = I_1 \cdot \ddot{\theta}_{s,1} \\ M_{s,2} = I_2 \cdot \ddot{\theta}_{s,2} \end{cases} \tag{1}$$

Secondly, the blood flow through the valve is calculated, which is governed by the conservation of mass and the Navier-Stokes equations. For the unsteady flow of an incompressible fluid, the differential equations to be solved are given by:

$$\nabla \cdot \vec{v} = 0 \tag{2a}$$

$$\rho \frac{\partial \vec{v}}{\partial t} + \rho \nabla \left(\vec{v}\vec{v} \right) = -\nabla p + \mu \nabla^2 \vec{v} + \rho \vec{g} \tag{2b}$$

(Hirt et al., 1997; Donea et al., 2004), in which $\vec{v}$ = flow velocity vector, ρ = fluid density, t = time, μ = dynamic viscosity and p = pressure. In the case of blood flow through a BMHV, it is usually assumed that the hinge axis is in the direction of gravity. Thus, the gravity has no effect on the moment about the hinge axis (Sotiropoulos et al., 2009) and, therefore, its influence (last term in Equation (2b)) is neglected.

Computational fluid dynamics (CFD) are used to solve Equation (2) for the entire fluid domain. From the resulting flow field, the pressure and viscous forces at the fluid-structure interface are derived. These forces are integrated at the fluid-structure interface giving the pressure and viscous moment $M_{f,i}$ about the hinge axis acting on the interface.

Finally, the (kinematic and dynamic) equilibrium equations at the fluid-structure interface need to be solved. The kinematic equilibrium states that the angular position of the fluid at the fluid-structure interface (i.e. $\theta_{f,i}$) should be equal to the angular position of the structural leaflet at the interface (i.e. $\theta_{s,i}$):

$$\begin{cases} \theta_{f,1} = \theta_{s,1} \\ \theta_{f,2} = \theta_{s,2} \end{cases} \tag{3}$$

Dynamic equilibrium also needs to be achieved. When the hinges of the valve are modeled as frictionless, the structural moment $M_{s,i}$ acting on each leaflet i should be equal to the pressure and viscous moment exerted by the flow, indicated by $M_{f,i}$:

$$\begin{cases} M_{f,1} - M_{s,1} \\ M_{f,2} = M_{s,2} \end{cases} \tag{4}$$

or with Equation (1):

$$\begin{cases} M_{f,1} = I_1 \cdot \ddot{\theta}_{s,1} \\ M_{f,2} = I_2 \cdot \ddot{\theta}_{s,2} \end{cases} \tag{5}$$

Both equations of equilibrium at the fluid-structure interface are solved using FSI methods. The subscripts s and f in Equation (5) are left out from here on. In the following, the pressure and viscous moment $M_{f,i}$ and the structural acceleration $\ddot{\theta}_{s,1}$ will thus respectively be referred to as "the moment M_i" and "the angular acceleration $\ddot{\theta}_i$". With this change in notation, Equation (5) becomes:

$$\begin{cases} M_1 = I_1 \cdot \ddot{\theta}_1 \\ M_2 = I_2 \cdot \ddot{\theta}_2 \end{cases} \tag{6}$$

In the remainder of this section, classifications of FSI methods used in literature to simulate a BMHV will be made, and the characteristics of each of the mentioned methods will be explained.

2.1 Fixed grid techniques versus moving grid techniques

A first classification concerns the kinematical description of the domain. For the structural problem, the motion is usually described by the Lagrangian method, where the computational grid moves with the material velocity. This is in contrast to a fluid domain, in which the motion is generally described by the Eulerian method and, therefore, the computational grid does not deform. In case of FSI, both methods can be combined in several approaches in order to describe the motion of the domain.

One approach is the "fixed grid" method, in which an immersed structure is allowed to "fictitiously" move through the Eulerian fluid grid in a Lagrangian way. The influence of the structure boundary on the fluid outside the structure is calculated by introducting body force sources into the Navier-Stokes equations, while keeping the velocity of the fictitiously overlapped fluid coupled to the structural velocity. Since the fluid grid is fixed, there is no need for remeshing and grid adaption. However, because the fluid-structure interface is not necessarily aligned with the spatial discretization and the data are, as such, interpolated, the flow field (and thus shear stresses) at this interface is not accurately calculated. Several fixed grid methods have been developed, such as the immersed boundary (IB) method, first proposed by Peskin (1972) for the simulation of heart valves. Borazjani et al. (2008) used the sharp interface CURVIB-method for simulating a BMHV. Other IB techniques were developed and used by Tai et al. (2007), De Tullio et al. (2009) and Xia et al. (2009). Also, the fictitious domain (FD) method can be used to simulate flexible heart valves (De Hart et al., 2000, 2003; Diniz dos Santos et al., 2008; Astorino et al., 2009). This fixed grid method uses Lagrange multipliers to impose the kinematic constraints. Van Loon et al. (2004) improved the accuracy of the FD method at the fluid-structure interface by proposing a local fluid grid adaption at the structure boundary.

Another approach is to use the arbitrary Lagrangian-Eulerian (ALE) method for the fluid domain. In this "moving grid" method, the fluid grid motion is driven by the motion of its boundaries, which are typically common boundaries of the moving fluid domain and the moving structure. This method introduces a fluid grid velocity $\vec{v}_g$ into the flow equations. When integrating Equation (2) over a fluid volume V, of which the surface S is moving with grid velocity $\vec{v}_g$ and has outward normal $\vec{n}$, Equation (2) becomes:

$$\frac{\partial}{\partial t}\int_V dV + \int_S \left(\vec{v} - \vec{v}_g\right)\cdot\vec{n}\, dS = 0 \tag{7a}$$

$$\frac{\partial}{\partial t}\int_V \rho\vec{v}\, dV + \int_S \rho\vec{v}\left(\vec{v} - \vec{v}_g\right)\cdot\vec{n}\, dS = -\int_S p\vec{n}\, dS + \int_S \mu\left(\nabla\vec{v} + \left(\nabla\vec{v}\right)^T\right)\cdot\vec{n}\, dS \tag{7b}$$

When $\vec{v}_g = \vec{v}$, this results in a purely Lagrangian description. When $\vec{v}_g = \vec{0}$, a purely Eulerian description is recovered. Moreover, the fluid grid velocity is called "arbitrary" because it does not have to correspond to the fluid velocity. However, when the grid deformation becomes too large, as is the case with BMHVs, this could deteriorate the grid quality. Therefore, local remeshing is needed between time-steps. The main advantage of the ALE approach is its accuracy, because the grid is aligned with the fluid-structure interface. However, the use of remeshing (and thus interpolation) introduces artificial diffusivity and can become expensive for complex three-dimensional geometries. Several studies have used the ALE approach to simulate the dynamics of the ATS Open Pivot™ Standard Heart Valve (Dumont et al., 2005, 2007), the St. Jude Medical™ BMHV (Penrose et al., 2002; Redaelli et al., 2004; Dumont et al., 2007; Guivier et al., 2007, 2009; Nobili et al., 2007, 2008; Choi et al., 2009; Hong et al., 2009), and other valve types (Makhijani et al., 1997; Vierendeels et al., 2005, 2007; Bang et al., 2006; Morsi et al., 2007).

2.2 Monolithic solver versus partitioned solver

Secondly, one can classify each FSI simulation by using a partitioned solver or a monolithic solver. In the monolithic approach, the entire FSI problem is simultaneously simulated by one solver.

This is in contrast to the partitioned approach, which solves the flow and the structural problem separately and, therefore, mostly uses different specialized solvers. The partitioned approach is used to simulate heart valves in Makhijani et al. (1997), Penrose et al. (2002), Redaelli et al. (2004), Dumont et al. (2005, 2007), Vierendeels et al. (2005, 2007), Bang et al. (2006), Guivier et al. (2007, 2009), Nobili et al. (2007, 2008), Morsi et al. (2007), Tai et al. (2007), Borazjani et al. (2008), Diniz dos Santos et al. (2008), Astorino et al. (2009), Choi et al. (2009), De Tullio et al. (2009), Hong et al. (2009) and, finally, Xia et al. (2009). In order to obtain the interaction between the fluid and the structure, data exchange at the fluid-structure interface and a coupling scheme between the separated solvers are needed. Unfortunately, not every coupling scheme converges quickly. The instability of coupling schemes without relaxation is analytically explained in Vierendeels et al. (2005) and Borazjani et al. (2008) for the case of BMHVs, and it is also demonstrated by the flow through arteries (Causin et al., 2005; Degroote et al., 2008, 2010). It is concluded that relaxation can be used to obtain stable and efficient approximations for the subsequent angular accelerations of the valve leaflets. Several coupling schemes with relaxation have thus been developed, and they can be divided into loose and strong coupling schemes.

In the loose coupling methods, only one coupling iteration is needed in each time-step, since the solution of the flow field at time-step n is used to calculate the angular accelerations of the leaflets for the next time-step n+1:

$$\ddot{\theta}_i^{n+1} = \left(1 - \omega_i^{n+1}\right) \cdot \ddot{\theta}_i^{n} + \omega_i^{n+1} \cdot \frac{M_i^n}{I_i} \tag{8}$$

A relaxation factor ($\omega_i^{n+1} < 1$) is necessary, since the scheme without relaxation ($\omega_i^{n+1} = 1$) is unstable (Causin et al., 2005; Vierendeels et al., 2005; Borazjani et al., 2008), as mentioned above. The loose coupling formulation is often used to simulate heart valves (Redaelli et al., 2004; Morsi et al., 2007; Nobili et al., 2007; Tai et al., 2007; Borazjani et al., 2008; Xia et al., 2009). It has the main benefit of a low computational cost because of the lack of a coupling iteration loop within each time-step. However, this lack implies that dynamic equilibrium at the fluid-structure interface (Equation (6)) is not necessarily achieved, which leads to unphysical oscillations in the leaflet movement and the flow and pressure field, as described in Annerel et al. (2011).

Dynamic equilibrium at the fluid-structure interface can be obtained by introducing a coupling iteration loop within each time-step, as is the case in the strong coupling methods. Generally, each of the strong coupling iterations follows the same pattern, as visualized in Fig. 2. At the beginning of each coupling iteration k of time-step n+1, the motion of the leaflets is computed from the angular accelerations $\ddot{\theta}_i^{n+1,k}$. The mesh is moved and the flow equations are solved. From the flow field, the moments $M_i^{n+1,k}$ are calculated. Finally, the convergence of the dynamic equilibrium at the fluid-structure interface, expressed by Equation (6), is checked. When this dynamic equilibrium is obtained, a new time-step is initiated. However, when dynamic equilibrium is not achieved, a new coupling iteration k+1 is initiated, and thus new angular accelerations $\ddot{\theta}_i^{n+1,k+1}$ need to be calculated. Therefore, introducing a coupling iteration loop requires, in each coupling iteration k of time-step n+1, a stable and efficient approximation of the angular accelerations for the next coupling iteration k+1.

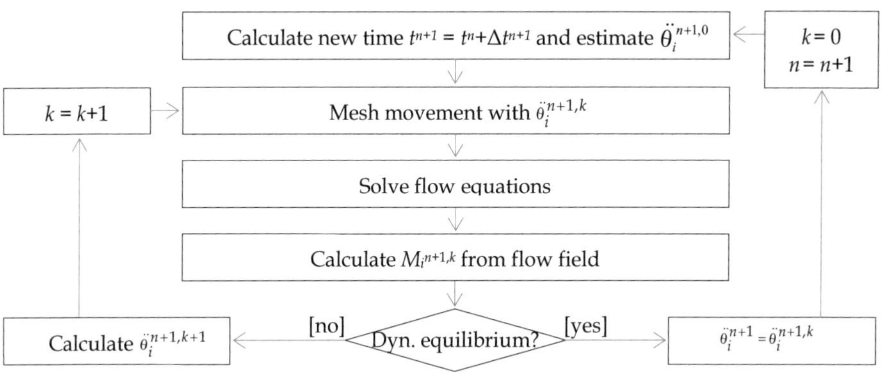

Fig. 2. Simplified flow chart of a strong FSI coupling algorithm with two degrees of freedom. n = time-step, k = coupling iteration step, i = leaflet number

A strong coupling scheme without relaxation can easily be proposed. From the moments of coupling iteration k in time-step n+1, the angular accelerations of the next coupling iteration k+1, i.e. $\ddot{\theta}_i^{n+1,k+1}$, can be calculated:

$$\ddot{\theta}_i^{n+1,k+1} = \frac{M_i^{n+1,k}}{I_i} \tag{9}$$

Unfortunately, such fixed-point iterations, also called Gauss-Seidel iterations without relaxation, are unstable for BMHVs (Vierendeels et al., 2005). Therefore, the scheme needs to be stabilized by using an appropriate prediction of the moments of the next coupling iteration k+1:

$$\ddot{\theta}_i^{n+1,k+1} = \frac{\hat{M}_i^{n+1,k+1}}{I_i} \tag{10}$$

with $\hat{M}_i^{n+1,k+1}$ denoting the predicted moment. Several methods are used in the literature to calculate a stable value for $\hat{M}_i^{n+1,k+1}$. Usually, this is achieved using a relaxation scheme, which leads to fixed-point iterations with relaxation ($\omega_i^{n+1,k} < 1$), also called the Gauss-Seidel coupling method with relaxation:

$$\hat{M}_i^{n+1,k+1} = \left(1-\omega_i^{n+1,k}\right)\cdot I_i\ddot{\theta}_i^{n+1,k} + \omega_i^{n+1,k}\cdot M_i^{n+1,k} \tag{11}$$

Inserted in Equation (10):

$$\ddot{\theta}_i^{n+1,k+1} = \left(1-\omega_i^{n+1,k}\right)\cdot \ddot{\theta}_i^{n+1,k} + \omega_i^{n+1,k}\cdot \frac{M_i^{n+1,k}}{I_i} \tag{12}$$

To simulate a BMHV in a partitioned way, several methods can be used to calculate an appropriate relaxation factor $\omega_i^{n+1,k}$ that stabilizes the solution process. In the following, using a fixed relaxation factor and a dynamic relaxation factor is discussed.

For the fixed relaxation factor, the factor value is kept constant during the entire simulation, as described in Le Tallec & Mouro (2001) for an industrial shock absorber valve:

$$\omega_i^{n+1,k} = \omega = Cst \tag{13}$$

Fixed relaxation was used to simulate the dynamics of a BMHV with a partitioned solver by Penrose et al. (2002), Nobili et al. (2007, 2008), Borazjani et al. (2008), De Tullio et al. (2009), and Hong et al. (2009). The main disadvantage of such a fixed relaxation is the lack of a physical meaning of the relaxation factor (Annerel et al., 2011). Therefore, the selection of an appropriate factor value is ad hoc and will be done primarily through trial-and-error, as noted by De Tullio et al. (2009).

For the dynamic relaxation factor, the factor value is updated in each coupling iteration of each time-step. Typically, the Aitken Δ^2 relaxation is used, as described in Irons et al. (1969), Mok et al. (2001), and Küttler et al. (2008). The Aitken Δ^2 relaxation updates the value of the factor in each coupling iteration of each time-step n+1:

$$\omega_i^{n+1,k} = \omega^{n+1,k} = -\frac{\left(\ddot{\boldsymbol{\theta}}^{n+1,k}-\ddot{\boldsymbol{\theta}}^{n+1,k-1}\right)^T\left(\boldsymbol{r}^{n+1,k}-\boldsymbol{r}^{n+1,k-1}\right)}{\left(\boldsymbol{r}^{n+1,k}-\boldsymbol{r}^{n+1,k-1}\right)^T\left(\boldsymbol{r}^{n+1,k}-\boldsymbol{r}^{n+1,k-1}\right)} \tag{14}$$

with

$$\ddot{\boldsymbol{\theta}}^{n+1,k} = \begin{bmatrix}\ddot{\theta}_1^{n+1,k}\\ \ddot{\theta}_2^{n+1,k}\end{bmatrix} \text{ and } \boldsymbol{r}^{n+1,k} = \begin{bmatrix}\dfrac{M_1^{n+1,k}}{I_1}-\ddot{\theta}_1^{n+1,k}\\ \dfrac{M_2^{n+1,k}}{I_2}-\ddot{\theta}_2^{n+1,k}\end{bmatrix} \tag{15}$$

Partitioned simulations of heart valves using the Aitken Δ^2 relaxation method are reported in Borazjani et al. (2008), Diniz dos Santos et al. (2008), and Astorino et al. (2009).

More recently, however, a (quasi-Newton) method with a dynamically changing relaxation matrix has been developed (Annerel et al., 2010; Dahl et al., 2010) and subsequently optimized in Annerel et al. (2011). The method is an extension of Vierendeels et al. (2005) and predicts the moments of the next coupling iteration (i.e. $\hat{M}_i^{n+1,k+1}$ in Equation (10)) through a linearization of the dynamic equilibrium. Thus, while taking into account the mutual interaction between the leaflets, Equation (6) is linearized for each coupling iteration k+1 of time-step n+1:

$$\begin{cases} M_1^{n+1,k} + \left(\dfrac{\partial M_1}{\partial \ddot{\theta}_1}\right)^{n+1,k} \left(\ddot{\theta}_1^{n+1,k+1} - \ddot{\theta}_1^{n+1,k}\right) + \left(\dfrac{\partial M_1}{\partial \ddot{\theta}_2}\right)^{n+1,k} \left(\ddot{\theta}_2^{n+1,k+1} - \ddot{\theta}_2^{n+1,k}\right) = I_1 \cdot \ddot{\theta}_1^{n+1,k+1} \\ M_2^{n+1,k} + \left(\dfrac{\partial M_2}{\partial \ddot{\theta}_1}\right)^{n+1,k} \left(\ddot{\theta}_1^{n+1,k+1} - \ddot{\theta}_1^{n+1,k}\right) + \left(\dfrac{\partial M_2}{\partial \ddot{\theta}_2}\right)^{n+1,k} \left(\ddot{\theta}_2^{n+1,k+1} - \ddot{\theta}_2^{n+1,k}\right) = I_2 \cdot \ddot{\theta}_2^{n+1,k+1} \end{cases} \quad (16)$$

The components of the Jacobian are the derivatives of the moments (exerted by the flow on the leaflets) with respect to changes in leaflet angular accelerations. This Jacobian is approximated with finite differences and is numerically calculated from the flow solver by variations of the leaflet angular accelerations. This method outperforms the fixed relaxation and Aitken Δ^2 relaxation in needed coupling iterations per time-step and CPU time (Annerel et al., 2010, 2011).

3. Insights into the general dynamics and flow fields of an aortic BMHV

The dynamics of a BMHV depend on passive movement. Therefore, the opening and closure of the leaflets are governed by the pressure gradients and flow fields in the heart and arteries (in case of atrioventricular valves) (Butany et al., 2003).
In the following, the kinematics and dynamics of a BMHV are discussed and obtained by numerical simulations in an axisymmetric geometry (Yoganathan et al., 2004; Borazjani et al., 2008; De Tullio et al., 2009; Sotiropoulos et al., 2009) and verified by experiments (Dasi et al., 2007). These discussed dynamics are also illustrated in the numerical simulations done in Section 4.

Opening phase

The contraction of the left ventricle at the beginning of systole induces an increase of the left ventricular pressure. Because of the resulting positive transvalvular pressure gradient, the flow starts to accelerate and induces the opening of the valve.
In a BMHV, the valve leaflets initially open with a large increase in angular acceleration (and related angular velocity). However, as the valve opens, the leaflets tend to align with the axial flow, and their local linear velocity tends to become orthogonal to the main flow stream lines, which produces a pressure moment that decreases the angular acceleration and lowers the angular velocity (De Tullio et al., 2009). This deceleration is beneficial because it results in a very small angular velocity of the leaflets when the leaflets reach the fully open position; therefore, it significantly lowers the impact forces at the blocking mechanism.
During the early leaflet opening phase, three jet flows are formed, with the roll-up of the valve housing shear layer into the aortic sinuses of Valsalva and the formation of two shear layers shed from the tips of the valve leaflets (Borazjani et al., 2008; De Tullio et al., 2009; Sotiropoulos et al., 2009). Subsequently, these leaflet shear layers break down and large-scale von Karman-like vortex shedding emerges (Sotiropoulos et al., 2009).

Fully open position

When the leaflets have reached the fully open position, the flow rate continues increasing until its maximum value at peak systole. Due to the acceleration of the flow, the formation of small-scale turbulence is prevented, and the bulk of the flow remains laminar (De Tullio et al., 2009). However, at peak systole, the flow starts to decelerate. Subsequently, the large-scale vortices in the sinuses of Valsalva and the leaflet shear layers rapidly undergo the transition to a small-scale turbulent state downstream of the valve (Borazjani et al., 2008; Sotiropoulos et al., 2009).

Closing phase

The valve leaflets start to close at the beginning of the steepest flow deceleration (De Tullio et al., 2009). Since the leaflets need to rotate over a large angle, some regurgitation occurs. The total volume of this reverse flow is denoted as the "closing volume" (as also described in Section 5).

During leaflet closure, the angular velocity of the leaflets keeps increasing until the closed position is reached. This gives rise to very large angular velocities (and thus stresses) when the leaflets impact the blocking mechanism at the fully closed position. Therefore, the closing kinematics are very different from those at the leaflet opening phase because the end of the opening occurs with small angular velocities, while at the end of the closing, the angular velocity attains peak value (De Tullio et al., 2009).

During the closing phase, the decelerating flow field is governed by small-scale eddies and turbulent vortices (Borazjani et al., 2008; Sotiropoulos et al., 2009).

Fully closed position

The leaflets reach the fully closed position at the negative peak of the flow rate (De Tullio et al., 2009). Due to the negative transvalvular pressure gradient when the leaflets are closed, flow leaks through the small gaps between the leaflets and through the gaps between the leaflets and valve casing (in particular, near the hinges), giving rise to squeezed jet flow. The total amount of this regurgitant flow is denoted as the "leakage volume" (see Section 5).

After valve closure, the turbulent structures in the flow slowly decay. Subsequently, the residual vortical structures are rapidly washed out at the beginning of a new cycle by the incoming accelerated flow when the valve reopens. (Borazjani et al., 2008; De Tullio et al., 2009; Sotiropoulos et al., 2009).

4. Three-dimensional strongly coupled partitioned FSI simulations of a BMHV

To illustrate the previous section, a BMHV is simulated in three different geometries. The used BMHV is a simplified model of the 25-mm ATS Open Pivot™ Standard Heart Valve in aortic position, with the orifice inner diameter measuring 20.8mm. The valve is simplified at the hinge regions by cutting away the blocking mechanism and hinges at the casing. Because of this simplification, the resulting opening velocity of the valve leaflets could become slightly overestimated since the additional counteracting moment created by the decelerated squeeze flows near the pivot hinge regions (i.e. the so-called pivot effect, as observed in the experiments in Feng et al. (1999)) is absent.

The valve is subsequently placed in three geometries. The first geometry consists of a rigid straight tube, as visualized in Fig. 3(*left*). The second geometry also consists of a rigid straight tube upstream of the valve, but rigid sinuses of Valsalva are added downstream of the valve. Such sinuses of Valsalva are anatomically present in the ascending aortic root and influence the valve closing (Grigioni et al., 2004). The sinuses of Valsalva are based on the geometry described in Reul et al. (1990) and are positioned symmetrically with respect to the leaflet rotation axes (Fig. 3(*middle*)). In the third geometry, the same sinuses of Valsalva are used, but they are placed asymmetrically (angle: 30°) with respect to the leaflet rotation axes in such a way that one of the leaflets directly faces one sinus (Fig. 3(*right*)).

For the geometries, the upstream tube has a diameter of 22mm and is 75mm long. The downstream geometry is 95mm long. The diameter of the downstream tube is 27.36 mm for the sinuses of Valsalva and 22mm for the straight tube.
These geometries are based on clinical practice, because when implanting the BMHV, the surgeon can choose to preserve the sinuses of Valsalva or to cut them away and replace the entire ascending aortic root (in the so-called Bentall procedure (Bentall et al., 1968)). Moreover, the surgeon can choose to position the valve symmetrically to the physiological sinuses of Valsalva, or to position it asymmetrically.
An unstructured fluid grid, consisting of approximately 800 000 tetrahedral cells, is generated in the geometries. Two cell layers are generated in the gap (which measures 0.1mm) between the leaflets and the casing near the hinge region. The ALE approach is followed, which means that the fluid grid follows the motion of the structure and subsequently needs an update to maintain good mesh quality. This update is done using a remeshing method and spring-based smoothing.

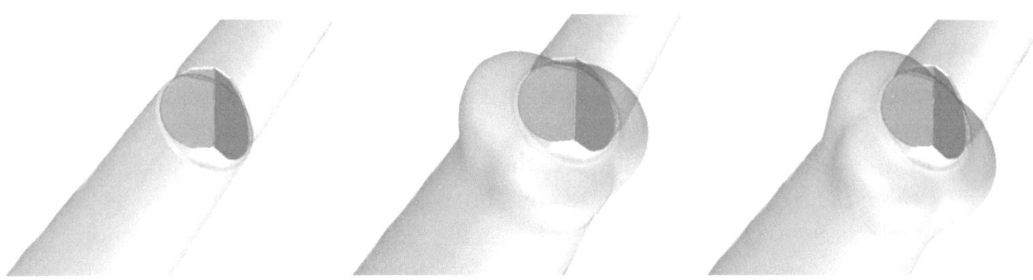

Fig. 3. Isometric view of the different geometries. *Left*: first geometry with straight tube. *Middle*: second geometry with symmetrically placed sinuses of Valsalva. *Right*: third geometry with asymmetrically positioned sinuses of Valsalva downstream of the valve

The dynamics of the BMHV are modeled by the strongly coupled partitioned quasi-Newton algorithm that was recently developed (Annerel et al., 2011). An inlet aortic flow pulse with a period of 1s (displayed in Fig. 4(*a*)) is imposed upstream and was previously used in Dumont et al. (2005, 2007) and Annerel et al. (2010, 2011). The flow pulse profile is uniform. A physiological pressure profile is imposed at the downstream outlet boundary. Note, however, that in a rigid geometry the pressure level does not affect the flow field since only the pressure gradient appears in the equations.
Blood is modeled as an incompressible Newtonian fluid with density and viscosity respectively equal to 1050kg/m^3 and 4E-3Pa·s (i.e. the high shear rate limit viscosity of blood). Although real blood is a heterogeneous non-Newtonian fluid, the modeling of blood as a homogeneous Newtonian fluid for high shear rates is widely agreed upon for flow in large arteries and valves (Paul et al., 2003; Sotiropoulos et al., 2009). Nevertheless, it is important to keep in mind that when studying low levels of shear stresses, for example in the recirculation regions and vortices in the wake, the non-Newtonian effects could become important and should be taken into account when assessing the hemodynamics of the valve (Sotiropoulos et al., 2009). In such cases it is valuable to model the blood as a non-Newtonian fluid as in the Cross and Carreau model (Cross, 1965; Carreau, 1972). However, modeling of the fine-flow features and the hemodynamics is beyond the scope of the described simulations and, therefore, a Newtonian blood model is used.

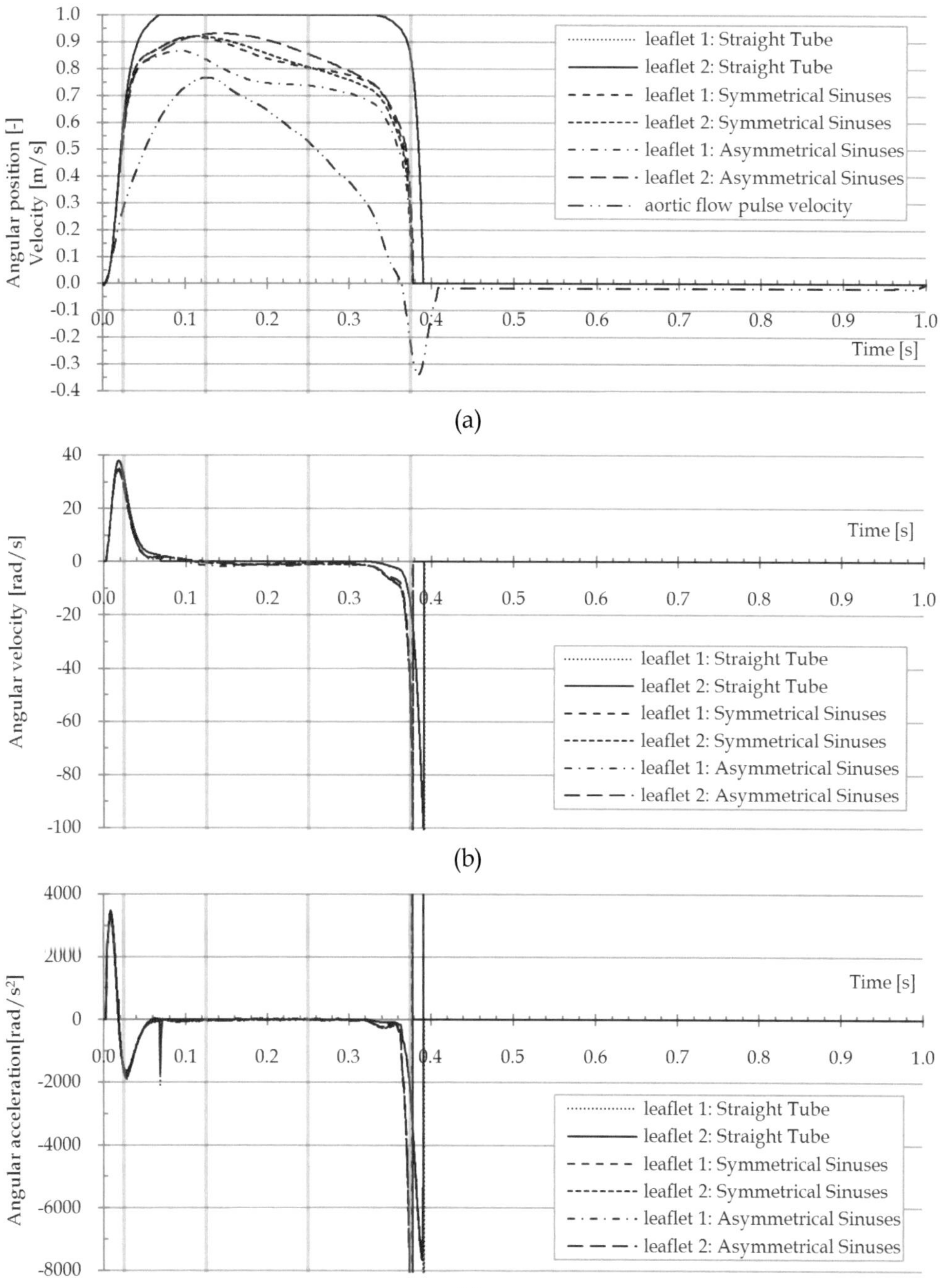

Fig. 4. Angular position of the leaflets (relative to maximal opening angle) and the aortic flow pulse velocity (*a*), angular velocity of the leaflets (*b*) and angular acceleration of the leaflets (*c*). The two leaflets of the geometry with the straight tube perform a complete symmetrical movement. The time levels at which the contours in Fig. 5 are shown are visualized by the vertical lines

No turbulence model is used, thus implying laminar flow. A no-slip boundary condition is applied at the walls. The valve is initially set in the closed position. The moment of inertia of one rigid valve leaflet about its rotation axis is equal to 9.94E-9kg·m^2.

The results of the simulations are depicted in Fig. 4 and Fig. 5. The angular positions of the leaflets are presented in Fig. 4(*a*), relative to the fully opened position. Therefore, 0 and 1 refer, respectively, to the fully closed and fully open position.

Although the valve leaflets open completely in the first geometry with the straight tube, the results show that this maximum opening position is not reached in both geometries with the sinuses of Valsalva. Such incomplete opening of the ATS Open Pivot™ Standard Heart Valve in a divergent geometry is explained by the greater sensitivity of the leaflet movement to the flow field compared with other BMHV designs, since the leaflets extend farther in the flow downstream of the orifice than is the case in other valve designs (Feng et al., 1999). Therefore, the valve does not open completely in the divergent transvalvular flow caused by the enlargement of the sinuses of Valsalva because the leaflets tend to align with the streamlines. In the straight tube, however, the valve leaflets open completely.

This incomplete opening also explains the difference in the closing phase between the geometries, since the valve in the sinuses of Valsalva geometries is closed sooner. This is because the leaflets in the straight tube reach the completely open position and therefore need to rotate over a greater angle in order to close. Hence, they have a greater closing volume (Feng et al., 2000). Nevertheless, the instant at which the leaflets start to close is approximately the same for both geometries.

Furthermore, for the asymmetrical geometry, the two leaflets show differences in movement. It can be understood that this asynchrony is triggered by the presence of the asymmetric geometry downstream of the valve (De Tullio et al., 2009; Hong et al., 2009). In the symmetrical geometries, there are no differences in movement between the two leaflets.

The velocity magnitudes at different time levels for the three geometries are shown in Fig. 5. Downstream of the valve, the three jet flows are clearly visible.

5. Design challenges

The ideal heart valve should have, among other things, a small drop in flow potential energy (i.e. small pressure drop over the valve and a high effective orifice area), a small retrograde flow, good hemodynamic properties, and high durability and safety in use.

In the remainder of this section, each of these design challenges will be discussed in detail.

Small regurgitation volume

Mechanical valves are characterized by a significant amount of regurgitant flow. This retrograde flow is the sum of the closing volume and the leakage flow (Yoganathan et al., 2004). The closing volume is the amount of reverse flow needed to let the leaflets rotate to the closed position. The leakage flow occurs during diastole, when the leaflets are in the closed position and blood flows back through the gaps of the valve due to the large negative pressure gradient over the valve.

The regurgitation volume V_{reg} (in ml) is typically measured by percentage ($\%reg$) of forward stroke volume SV_{fwd} (in ml), as described in Verdonck et al. (2002):

$$\%reg = \frac{V_{reg}}{V_{reg} + SV_{fwd}} \tag{17}$$

Since the regurgitation lowers the net cardiac output and therefore enlarges the workload of the heart, its percentage should be minimized when designing heart valves.

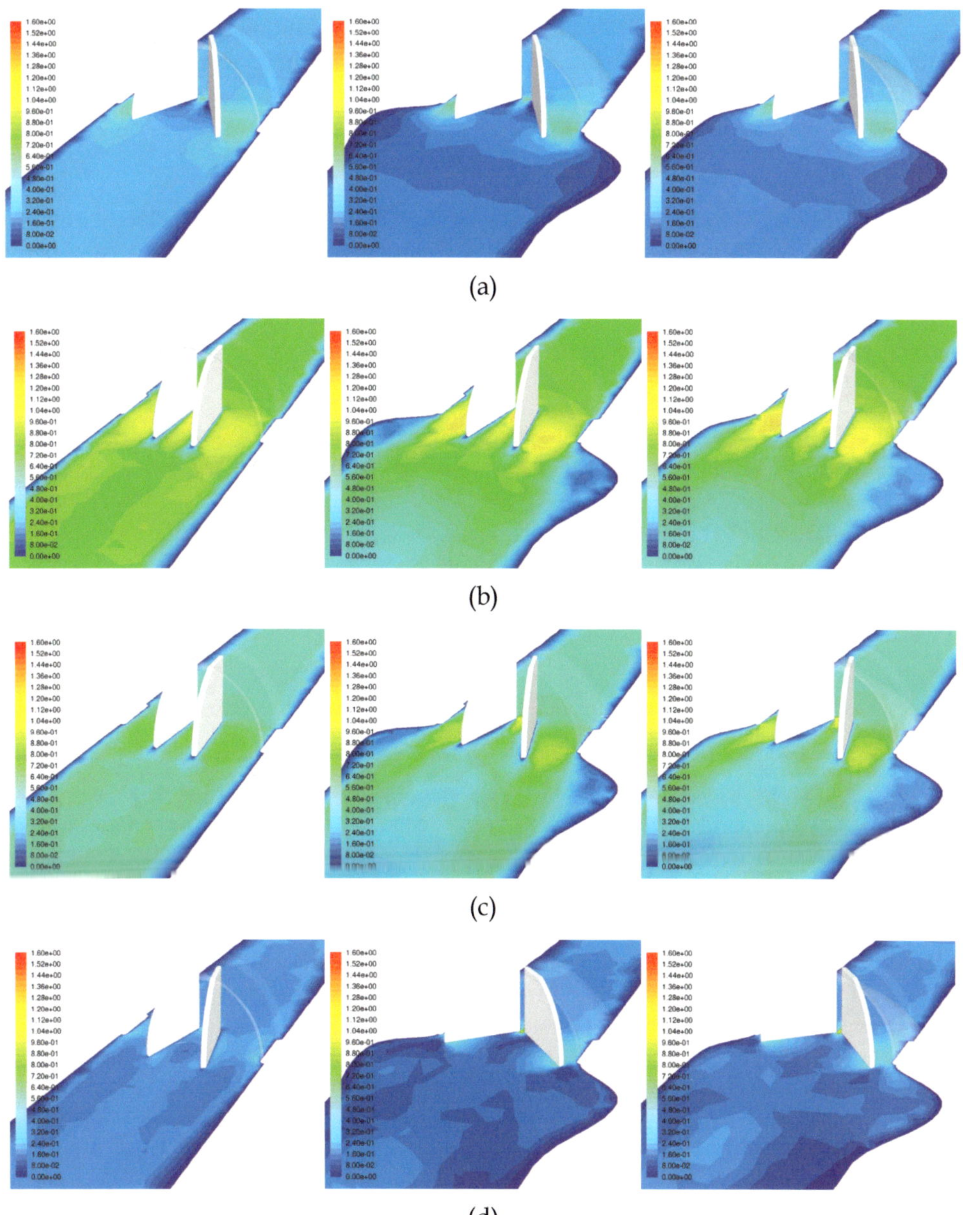

Fig. 5. Velocity Magnitude Contours in m/s visualized on a longitudinal section perpendicular to the leaflet rotation axes, for the geometry with the straight tube (*left*), the symmetrically placed sinuses of Valsalva (*middle*) and the asymmetrical sinuses of Valsalva (*right*). The plots are taken at t = 0.025s (*a*), t = 0.125s (*b*), t = 0.250s (*c*), and t = 0.375s (*d*), represented by the vertical lines in Fig. 4

Low transvalvular pressure gradient (TPG)

The transvalvular pressure gradient (TPG) is related to the drop in pressure that is needed for viscous blood to flow through the valve (Yoganathan et al., 2004). This forward pressure difference $\Delta p_{Doppler}$ (in mmHg) can be derived from a simplified form of the Bernoulli equation and the mean (Doppler) velocity V_{mean} (in m/s) during forward flow (Verdonck et al., 2002):

$$\Delta p_{Doppler} = 4V_{mean}^2 \tag{18}$$

The TPG is a measure of valve efficiency (Yoganathan et al., 2004). The workload on the left ventricle is directly related to the magnitude of this pressure difference, because when the magnitude of the TPG increases, an increasing systolic pressure in the left ventricle is needed to drive flow forward into the aorta. Therefore, the TPG should be minimized when designing valve prostheses (Yoganathan et al., 2004).

High effective orifice area (EOA)

Because the TPG is heavily dependent on the flow rate, another less flow-rate-dependent parameter is more commonly used as a measure for the quality of the valve, namely the effective orifice area (EOA).

Several formulations of the EOA (in cm^2) can be defined, of which the Gorlin equation is mostly used (Baumgartner et al., 1992; Yoganathan et al., 1984). It is based on the fundamental hydraulic law of flow through an orifice and couples the flow through the valve orifice to the Doppler pressure gradient over the valve (Verdonck et al., 2002):

$$EOA = \frac{Q_{fwd,mean}}{51.6\sqrt{\Delta p_{Doppler}}} \tag{19}$$

where $Q_{fwd,mean}$ is the mean forward flow rate (in cm^3/s). The constant 51.6 accounts for gravity and unit conversions (Baumgartner et al., 1992; Verdonck et al., 2002; Yoganathan et al., 2007).

The EOA is a measure for valve quality because it assesses the severity of the stenosis formed by the presence of the valve and thus the degree to which the prosthesis obstructs the blood flow (Yoganathan et al., 2004). A large EOA corresponds to a smaller pressure drop and thus to a smaller energy loss (Yoganathan et al., 2004). Therefore, when designing a valve prosthesis, the resulting EOA should be maximized.

Moreover, the EOA can be used to compare the efficiency of various valve designs, because it is a better index of valve function than is TPG alone (Zoghbi et al., 2009). However, to get a normalized value, the EOA should be made independent of the valve size by dividing it by the valve sewing ring area A_{sew}. This results in the performance index (PI), which provides a measure of the valve's resistance characteristics normalized to valve size (Yoganathan et al., 2004, 2007):

$$PI = \frac{EOA}{A_{sew}} \tag{20}$$

Therefore, the parameter PI can be used to fairly compare the efficiency of various artificial valves.

Good hemodynamic properties

One of the most challenging aspects in valve design is the improvement of hemocompatibility. Because the cardiovascular system is a closed circulatory system, damage to the blood cells can accumulate each time blood passes through the valve, which leads to an increased risk for platelet activation and hemolysis of the red blood cells (erythrocytes). This could result in clinical complications such as thromboembolisms and valve stenosis.

Blood cells can become damaged by non-physiological flow patterns or by contact with artificial materials (Paul et al., 2003). Therefore, to optimize blood flow through the valve, one should minimize the production of shear stresses and turbulence in the flow and avoid any flow stagnation and separation in the vicinity of the valve (Yoganathan et al., 2004). Moreover, the valve should be composed of (or coated with) biocompatible materials. Therefore, mostly pyrolytic carbon is used.

Durability and failure-safe design

Structural wear and fatigue of the valve can deteriorate the valve material and can cause severe valve failure.

Moreover, cavitation, which leads to erosion and pitting, can occur in BMHVs. Such cavitation-induced erosion and pitting were first related to BMHVs in the 1980s after observation of a series of severe leaflet escapes of the Edwards-Duromedics bileaflet valve (Mastroroberto et al., 2000; Johansen, 2004). It was seen that the hard, but brittle, pyrolytic carbon can become subject to cavitation-induced fatigue leading to a transverse fracture of the leaflet or a leaflet fracture near the pivot mechanism (Klepetko et al., 1989).

Later, leaflet escape in the same (but revised) bileaflet valve type was observed in mitral (Hemmer et al., 2000; Mert et al., 2003) and aortic position (Christiansen, 2001).

Therefore, for a durable and failure-safe design, the structural wear and fatigue potential should be minimized along with a minimization of the formation of cavitation bubbles.

Design challenges and BMHVs

Although current aortic BMHVs show a higher EOA and a higher PI compared with other artificial heart valve designs, such as the caged ball valve, the tilting disc valve, and the (non)stented bioprostheses (Yoganathan et al., 2004), some major design challenges concerning the hemodynamics and the durability need to be resolved. Moreover, BMHVs have a larger regurgitant volume than other artificial valves (Yoganathan et al., 2004).

In the remainder of this section, the hemodynamics and the cavitation of the BMHV are discussed in detail, with special interest to the flow near the hinges.

5.1 Blood damage and BMHVs

When blood flows through artificial devices, blood particulates can become damaged and initiate a cascade of events leading to coagulation and the formation of thrombi. Therefore, when a BMHV is implanted, the patient is required to take lifelong anticoagulation therapies (Paul et al., 2003; Bluestein et al., 2004; Dasi et al., 2009; Morbiducci et al., 2009).

Blood trauma can occur via several mechanisms, depending on the type of damaged blood cell. In the past, the fragmentation and damaging of erythrocytes was experimentally quantified, since this leads to hemolysis (Sutera et al., 1975; Paul et al., 2003). In recent years, however, platelet activation is believed to be the major underlying formation mechanism for thromboembolic complications in the flow past mechanical heart valves (Bluestein, 2004; Morbiducci et al., 2009).

The amount of blood damage depends primarily on the cumulative effect of the magnitude and the duration (the exposure time) of the applied force. Critical values of both factors can be exceeded by flow-dependent and non-flow-dependent causes (Paul et al., 2003).
The non-flow-dependent causes are the contact with artificial surfaces, which can be eliminated by using biocompatible materials. Therefore, pyrolytic carbon is commonly used for BMHVs because of its strength and high durability (Chandran et al., 2010) and good biocompatible properties (Johansen, 2004).
The flow-dependent causes are believed to originate from non-physiological flow patterns. However, despite many research efforts, the exact mechanisms underlying these flow-induced thromboembolic complications are still poorly understood (Bluestein, 2004). It is believed that the presence of elevated shear stresses in the flow is the most important platelet-damaging effect. Three non-physiological flow patterns can be distinguished.
Firstly, the squeeze flows observed as leakage flow when the leaflets are completely closed during diastole are of specific interest. Some leakage flow near the hinges is beneficial because it washes out the hinge regions and prevents flow stagnation and the development of thrombosis. However, the high-flow-velocity gradients can become too large, which causes elevated shear stresses and related platelet activation (Yoganathan et al., 2004).
Secondly, regions of flow separation, recirculation, and stagnation promote the deposition of damaged blood cells and increase the formation of thrombi (Yoganathan et al., 2004).
Finally, the shear layers surrounding the leaflets and the wake also expose the platelets to elevated shear stresses and lead them towards entrapment in the shed vortices of the wake (Bluestein et al., 2002).
Several studies used numerical methods to calculate the accumulated platelet activation when the blood flows through a BMHV. In the past, the valve leaflets were kept in a fixed position throughout the cardiac cycle due to the computational cost (Bluestein et al., 2002; Alemu et al., 2007; Dumont et al., 2005, 2007). More recently, however, Morbiducci et al. (2009) combined numerical FSI simulations with a numerical blood damage model. They reported that platelet activation is lower at early systole than at late systole and that the spanwise vorticity has a greater influence on the activation of platelets than does the streamwise vorticity.
A critical value for accumulated shear stress above which platelets are considered activated is, for example, given by the Hellums activation threshold criterion, i.e. $3.5 Ns/m^2$ (Hellums et al., 1987; Dumont et al., 2007).

5.2 Cavitation and BMHVs

Cavitation is the formation of voids or gas bubbles in liquids caused by a local reduction of the pressure to below that of vapor pressure. However, as soon as the surrounding pressure increases above vapor pressure, the formed bubbles will rapidly implode, which produces devastating shockwaves in the surrounding fluid (Johansen, 2004).
Several fluid mechanisms can lead to a pressure drop below vapor pressure in the blood flow during the closing phase of a BMHV. Firstly, squeeze flows are considered a contributing factor to the initation of cavitation. Such squeeze jets are formed at the very instant before leaflet closing, when the blood between the leaflets and valve casing is accelerated through the narrowing gap. This creates a high velocity jet flow with a large pressure gradient. The pressure can locally fall below vapor pressure, thus leading to cavitation (Bluestein et al., 1994; Johansen, 2004). Secondly, large vortices can be shed from the leaflet tips during the closing of the leaflets and during regurgitation. Towards the core of these vortices, the pressure decreases and the flow velocity increases. Therefore, the

conditions for cavitation can be reached in these vortex cores (Avrahami et al., 2000; Johansen, 2004). Finally, the formation of cavitation bubbles can also be augmented by the sudden stop of the valve leaflets as they impact the casing, often referred to as "water hammer cavitation"(Lee et al., 2002; Johansen, 2004).

It is believed that in BMHVs none of these mechanisms alone but solely their combined interaction can initiate and augment cavitation. Moreover, valves with very stiff leaflets, closing at high velocity and decelerating rapidly (due to the impact at the blocking mechanism of the casing), are more prone to cause cavitation than valves with flexible leaflets that are gently decelerated (Zapanta et al., 1998; Johansen, 2004).

Although the formation of cavitation bubbles in the blood flow through a BMHV is an extremely rare phenomenon, it is undesirable because the shockwaves produced during the implosion of the cavitation bubbles can create high-velocity microjets. These microjets can deteriorate the valve structures as well as the nearby blood cells, thus leading to severe thromboembolic complications and valve failures (Johansen, 2004).

Cavitation-induced material deterioration of a BMHV was first related to BMHVs in the 1980s after several leaflet escapes of the Edwards-Duromedics bileaflet valve, as described above (Mastroroberto et al., 2000; Johansen, 2004). It was observed that the impingement of high-velocity microjets can cause erosion and pitting when it impacts the structural surfaces. Lee et al. (2002) reported the appearance of cavitation-induced erosion pits in regions where squeeze flow occurred immediately before valve closure. Moreover, the study indicated that the number of pits was closely related to the magnitude of the pressure drop caused by the water hammer phenomenon.

6. Conclusion

Each year, replacing failing aortic heart valves with mechanical heart valves saves thousands of human lives.

However, modern BMHVs are still far from perfect and still face major design challenges. Most of these design challenges involve the hemodynamic properties of the valve and are thus directly related to the blood flow. Therefore, a thorough understanding of the blood flow is required for design optimization.

Current numerical simulation techniques can provide such valuable information and are considered crucial for gaining insights into the blood flow and assessing the performance of future valve prototypes.

The numerical simulations discussed in this chapter illustrate the incomplete opening of the aortic ATS Open Pivot™ Standard Heart Valve in a diverging geometry. Moreover, asymmetrically placed sinuses of Valsalva induce an asymmetrical movement of the valve leaflets.

7. Acknowledgment

Sebastiaan Annerel gratefully acknowledges a BOF-grant (Special Research Fund) from Ghent University Association.

8. References

Akutsu, T. & Higuchi, D. (2001). Flow analysis of the bileaflet mechanical prosthetic heart valves using laser Doppler anemometer: effect of the valve designs and installed orientations to the flow inside the simulated left ventricle. *J Artif Organs*, Vol. 4, pp. 113-125.

Alemu, Y. & Bluestein, D. (2007). Flow-induced platelet activation and damage accumulation in a mechanical heart valve: numerical studies. *Artific Organs*, Vol. 31, No. 9, pp. 677-688.

Aljassim, O., Svensson, G., Houltz, E. & Bech-Hanssen, O. (2008). Doppler-catheter discrepancies in patients with bileaflet mechanical prostheses or bioprostheses in the aortic valve position. *Am J Cardiol*, Vol. 2008, pp. 1383-1389.

Annerel, S., Degroote, J., Claessens, T. & Vierendeels, J. (2010). Evaluation of a new implicit coupling algorithm for the partitioned fluid-structure interaction simulation of bileaflet mechanical heart valves. *IOP Conf Ser: Mater Sci Eng*, Vol. 10, 012124.

Annerel, S., Degroote, J., Claessens, T., *et al.* (2011). A fast strong coupling algorithm for the partitioned fluid-structure interaction simulation of BMHVs. *Comput Method Biomec*, In press.

Aoyagi, S., Arinaga, K., Fukunaga, S., Tayama, E., Kosuga, T. & Akashi, H. (2006). Leaflet movement of the ATS Valve in the aortic position: unique behavior observed in 19-mm valves. *Ann Thorac Surg*, Vol. 82, pp. 853-857.

Aslam, A.K., Aslam, A.F., Vasavada, B. & Khan, I.A. (2007). Prosthetic heart valves: types and echocardiographic evaluation. *Int J Cardiol*, Vol. 122, pp. 99-110.

Astorino, M., Gerbeau, J.-F., Pantz, O. & Traoré, K.-F. (2009). Fluid-structure interaction and multi-body contact: application to aortic valves. *Comput Methods Appl Mech Engrg*, Vol. 198, pp. 3603-3612.

Avrahami, I., Rosenfeld, M., Einav, S., Eichler, M. & Reul, H. (2000). Can vortices in the flow across mechanical heart valves contribute to cavitation? *Med Biol Eng Comput*, Vol. 38, pp. 93-97.

Bang, J.S., Yoo, S.M. & Kim, C.N. (2006). Characteristics of pulsatile blood flow through the curved bileaflet mechanical heart valve installed in two different types of blood vessels: velocity and pressure of blood flow. *ASAIO J*, Vol. 52, pp. 234-242.

Baumgartner, H., Khan, S.S., DeRobertis, M., Czer, L.S. & Maurer, G. (1992). Doppler assessment of prosthetic valve orifice area. An in vitro study. *Circulation*, Vol. 85, pp. 2275-2283.

Bech-Hanssen, O., Caidahl, K., Wallentin, I., Ask, P. & Wranne, B. (2001). Assessment of effective orifice area of prosthetic aortic valves with Doppler echocardiography: An in vivo and in vitro study. *J Thorac Cardiovasc Surg*, Vol. 122, pp. 287-295.

Bentall, H. & De Bono, A. (1968). A technique for complete replacement of the ascending aorta. *Thorax*, Vol. 23, pp. 338-339.

Bluestein, D., Einav, S. & Hwang, N.H.C. (1994). A squeeze flow phenomenon at the closing of a bileaflet mechanical heart valve prosthesis. *J Biomech*, Vol. 27, No. 11, pp. 1369-1378.

Bluestein, D., Li, Y.M. & Krukenkamp, I.B. (2002). Free emboli formation in the wake of bi-leaflet mechanical heart valves and the effects of implantation techniques. *J Biomech*, Vol. 35, pp. 1533-1540.

Bluestein, D. (2004). Research approaches for studying flow-induced thromboembolic complications in blood recirculating devices. *Expert Rev. Med Devices*, Vol. 1, No. 1, pp. 65-80.

Borazjani, I., Ge, L. & Sotiropoulos, F. (2008). Curvilinear immersed boundary method for simulating fluid structure interaction with complex 3D rigid bodies. *J Comput Phys*, Vol. 227, No. 16, pp. 7587-7620.

Browne, P., Ramuzat, A., Saxena, R. & Yoganathan, A.P. (2000). Experimental investigation of the steady flow downstream of the St. Jude bileaflet heart valve: A comparison between laser Doppler velocimetry and particle image velocimetry techniques. *Ann Biomed Eng*, Vol. 28, No. 1, pp. 39-47.

Butany, J., Ahluwalia, M.S., Munroe, C., *et al.* (2003). Mechanical heart valve prostheses: identification and evaluation (erratum). *Cardiovasc Pathol*, Vol. 12, pp. 322-344.

Carreau, P. (1972). Rheological equations from molecular network theories. *Trans Soc Rheol*, Vol. 16, No.1, pp. 99–127.

Causin, P., Gerbeau, J.-F. & Nobile, F. (2005). Added-mass effect in the design of partitioned algorithms for fluid-structure problems. *Comput Methods Appl Mech Engrg*, Vol. 194, pp. 4506-4527.

Choi, C.R. & Kim, C.N. (2009). Numerical analysis on the hemodynamics and leaflet dynamics in a bileaflet mechanical heart valve using a fluid-structure interaction method. *ASAIO J*, Vol. 55, No. 5, pp. 428-437.

Christiansen, S., Scheld, H.H. & Hammel, D. (2001). Leaflet escape in a Tekna valve in aortic position. *Ann Thorac Surg*, Vol. 71, p. 761.

Cross, M. (1965). Rheology of non-Newtonian fluids: a new flow equation for pseudoplastic systems. *J Colloid*, Vol. 20, pp. 417–437.

Dahl, S.K., Vierendeels, J., Degroote, J., Annerel, S., Hellevik, L.R. & Skallerud, B. (2010). FSI-simulation of asymmetric mitral valve dynamics during diastolic filling. *Comput Method Biomec*, DOI: 10.1080/10255842.2010.517200.

Dasi, L.P., Ge, L., Simon, H.A., Sotiropoulos, F. & Yoganathan, A.P. (2007). Vorticity dynamics of a bileaflet mechanical heart valve in an axisymmetric aorta. *Phys Fluids*, Vol. 19, 067105.

Dasi, L.P., Simon, H.A., Sucosky, P. & Yoganathan, A.P. (2009). Fluid mechanics of artificial heart valves. *Clin Exp Pharmacol Physiol*, Vol. 36, pp. 225-237.

Degroote, J., Bruggeman, P., Haelterman, R. & Vierendeels, J. (2008). Stability of a coupling technique for partitioned solvers in FSI applications. *Comput Struct*, Vol. 86, pp. 2224-2234.

Degroote, J., Annerel, S. & Vierendeels, J. (2010). Stability analysis of Gauss-Seidel iterations in a partitioned simulation of fluid-structure interaction. *Comput Struct*, Vol. 88, pp. 263-271.

De Hart, J., Peters, G.W.M., Schreurs, P.J.G. & Baaijens, F.P.T. (2000). A two-dimensional flui-structure interaction model of the aortic value. *J Biomech*, Vol. 33, pp. 1079-1088.

De Hart, J., Peters, G.W.M., Schreurs, P.J.G. & Baaijens, F.P.T. (2003). A three-dimensional computational analysis of fluid–structure interaction in the aortic valve. *J Biomech*, Vol. 36, pp. 103–112.

De Tullio, M.D., Cristallo, A., Balaras, E. & Verzicco, R. (2009). Direct numerical simulation of the pulsatile flow through an aortic bileaflet mechanical heart valve. *J Fluid Mech*, Vol. 622, pp. 259-290.

Diniz dos Santos, N.D., Gerbeau, J.-F. & Bourgat, J.-F. (2008). A partitioned fluid-structure algorithm for elastic thin valves with contact. *Comput Methods Appl Mech Engrg*, Vol. 197, pp. 1750-1761.

Donea, J., Huerta, A., Ponthot, J.-P. & Ferran A.R. (2004). Chapter 14 Arbitrary Lagrangian-Eulerian Methods, In: *Encyclopedia of Computational Mechanics, Volume 1: Fundamentals*. E. Stein, R. de Borst, J.R. Hughes (Eds.), John Wiley & Sons, ISBN:0-470-84699-2.

Dumont, K., Segers, P., Vandenberghe, S., Van Nooten, G. & Verdonck, R. (2002). Omnicarbon 21 mm aortic valve prosthesis: in vitro hydrodynamic and echo-doppler study. *Int J Artif Organs*, Vol. 25, pp. 783-790.

Dumont, K., Vierendeels, J., Segers, P., Van Nooten, G. & Verdonck, P. (2005). Predicting ATS Open Pivot Heart Valve performance with computational fluid dynamic. *J Heart Valve Dis*, Vol. 14, pp. 393-399.

Dumont, K., Vierendeels, J., Kaminsky, R., Van Nooten, G., Verdonck, P. & Bluestein, D. (2007). Comparison of the hemodynamic and thrombogenic performance of two bileaflet mechanical heart valves using a CFD/FSI model. *J Biomech Eng*, Vol. 129, pp. 558-565.

Feng, Z., Umezu, M., Fujimoto, T., *et al.* (1999). Analysis of ATS leaflet behaviour by in vitro experiment. *J Artif Organs*, Vol. 2, pp. 46-52.

Feng, Z., Umezu, M., Fujimoto, T., Tsukahara, T., Nurishi, M. & Kawaguchi, D. (2000). In vitro hydrodynamic characteristics among three bileaflet valves in the mitral position. *J Artif Organs*, Vol. 24, No. 5, pp. 346-352.

Feng, Z., Nakamura, T., Fujimoto, T. & Umezu, M. (2001). Influence of valve size on the hydrodynamic performance of the ATS valve. *J Artif Organs*, Vol. 4, pp. 303-307.

Grigioni, M., Daniele, C., D'Avenio, G., *et al.* (2004). Innovative technologies for the assessment of cardiovascular medical devices: state-of-the-art techniques for artificial heart valve testing. *Expert Rev Med Devices*, Vol. 1, No. 1, pp. 81-93.

Guivier, C., Deplano, V. & Pibarot, P. (2007). New insights into the assessment of the prosthetic valve performance in the presence of subaortic stenosis through a fluid-structure interaction model. *J Biomech*, Vol. 40, pp. 2283-2290.

Guivier-Curien, C., Deplano, V. & Bertrand, E. (2009). Validation of a numerical 3-D fluid-structure interaction model for a prosthetic valve based on experimental PIV measurements. *Med Eng Phys*, Vol. 31, pp. 986-993.

Hellums, J., Peterson, D., Stathopoulos, N., Moake, J. & Giorgio, T. (1987). Studies on the mechanisms of shear-induced platelet activation, Springer-Verlag, New York.

Hemmer, W.B., Doss, M., Hannekum, A. & Kapfer, X. (2000). Leaflet escape in a TEKNA and an original duromedics bileaflet valve. *Ann Thorac Surg*, Vol. 69, pp. 942-944.

Hirt, C.W., Amsden, A.A. & Cook, J.L. (1997). An arbitrary Lagrangian-Eulerian computing method for all flow speeds. *J Comput Phys*, Vol. 135, pp. 203-216.

Hufnagel, C.A., Harvey, W.P., Rabil, P.J. & McDermott, T.F. (1954). Surgical correction of aortic insufficiency. *Surgery*, Vol. 35, pp. 673–683.

Irons, B.M. & Tuck, R.C. (1969). A version of the Aitken accelerator for computer iteration. *Int J Numer Meth Eng*, Vol. 1, pp. 275-277.

Johansen, P. (2004). Mechanical heart valve cavitation. *Expert Rev Med Devices*, Vol. 1, No. 1, pp. 95-104.

Kaminsky, R., Kallweit, S., Weber, H.-J., Claessens, T., Jozwik, K. & Verdonck, P. (2007). Flow visualization through two types of aortic prosthetic heart valves using stereoscopic high-speed particle image velocimetry. *Artif Organs*, Vol. 31, No. 12, pp. 869-879.

Kelly, S., Verdonck, P., Vierendeels, J., Riemslagh, K., Dick, E. & Van Nooten, G. (1999). A three-dimensional analysis of flow in the pivot regions of an ATS bileaflet valve. *Int J Artif Organs*, Vol. 22, pp. 754-763.

Klepetko, W., Moritz, A., Mlczoch, J., Schurawitzki, H., Domanig, E. & Wolner, E. (1989). Leaflet fracture in Edwards-Duromedics bileaflet valves. *J Thorac Cardiovasc Surg*, Vol. 97, No. 1, pp. 90-94.

Küttler, U. & Wall, W.A. (2008). Fixed-point fluid-structure interaction solvers with dynamic relaxation. *Comput Mech*, Vol. 43, pp. 61-72.

Lee, H., Yamamoto, K., Kudo, N., Shimooka, T., Mitamura, Y. & Yuhta, T. (2002). Examination of cavitation-induced surface erosion pitting of a mechanical heart valve using closing velocities. *J Artif Organs*, Vol. 5, pp. 193–199.

Le Tallec, P. & Mouro, J. (2001). Fluid structure interaction with large structural displacements. *Comput Methods Appl Mech Engrg*, Vol. 190, pp. 3039-3067.

Makhijani, V.B., Yang, H.Q., Dionne, P.J. & Thubrikar, M.J. (1997). Three-dimensional coupled fluid–structure simulation of pericardial bioprosthetic aortic valve function. *ASAIO J*, Vol. 43, No. 5, pp. M387–M392.

Masson, C. & Rieu, R. (1998). Time-frequency analysis of the noise produced by the closing of artificial heart valves: an in vitro study. *Med Eng Phys*, Vol. 20, pp. 418-431.

Mastroroberto, P., Chello, M., Bevacqua, E., Cirillo, F. & Covino, E. (2000). Duromedics original prosthesis: what do we really know about diagnosis and mechanism of leaflet escape? *Can J Cardiol*, Vol. 16, No. 10, pp. 1269-1272.

Mert, K., Ozkara, A. & Hatemi, A. (2003). Leaflet escape in a revised Edwards-Duromedics mitral prosthesis. *J Heart Valve Dis*, Vol. 12, No. 4, pp. 513-515.

Mok, D.P., Wall, W.A. & Ramm, E. (2001). Accelerated iterative substructuring schemes for instationary fluid-structure interaction. In: *Computational Fluid and Solid Mechanics*, K. Bathe (Ed.), Elsevier, pp. 1325-1328.

Morbiducci, U., Ponzini, R., Nobili, M., *et al.* (2009). Blood damage safety of prosthetic heart valves. Shear-induced platelet activation and local flow dynamics: a fluid-structure approach. *J Biomech*, Vol. 42, pp. 1952-1960.

Morsi, Y.S., Yang, W.W., Wong, C.S. & Das, S. (2007). Transient fluid-structure coupling for simulation of a trileaflet heart valve using weak coupling. *J Artif Organs*, Vol. 10, pp. 96-103.

Nobili, M., Passoni, G. & Redaelli, A. (2007). Two fluid-structure approaches for 3D simulation of St. Jude Medical bileaflet valve opening. *J Appl Biomater Biom*, Vol. 5, pp. 49-59.

Nobili, M., Morbiducci, U., Ponzini, R., *et al.* (2008). Numerical simulation of the dynamics of a bileaflet prosthetic heart valve using a fluid-structure interaction approaches. *J Biomech*, Vol. 41, pp. 2539-2550.

Paul, R., Apel, J., Klaus, S., Schügner, F., Schwindke, P. & Reul, H. (2003). Shear stress related blood damage in laminar Couette flow. *Artif Organs*, Vol. 27, No. 6, pp. 517-529.

Penrose, J.M.T. & Staples, C.J. (2002). Implicit fluid-structure coupling for simulation of cardiovascular problems. *Int J Numer Meth Fl*, Vol. 40, pp. 467-478.

Peskin, C. (1972). Flow patterns around heart valves: a numerical method. *J Comput Phys*, Vol. 10, pp. 252-271.

Redaelli, A., Bothorel, H., Votta, E., *et al.* (2004). 3-D Simulation of the St. Jude medical bileaflet valve opening process: fluid-structure interaction study and experimental validation. *J Heart Valve Dis*, Vol. 13, pp. 804-813.

Reul, H., Vahlbruch, A., Giersiepen, M., Schmitz-Rode, Th., Hirtz, V. & Effert, S. (1990). The geometry of the aortic root in health, at valve disease and after valve replacement. *J Biomech*, Vol. 23, pp. 181-191.

Sezai, A., Umeda, T., Hata, M., *et al.* (2009). A transesophageal echocardiographic and cine-fluoroscopic evaluation of an ATS prosthetic valve opening. *Surg Today*, Vol. 39, pp. 300-305.

Sotiropoulos, F. & Borazjani, I. (2009). A review of state-of-the-art numerical methods for simulating flow through mechanical heart valves. *Med Biol Eng Comput*, Vol. 47, pp. 245-256.

Sutera, S.P. & Mehrjardi, M.H. (1975). Deformation and fragmentation of human red blood cells in turbulent shear flow. *Biophys J*, Vol. 15, pp. 1-10.

Tai, C.H., Liew, K.M. & Zhao, Y. (2007). Numerical simulation of 3D fluid-structure interaction flow using an immersed object method with overlapping grid, *Comput Struct*, Vol. 85, pp. 749-762.

Van Loon, R., Anderson, P.D., de Hart, J. & Baaijens, F.P.T. (2004). A combined fictitious domain/adaptive meshing method for fluid-structure interaction in heart valves. *Int J Numer Meth Fl*, Vol. 46, pp. 533-544.

Verdonck, P. (2002). The role of computational fluid dynamics for artificial organ design. *Artif Organs*, Vol. 26, pp. 569-570.

Verdonck, P., Dumont, K., Segers, P., Vandenberghe, S. & Van Nooten, G. (2002). Mock loop testing of On-X prosthetic mitral valve with Doppler echocardiography. *Artif Organs*, Vol. 26, pp. 872-878.

Vierendeels, J., Dumont, K., Dick, E. & Verdonck, P. (2005). Analysis and stabilization of fluid-structure interaction algorithm for rigid-body motion. *AIAA J*, Vol. 43, pp. 2549-2557.

Vierendeels, J., Dumont, K. & Verdonck, P. (2008). A partitioned strongly coupled fluid-structure interaction method to model heart valve dynamics. *J Comput Appl Math*, Vol. 215, pp. 602-609.

Xia G.H., Zhao, Y. & Yeo, J.H. (2009). Parallel unstructured multigrid simulation of 3D unsteady flows and fluid-structure interaction in mechanical heart valve using immersed membrane method. *Comput Fluids*, Vol. 38, No. 1, pp. 71-79.

Yin, W., Krukenkamp, I.B., Saltman, A.E., *et al.* (2006). Thrombogenic performance of a St.Jude bileaflet mechanical heart valve in a sheep model. *ASAIO J*, Vol. 52, pp. 28-33.

Yoganathan, A.P., Chaux, A., Gray, R., *et al.* (1985). Bileaflet, tilting disc and porcine aortic valve substitutes: in vitro hydrodynamic characteristics. *J Am Coll Cardiol*, 3 Vol. 3, No. 2, pp. 313-320.

Yoganathan, A.P., He, Z. & Jones, S.C. (2004). Fluid mechanics of heart valves. *Annu Rev Biomed Eng*, Vol. 6, pp. 331-362.

Yoganathan, A.P., Chandran, K.B. & Sotiropoulos, F. (2005). Flow in prosthetic heart valves: state-of-the-art and future directions. *Ann Biomed Eng*,. Vol. 33, No. 12, pp. 1689-1694.

Yoganathan, A.P. & Travis, B.R. (2007). Chapter 24 Fluid dynamics of prosthetic valves, In: *The Practice of Clinical Echocardiography*, Third Edition, Otto C.M., Saunders Elsevier, ISBN: 978-1-4160-3640-1, pp. 552-577.

Zapanta, C.M., Stinebring, D.R., Deutsch, S., Geselowitz, D.B. & Tarbell, J.M. (1998). A comparison of the cavitation potential of prosthetic heart valves based on valve closing dynamics. *J Heart Valve Dis*, Vol. 7, No. 6, pp. 655-667.

Zoghbi, W.A., Chambers, J.B., Dumesnil, J.G., *et al.* (2009). Recommendations for evaluation of prosthetic valves with echocardiography and Doppler ultrasound. *J Am Soc Echocardiogr*, Vol. 22, No. 9, pp. 975–1014.

Part 2

General Consideration of Aortic Valve Disease

3

Aortic Valve Disease from Etiology to Bedside

Shahab Shahrzad and Samira Taban
Shiraz University of Medical Science,
Cardiology Department, Cardiology Research Center,
Iran

1. Introduction

Aortic valve is located in the outflow tract of left ventricle (LV), the systemic ventricle, and it should provide LV with an open tract during systolic period in order to have a perfect tissue perfusion with the least energy consumed by LV, and a closed tract during diastole to prevent blood regurgitation from systemic circulation to LV in diastole to avoid acute and late consequences of LV volume overloading.

Aortic valve diseases are mostly asymptomatic for a long period of time. This may culminate in irreversible LV damage before diagnosis.

Nowadays aortic valve replacement (AVR) for aortic stenosis is the most frequent cause of cardiac valvular surgery, because most of the mitral valve procedures are performed precutaneously.

1.1 Aortic root anatomy

Aorta is mainly composed of two parts: abdominal and thoracic, before it bifurcates to two common iliac arteries. The thoracic aorta is divided to three parts. The first one is ascending aorta which extends from aortic root to the arch of aorta and has no branches. The arch is the second part which has three main branches. Brachiocephalic artery, Left common carotid artery and left subclavian artery. After the last branch the descending aorta begins which extends inferiorly and passes through diaphragm where it turns to the abdominal aorta.

Left ventricle connects to ascending aorta via aortic root which provides the supporting structures for the leaflets of the aortic valve and the heart (Anderson 2000), and forms the bridge between the left ventricle and the ascending aorta. There is still no consensus as how best to describe the components of the root (Antunes 2005). The root itself, surrounding and supporting the leaflets, has length in that it extends from the basal attachments of the leaflets within the left ventricle to the ascending aorta (Anderson 2007). The very proximal part of aorta after leaflets is somehow dilated and is named sinus of valsalva. Its function is to support the leaflets and also right and left coronary arteries arise from this part of aorta. The tubular portion of ascending aorta is just after sinus of valsalva and the junction of this two parts is named sinotubular junction. (Figure 1, 2). The aortic valve itself is composed of three leaflets which attach to the aortic root like a crown (Figure 3). This crown like structure is essential for the function of the valve and in some congenital disorders of the valve such as bicuspid aortic valve restoration of this structure will result in better valvular function (Pretre et al., 2006). The aortic ring is the part that these leaflets attach to. These leaflets

attachment vary in the way that some of them attach to the muscular part of LV and some of them to the fibrinous part of the ring (Anderson 2000)
In conclusion the left ventricular blood goes to left ventricular outflow tract which ends in aortic root which is composed of aortic valve, aortic ring, sinus of valsalva and the sinotubular junction.

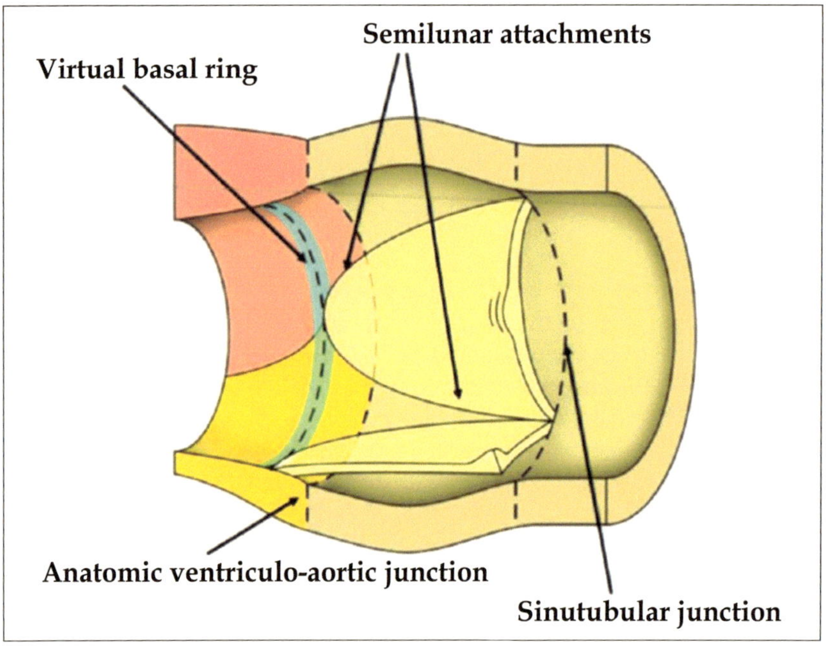

(Reproduced from Robert H. Anderson. The surgical anatomy of the aortic root. doi:10.1510/mmcts. 2006.002527 with permission.)

Fig. 1. The anatomy of Aortic Root

2. Aortic stenosis

2.1 Definition

Aortic stenosis (AS) means obstruction in left ventricular outflow tract (LVOT). It can be easily divided to three categories: subvalvular AS, valvular AS and supra valvular AS. Valvular AS is the most common cause of LVOT obstruction. Sub valvular AS comprises hypertrophic obstructive cardiomyopathy and sub aortic web. These two entities are almost always congenital but may show themselves later in the life. Supra valvular aortic stenosis is mainly part of complex congenital anomalies such as William syndrome that is associated with hypercalcemia. Valvular aortic stenosis is the mainstay of this article. It's a slowly progressive disease which progresses over time and causes a gradually aggravating LVOT obstruction. In an adult the average aortic valve area is about 4^{cm2} and the normal aortic valve area should be at least 2^{cm2}. Areas less than that are defines as aortic stenosis. There are some other definition criteria by echocardiography or cardiac catheterization. Aortic flow peak gradient more than 20 ^{mmHg} in echocardiography (Baumgartner 2009) (Bonow 2006 ACC AHA guidelines) or in left side catheterization is also defined as AS. But the best definition is always the surface area of the valve because these gradients can be influenced

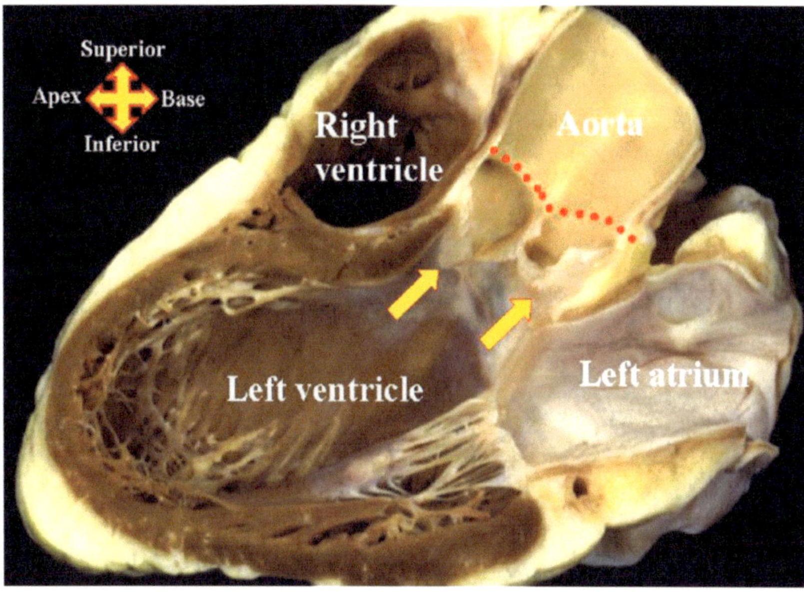

(Reproduced from Robert H. Anderson. The surgical anatomy of the aortic root. doi:10.1510/mmcts.2006.002527 with permission.)

Fig. 2. The anatomy of Aortic Root

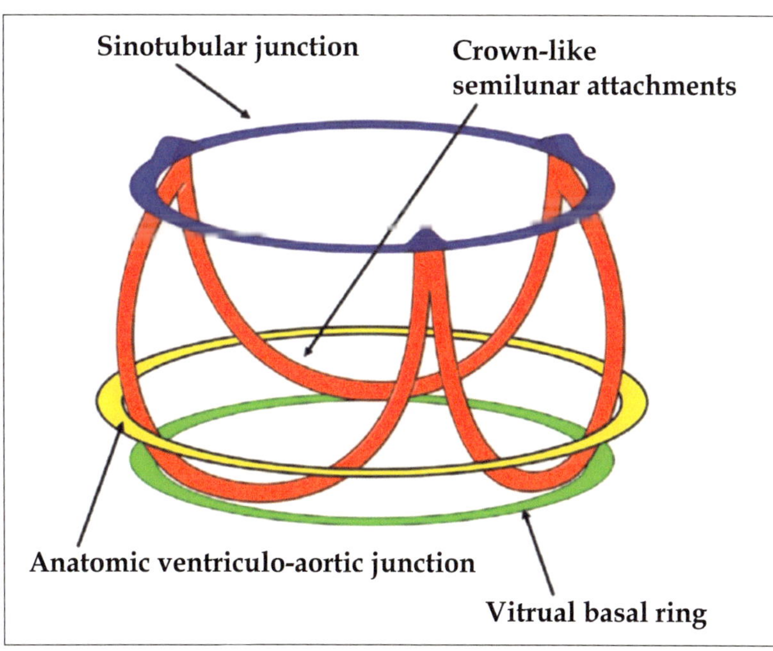

(Reproduced from Robert H. Anderson. The surgical anatomy of the aortic root. doi:10.1510/mmcts.2006.002527 with permission.)

Fig. 3. The anatomy of Aortic Root

by the cardiac output of the patient. In a normal man with anemia the cardiac output is increased to compensate for the decreased oxygen carrying capacity of the blood. This can cause increase in flow velocity across the valve and the overestimation of the gradient and a false diagnosis of an AS or overestimation of the AS severity. On the other hand in a patient with severe AS and advanced LV dysfunction the left ventricle do not have enough power to pump the blood across the valve and the trans-valvular jet velocity and gradient will be falsely low. This can have therapeutic importance because if these kind of patients are not diagnosed as AS their only option is medical therapy with limited outcome but with the proper diagnosis and alleviation of LVOT obstruction LV function will restore although partially (Bonow 2006 ACC AHA guidelines).

2.2 Etiology

AS is the most common valvular heart disease in human (Kurtz 2010). Most cases of adult aortic stenosis are caused by calcification of normal tricuspid or bicuspid aortic valve (Bonow 2006 ACC AHA guidelines). These are most commonly seen in elderly and those older than 65. The third most common cause of AS is rheumatic heart disease which is highly associated whit mitral valve disease as well. There are couple of other etiologies for AS which are all rare, they include homozygous familial hypercholesterolemia, congenital heart disease (other than bicuspid aortic valve such as unicuspid aortic valve), radiation induced aortic stenosis.

2.2.1 Calcific degenerative aortic stenosis (CDAS)

This is the most common cause of aortic stenosis. This is also called senile degenerative aortic sclerosis and stenosis, but the pathophysiology of this disease is not an irreversible simple age related degenerative disorder. On the other hand Calcific AS is an active disease process characterized by lipid accumulation, inflammation, and calcification, with many similarities to atherosclerosis (Bonow 2006 ACC AHA guidelines)(Kurtz 2010). CDAS is started by accumulation of lipid particles and oxidized low density lipoprotein (LDL) in aortic leaflets just like precursors of atherosclerosis plaque. This particles and their oxidative products cause activation of local lymphocytes and macrophages and production of angiotensin II, which all ultimately convert leaflet fibroblasts to osteoblasts which are the cells that produce bony and calcific structure. These cells are responsible for calcium deposition in CDAS. These changes start from the base of the leaflet and extend to their tip but no leaflet and commissural fusion happens like the one seen in rheumatic heart disease. These changes resulted in emergence of therapeutic medical ideas for treatment of AS. The most important of them are STATINs which are lipid lowering agents. Unfortunately clinical trials have not showed any benefit in reversing CDAS by STATINs. Chan KL et al., (2010) studied this concept and their result was that Cholesterol lowering with rosuvastatin 40 mg did not reduce the progression of AS in patients with mild to moderate AS; thus, statins should not be used for the sole purpose of reducing the progression of AS. The main reason may be the advanced degenerated calcific nature of the disease. These changes are very similar to those that occurs in vascular atherosclerosis and actually they have similar risk factors, both are more prevalent in patients whit diabetes mellitus, hypertension, hyperlipidemia and renal failure. CDAS is accelerated in patients with intrinsic aortic valve disease such as bicuspid aortic valve.

2.2.2 Bicuspid aortic valve

This is the most common congenital cause of AS and the most common cause of AS in neonates and the most common cause of CDAS in those younger than 60. Bicuspid aortic valve can be associated with sever aortic regurgitation but most commonly it is associated with AS before 60. Also it is associated with diseased aortic wall which can culminate in aortic aneurysm as well as aortic dissection(Roberts 1970). Most of the time replacement of aortic root is indicated during operation of the valve in bicuspid valve patients. Some have reported the repair of the valve and restoration of normal crown structure of the aorta as the surgical therapeutic modality for bicuspid aortic valve(Pretre et al., 2006)

2.2.3 Rheumatic AS

It is the third common cause of AS. Its prevalence is decreasing because of increasing proper management of streptococcal pharyngitis. It's almost always associated with some amount of aortic regurgitation and mitral stenosis. In fact rheumatic fever only involves aortic valve in one third of the patients. It most commonly involves tip of aortic leaflets with thickening, commissural fusion and finally calcification which causes doming of the valve in echocardiography. It is important to remember to evaluate the mitral valve in every patients with rheumatic AS(Bonow 2006 ACC AHA guidelines)(Kurtz 2010).

2.3 Pathophysiology of LV changes induces by AS

AS is the most common cause of LV outflow tract (LVOT) obstruction.It progresses slowly over the time, so the LV can compensate for the pathologic changes that it can cause. AS causes increases resistant in LVOT and the after load of the LV (which is the force that the LV contracts against). This results in increased wall stress of LV. Wall stress is equal to pressure of LV multiplied by radius of LV divided by wall thickness of LV:

$$\text{Wall stress} = \text{Pressure} \times \text{radius} / (2 \times \text{wall thickness})$$

Increased wall stress can cause ischemia and ultimately myocardial damage. LV increases its own thickness by hypertrophy to compensate the increase in wall stress. This can compensate for the increase in after load and LV ejection fraction(LVEF) remains in normal range. But if the amount of hypertrophy is less than enough the LVEF will decrease , this is called after load mismatch and can be corrected by alleviating the obstruction in LVOT. On the other hand in some patients the decrease LVEF is due to intrinsic myocardial damage. In these patients even aortic valve replacement cannot increase the LV function. Increased LV thickness and hypertrophy is not all physiologic and has some negative effects on the myocardium. First of all the hypertrophied myocardium has less coronary blood flow reserve(Marcus 1982) that exposes it to ischemia specially during exercise. Then is the fact that the hypertrophied myocardium is more sensitive to a constant level of ischemia compared to normal myocardium. The final problem is over hypertrophy which is almost exclusively seen in old women. This can cause even high LVEF but conversely is associated with high operative mortality(Bonow 2006 ACC AHA guidelines). In the majority of AS patients the final step is the time that LV hypertrophy cannot compensate for increased after load and LV Dysfunction ensues. This is the step that the patient finally becomes symptomatic. That's why a patient with AS has a good prognosis till he or she is asymptomatic, and stays symptom free for a long time, but as soon as the symptoms emerge the prognosis of the disease worsens and progresses rapidly by LV failure.

2.4 Sign and symptoms

Unfortunately AS is asymptomatic for a long period of time. AS symptoms is mainly due to 3 physiologic phenomena: cardiac ischemia, elevated LV filling pressure, and decreased cardiac output (Kurtz 2010). The first symptom in most cases is dyspnea in exertion. The dyspnea progresses over time and the more the disease progresses the less will become the level of the activity that the patient can take without dyspnea. Finally the patient will have dyspnea at rest. All three mentioned phenomena's are responsible for dyspnea. The second common sign is chest pain which is again seen in specially on activity. The cause of the chest pain is multi-factorial. Half of them have coronary artery disease (CAD) which can cause the chest pain. In those without CAD the chest pain caused by increased demand because of LV hypertrophy and decreased aortic pressure because of the AS itself. Also as mentioned decreased coronary flow reserve can cause real ischemia in AS. Syncope specially during activity is the third common symptom and is caused because of low cardiac output , and decreased cerebral perfusion. Other causes of syncope are inappropriate vasodilatation because of abnormal myocardial receptor activation (reflex mediated syncope) and rarely arrhythmias. Sudden cardiac death usually happens in 1% of patients and occurs mostly in those with other symptoms and not as the first presentation. Peripheral embolization and heart failure are rarer symptoms of AS and are mostly seen in final stages of the disease. There is a very special symptom in AS patients that happens because of vascular dysplasia. AS patients can have angiodysplasia in their right colon. the exact reason of this vascular abnormality is not known but it can be due to increased shearing stress and platelet activation. This problem is associated with gastrointestinal bleeding and is relieved after AS is corrected. Although the patient may have no symptom, in physical examination we can find couple of symptoms that can relive the problem. The peripheral pulses and cardiac auscultation are the main targets in physical examination. The best pulse to evaluate is carotid pulse. It becomes narrow and the time to the peak pressure increases. this is called pulsus parvus et tardus. In cardiac auscultation a mid-systolic ejection murmur which is crescendo decrescendo can be heard in right second intercostals space which radiates to the right side of the neck. Also aortic ejection click can be heard in those patients whose valve is not heavily calcified. Heavy calcification of the valve can decrease the doming of the valve which is the main cause of the ejection click. The severity of the murmur although helpful in assessing the severity of AS, can be influenced by the level of cardiac output and be misleading.

2.5 Evaluation of patients with AS

The evaluation begins with meticulous history taking and physical examination. The quality of pulses, second heart sound, systolic murmur and peripheral signs of heart failure are used for diagnosis and determining the severity and prognosis of the disease. Narrow pulse pressure and systolic murmur of grade III or more and signs of heart failure are usually associated with severe AS, although the severity of the murmur can be influenced by the level of the cardiac output (it increases with increased cardiac output like anemia). Symptoms of the patient are very important because even in the presence of normal LV function emergence of symptoms are strong indication for aortic valve replacement (Bonow 2006 ACC AHA guidelines)(Kurtz 2010). It is important to obtain specific history for dyspnea and exercise intolerance as the patient may ignore them because of the chronic nature of the disease. Electrocardiography (ECG) is the next tool to evaluate the patient, which shows LV hypertrophy, abnormal ST-T changes, arrhythmias, atrio-ventricular and inter-ventricular conduction abnormalities. Inter-ventricular conduction delay specially left bundle branch block is mostly seen in advanced myocardial dysfunction. ECG is primarily important in diagnosing the associated cardiac problems such as ischemic heart disease, and all of the findings that can be seen in AS are neither specific nor sensitive. Echocardiography is the most commonly used and the most practical mean of diagnosing and evaluation the severity of AS and associated conditions. There are multiple echocardiographic modalities such as 2D imaging, Doppler mode and color Doppler mode for this purpose (Table 1). The aortic valve area can be measured by 2-D echocardiography via parasternal short axis view of the aorta. Also Doppler echocardiography can measure the valve area by continuity equation. This is based on the rule that the amount of blood that passes the LVOT is equal the blood that crosses the aortic valve.

$$\text{Aortic valve area} = \text{LVOT VTI} \times \text{LVOT AREA} / \text{Aortic valve VTI}$$

Where VTI is velocity time integral and can be calculated easily by Doppler echocardiography. The easiest and most commonly used method is assessing trans valvular flow velocity and gradient. AS then can be categorized to mild, moderate and severe. (Table 1) Other imaging tools such as CT scan and MRI are also useful. They can specially evaluate the ascending aorta that can be dilated and aneurismal in AS. Cardiac catheterization is almost always used when the previously mentioned modalities fail to accomplish the diagnosis or when there are conflicts between them.

	Aortic Stenosis		
Indicator	Mild	Moderate	Severe
Jet velocity (m per second)	Less than 3.0	3.0–4.0	Greater than 4.0
Mean gradient (mm Hg)*	Less than 25	25–40	Greater than 40
Valve area (cm^2)	Greater than 1.5	1.0–1.5	Less than 1.0
Valve area index (cm^2 per m^2)			Less than 0.6

Table 1. Assessment of AS severity by echocardiography (Source: American Heart Association, Inc.)

2.6 Medical management of patients with AS

AS does not have a medical treatment, but the medical follow up is very important before AVR to determine the perfect time of operation according to guideline and charts, and post AVR for proper anticoagulation and complication management. Periodic echocardiographic and clinical evaluation of the patients with AS is the main nonsurgical management of AS patients. This intervals are determined by the severity of AS and patients symptoms. Those with mild AS should be evaluated every 3-5 years, patients with moderate AS every 1-2 years and severe AS should be evaluated yearly. Also pregnant women and those who become symptomatic should have prompt evaluation (Bonow 2006 ACC AHA guidelines) (Kurtz 2010). Other major medical therapy targets associated risk factors such as hypertension, hyperlipidemia and diabetes mellitus. Endocarditis prophylaxis is no longer needed for AS patients because the risk of infection is low. Many investigators have tried to find a way to delay or even reverse the progression of AS. There are couple of reports that some drugs such as STATINs may have some effect in slowing the progression of AS, but most studies have failed to show any effect. Rosenhek et al., (2004) compared the effect of angiotensin converting enzyme inhibitors (ACEIs) with statins in reducing AS progression. According to their study ACEIs do not appear to slow AS progression. However, statins significantly reduce the hemodynamic progression of both mild-to-moderate and severe AS, an effect that may not be related to cholesterol lowering. On the other hand Chan et al., (2010) reported that Cholesterol lowering with rosuvastatin 40 mg did not reduce the progression of AS in patients with mild to moderate AS.

2.7 Endovascular management of patients with AS

This method is mostly used during childhood according to specific guidelines and with specific methods. In adults this procedure has little value because of high risk of complication, procedure failure and high rates of recurrence on the contrary in childhood the valve is more pliable and the success rate of the procedure is high, so precutaneous aortic valvoplasty is the standard procedure for treatment of AS in childhood. Nevertheless precutaneous balloon valvoplasty can be performed in highly selected adult patients such as those with very high surgical risk and also as a bridge to AVR in those with decompensated condition. Although it cannot replace for standard AVR procedure (springing 1995)(Webb 2006). The other option is precutaneous valve replacement. Three different methods are available but all of them are associated with high mortality and morbidity and are not routinely performed.

- **Class I:** Conditions for which there is evidence for and/or general agreement that the procedure or treatment is beneficial, useful, and effective.
- **Class II:** Conditions for which there is conflicting evidence and/or a divergence of opinion about the usefulness/efficacy of a procedure or treatment.
  - **Class IIa:** Weight of evidence/opinion is in favour of usefulness/efficacy.
  - **Class IIb:** Usefulness/efficacy is less well established by evidence/opinion.
- **Class III:** Conditions for which there is evidence and/or general agreement that the procedure/treatment is not useful/effective and in some cases may be harmful.

Table 2. Definition of multiple classes (Source: American Heart Association, Inc.)

2.8 Surgical management of AS

Aortic valve repair for AS is almost never done because of high rate of failure therefore AVR is the standard management of AS. Although Pretre et al., (2006) reported repair of bicuspid aortic valve and restoration of normal anatomical crown like structure, AVR is still the procedure of choice for AS patients. The timing and indication of surgery is determined through specific guidelines (Figure 4 and Table 2). the most important issues in this manner are patients symptoms and LVEF. Symptomatic patients or those with LVEF less than 50% should undergo AVR. There are multiple kinds of prosthetic valve. Each kind has its own properties. Selection of the prosthetic valve is also done via the guidelines. Aortic root size is the other important issue that should be considered before operation. Aortic root size should be exactly determined with CT scan or MR. Aortic root more than 4.5 cm specially in those with bicuspid aortic valve or marfan syndrome is an indication for aortic root replacement. This operation is called Bental operation and involves a metallic prosthesis sewed in a Dacron artificial ascending aorta that is replaced for aortic root (Hiratzka 2010).

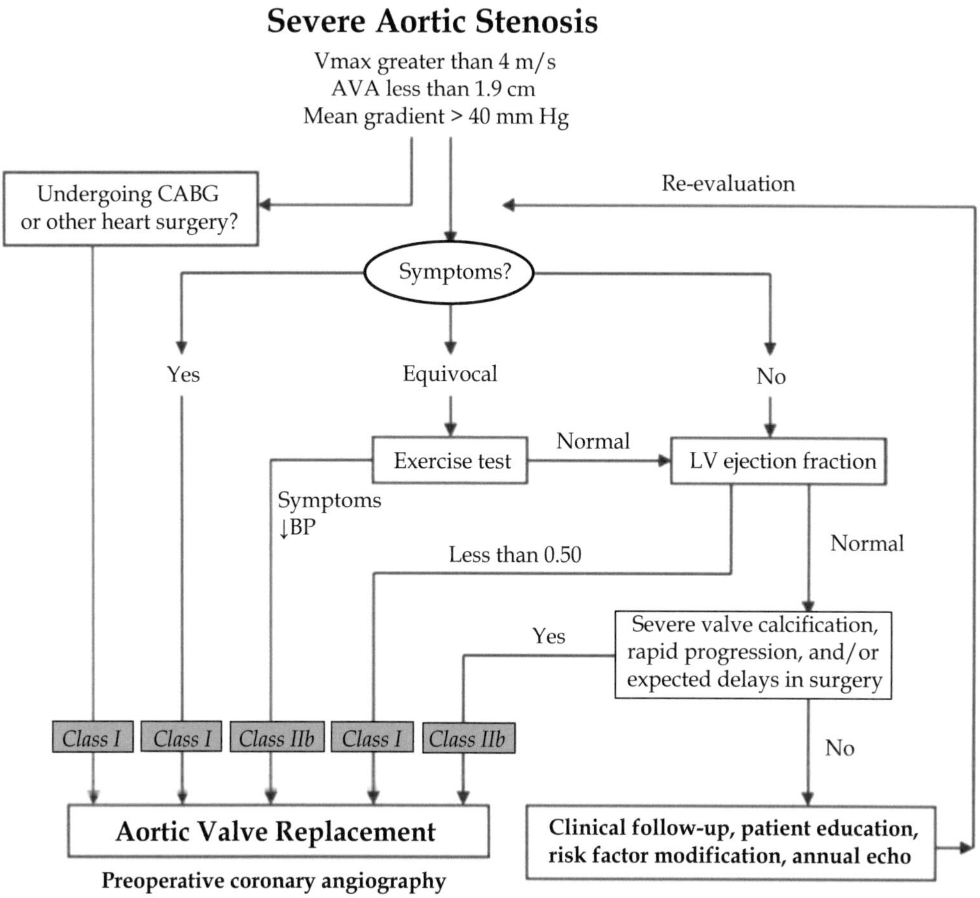

Fig. 4. Timing of operation in AS patients (Source: American Heart Association, Inc.)

2.9 Natural course of AS

Frank S et al (1973) studied the natural history of the patients with severe AS who did not undergo AVR. He showed that during a 10 year follow up 90% of the patients will die without surgical intervention. He also found that those with combination of symptoms such as dyspnea. Angina and syncope has the worst prognosis. Aortic stenosis has good prognosis when it's asymptomatic and its mortality rate is almost the same as those without AS. But as soon as it gets symptomatic the survival is only about 2-3 years without treatment. The mean survival is 5, 3, 2 years for angina, syncope and heart failure respectively (Kurtz 2010). With operation in perfect time the survival will remain good. After operation patients should be evaluated by history and physical examination yearly.

3. Aortic insufficiency

3.1 Definition

Inability of aortic valve to withhold regurgitation of blood from aorta to LV in diastole is defined as aortic insufficiency (AI) or aortic regurgitation. It is not as prevalent as AS but it can be seen in at least 75% of patients with CDAS. The main difference of AS and AI is that AS imposes a systolic pressure over load to the LV, in contrast to AI that mainly increases the diastolic LV load. Thus LV dilatation during asymptomatic period is more prevalent in AI.

3.2 Etiology

It can be divided into problems of the valve itself and those that are due to aortic root dilatation(Bonow 2006 ACC AHA guidelines). Diseases that involve the aortic valve itself cause AI by disturbing the normal motion or normal coaptation of the leaflets. These include, congenital abnormalities of the aortic valve (most notably bicuspid valves), calcific degeneration, rheumatic disease, infective endocarditis, systemic hypertension, myxomatous degeneration. Anorectic drugs radiation and trauma are rare valvular causes of AI. Nowadays aortic root diseases are responsible for at least 50% of cases of aortic insufficiency (AI). It can be caused by systemic disorders such as hypertension or marfan syndrome or can be idiopathic. One interesting cause of AI is consumption of anorectic medications which can cause AI by damaging the valve itself. Most causes of AI cause a chronic disease that can be asymptomatic for even decades but some etiologies can cause acute sever AI that can be even fatal if left untreated. They include infective endocarditis, trauma and aortic dissection. Moaref et al. (2009) reported a case of acute aortic regurgitation due to acquired aorto-ventricular tunnel as a complication of infective endocarditis.

3.3 Pathophysiology of acute AI

In acute severe AR, the sudden large regurgitant volume is imposed on a left ventricle of normal size that has not had time to accommodate the volume overload. With an abrupt increase in end-diastolic volume, the ventricle operates on the steep portion of a normal diastolic pressure-volume relationship, and LV end-diastolic and left atrial pressures may increase rapidly and dramatically. The Frank-Starling mechanism is used, but the inability of the ventricle to develop compensatory chamber dilatation acutely results in a decrease in forward stroke volume. Although tachycardia develops as a compensatory mechanism to maintain cardiac output, this is often insufficient. Hence, patients frequently present with pulmonary edema or cardiogenic shock. Acute AR creates especially marked hemodynamic changes in patients with pre-existing pressure overload hypertrophy, in whom the small, noncompliant LV cavity is set on an even steeper diastolic pressurevolume relationship and has reduced preload reserve. Examples of this latter situation include aortic dissection in patients with systemic hypertension, infective endocarditis in patients with pre-existing AS, and acute regurgitation after balloon valvotomy or surgical commissurotomy for congenital AS (Bonow 2006 ACC AHA guidelines).

3.4 Pathophysiology of chronic AI

The left ventricle responds to the volume load of chronic AR with a series of compensatory mechanisms, including an increase in end-diastolic volume, an increase in chamber compliance that accommodates the increased volume without an increase in filling pressures, and a combination of eccentric and concentric hypertrophy. The greater diastolic volume permits the ventricle to eject a large total stroke volume to maintain forward stroke volume in the normal range. This is accomplished through rearrangement of myocardial fibers with the addition of new sarcomeres and development of eccentric LV hypertrophy (Grossman 1975). As a result, preload at the sarcomere level remains normal or near normal, and the ventricle retains its preload reserve. The enhanced total stroke volume is achieved through normal performance of each contractile unit along the enlarged circumference (Ross 1972). Thus, LV ejection performance is normal, and ejection phase indexes such as ejection fraction and fractional shortening remain in the normal range. However, the enlarged chamber size, with the associated increase in systolic wall stress, also results in an increase in LV afterload and is a stimulus for further hypertrophy (Grossman 1975). Thus, AR represents a condition of combined volume overload and pressure overload. As the disease progresses, recruitment of preload reserve and compensatory hypertrophy permit the ventricle to maintain normal ejection performance despite the elevated afterload (Ricci 1982). The majority of patients remain asymptomatic throughout this compensated phase, which may last for decades. Vasodilator therapy has the potential to reduce the hemodynamic burden in such patients. For purposes of the subsequent discussion, patients with normal LV systolic function will be defined as those with normal LV ejection fraction at rest. It is recognized that other indices of LV function may not be "normal" in chronic severe AR and that the hemodynamic abnormalities noted above may be considerable. It is also recognized that the transition to LV systolic dysfunction represents a continuum and that there is no single hemodynamic measurement that represents the absolute boundary between normal LV systolic function and LV systolic dysfunction. In a large subset of patients, the balance between afterload excess, preload reserve, and hypertrophy cannot be maintained indefinitely. Preload reserve may be exhausted, and/or the hypertrophic response may be inadequate, so that further increases in afterload result in a reduction in ejection fraction, first into the low normal range and then below normal. Impaired myocardial contractility may also contribute to this process. Patients often develop dyspnea at this point in the natural history. In addition, diminished coronary flow reserve in the hypertrophied myocardium may result in exertional angina. However, this transition may be much more insidious, and it is possible for patients to remain asymptomatic until severe LV dysfunction has developed. LV systolic dysfunction (defined as an ejection fraction below normal at rest) is initially a reversible phenomenon related predominantly to afterload excess, and full recovery of LV size and function is possible with AVR. With time, during which the ventricle develops progressive chamber enlargement and a more spherical geometry, depressed myocardial contractility predominates over excessive loading as the cause of progressive systolic dysfunction. This can progress to the extent that the full benefit of surgical correction of the regurgitant lesion, in terms of recovery of LV function and improved survival, can no longer be achieved AS (Bonow 2006 ACC AHA guidelines).

3.5 Signs and symptoms

Similar to AS, AI is also asymptomatic for a long time, and at the time of diagnosis many of them have dilated LVs with severe dysfunction. The first sign is almost always exercise intolerance, followed by chest pain sudden cardiac death, syncope and heart failure. Such as AS symptoms are most commonly seen during exercise, but exceptionally the chest pain can be seen during sleep. The reason is the bradycardia during sleep. Bradycardia will increase the diastolic time during a cardiac cycle. The more the diastolic interval the more the regurgitant volume (because the regurgitation of the blood occurs in diastolic interval). The reason of angina is coronary artery disease in a fraction of patients but even in the absence of coronary artery disease angina can be seen. In these patients the reason of angina is decreased coronary flow reserve because of decreased driving pressure (low aortic diastolic pressure) and increased LV diastolic pressure (Nitenberg 1988). As in AS sudden cardiac death is more prevalent in symptomatic patients. In physical examination there are couples of sings that can help in diagnosis of AI and almost all of them are because of high stroke volume. Bounding pulse is the vigorous large pulses that can be palpated in sever AI and is because of high cardiac output and low diastolic pressure. Muller sign is the pulsation of uvula with each heart beat and is again because of high cardiac output. De Musset's sign is the bobbing motion of the head with the heart beat. Becker's sign is the pulsation of retinal vessels with beating heart. These peripheral signs are seen in chronic sever AI and are absent in acute AI, because they are the result of high stroke volume and cardiac output. In chronic AI the heart has the time to compensate and can pump the extra amount of blood that has been regurgitated to LV in diastole, but in acute severe AI the LV will fail suddenly and the stroke volume will remain the same or even decrease, so these sings would be absent. The cardiac auscultation of patients with AI will show a diastolic murmur that starts from early diastole in a decrescendo manner and regarding the severity of AI and its chronicity it will extend throughout the diastole. In acute severe AI the murmur will end soon in middle of diastole, but in chronic severe AI it will extend to the end of diastolic time.

3.6 Evaluation of patients with AI

The evaluation begins with seeking the history of any disease that can be associated with AI and also looking for subtle symptoms of AI such as nocturnal chest pain and heart failure. It is very important to be able to diagnose AI in physical examination because AI will remain silent for many years and finally it will be emerged as an irreversible LV dysfunction when the therapy will have little effect. There are great amount of signs in the physical examination of a patient with AI such as Muller sign, Becker sign. They can be used for diagnosis and determining the severity of the problem. ECG showed eccentric LV hypertrophy with atrioventricular and interventricular (specially in LV dysfunction) conduction abnormalities. These ECG findings are neither specific nor sensitive. CXR shows huge cardiomegally with aortic dilatation. In patients with AS the ascending aorta will be dilated but in AI the entire aorta is dilated. Also in AS the rate of aortic valve calcification is higher, which can be seen in CXR. Echocardiography is again the most frequent way of diagnosing and evaluating AI which is done via its divers modalities (Table 2).All of the patients with AI should undergo serial echocardiography with specific intervals in order to prevent the irreversible LV damage (Figure 5). As soon as the time the symptoms begin or the LV dilates or the LV dysfunction starts surgical treatment is indicated. CT scan and MRI are also used in this matter specially when evaluation of the aorta itself is also needed. They can precisely measure the size of the aortic root and ascending aorta. These sizes are extremely important when the surgery is planned, because the ascending aorta may be replaced as well. Cardiac catheterization is reserved for those cases which need further evaluation after previously mentioned modalities.

	Aortic Regurgitation		
	Mild	Moderate	Severe
Qualitative			
Angiographic grade	1+	2+	3–4+
Color Doppler jet width	Central jet, width less than 25% of LVOT	Greater than mild but no signs of severe AR	Central jet, width greater than 65% LVOT
Doppler vena contracta width (cm)	Less than 0.3	0.3–0.6	Greater than 0.6
Quantitative (cath or echo)			
Regurgitant volume (ml per beat)	Less than 30	30–59	Greater than or equal to 60
Regurgitant fraction (%)	Less than 30	30–49	Greater than or equal to 50
Regurgitant orifice area (cm^2)	Less than 0.10	0.10–0.29	Greater than or equal to 0.30
Additional essential criteria			
Left ventricular size			Increased

Table 3. Echocardiographic evaluation of AI severity (Source: American Heart Association, Inc.)

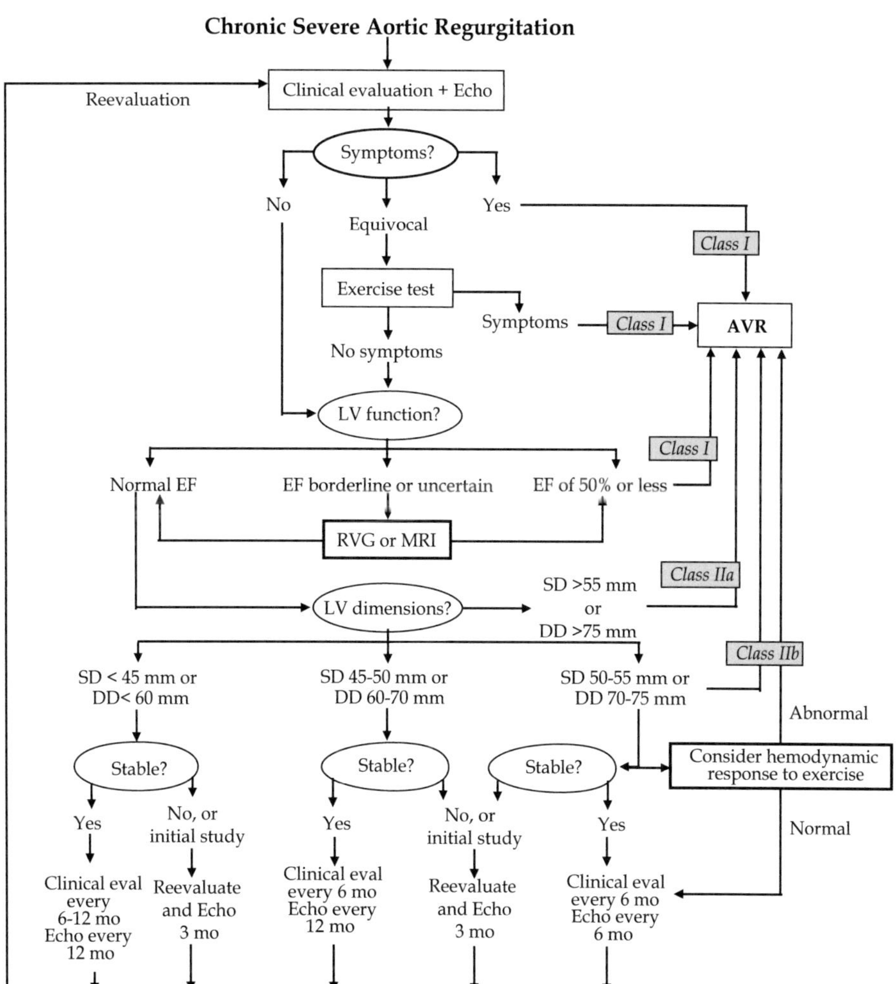

Fig. 5. Management of patients with severe AI (Source: American Heart Association, Inc.)

3.7 Medical treatment of AI

There is a great controversy in this field. Some believe that amlodipine can postpone the time of surgery or preserve the LV function during a 6 months period of time. Most specialists believe that there is no proper medical therapy for AI except in those with high operative mortality and those with advanced LV dysfunction as a part of heart failure management. In these patients specially vasodilators are indicated. Meticulous medical follow up is needed before and after AVR as in aortic stenosis. In those with advanced LV dysfunction and high risk for surgery medical treatment with the same medications as other heart failure patients is started. The exception are those drugs that decrease the heart rate because they can prolong the diastolic time and as the result the regurgitant volume.

3.8 Endovascular therapy of AI

There has been a great advance in this field in recent years, and developing techniques of precutaneous AVR are developing which is done in selected patients. But more advances is this field is needed and its not performed routinely because of high failure rate.

3.9 Surgical therapy of AI

This is the mainstay of management of AI and the timing of operation is determined through specific guidelines (Figure 5). This timing is performed specially with determining the size of the LV as well as its function. The other important issue is the symptoms of the patient. Operation is indicated when the patient becomes symptomatic. Aortic valve repair is reserved for specific situation such as myxomatous valve disease, traumatic or infective cases. It is not performed it most of the patients because of its failure rate. AVR is the most common procedure used with or without root replacement (Bental procedure). Root replacement is indicated in those patients that have dilated or dissected root. Selection of the valve can be done via specific guidelines. After AVR the dilatation and dysfunction of the LV will be reversed if the operation is performed on the proper time. Short-term and long-term improvement in left ventricular systolic function after operation is related significantly to the early reduction in left ventricular dilatation arising from correction of left ventricular volume overload. Moreover, late improvement in ejection fraction occurs commonly in patients with an early increase in ejection fraction after valve replacement but is unlikely to occur in patients with no change in ejection fraction during the first 6 months after operation (Bonow 2006 ACC AHA guidelines)(Bonow 1983)(Bonow 1988)(Bonow 1984).

3.10 Natural course of AI

As in AS the patients with AI have a good prognosis until they are asymptomatic (Tornos 1995). Also the LV function and the size of the LV are important prognostic factors. Decreased LV contractility and dilated LV are predictors of poor prognosis, so small LV sizes and normal ejection fraction show good long term and post operative survivals. But in patients who become symptomatic the prognosis worsens rapidly and the expected survival is about 2 to 4 years in these patients if surgical intervention is not performed. But even in these patients if the AVR is performed in the proper time the survival and prognosis is excellent. Bonow et al.,(1988) reported that in asymptomatic patients with normal left ventricular function, death is rare, and less than 4% per year require aortic valve replacement because symptoms or left ventricular dysfunction develop. When aortic valve replacement is delayed until symptoms or left ventricular dysfunction develop, postoperative survival is excellent, and left ventricular size and function improve postoperatively. Hence, "prophylactic" aortic valve replacement to preserve left ventricular function should not be performed in asymptomatic patients with severe aortic regurgitation and normal left ventricular function.

4. Aortic valve prosthesis

They can be mainly classified into two types: Metallic (Figure 6) and Bioprosthetic (Figure 7).

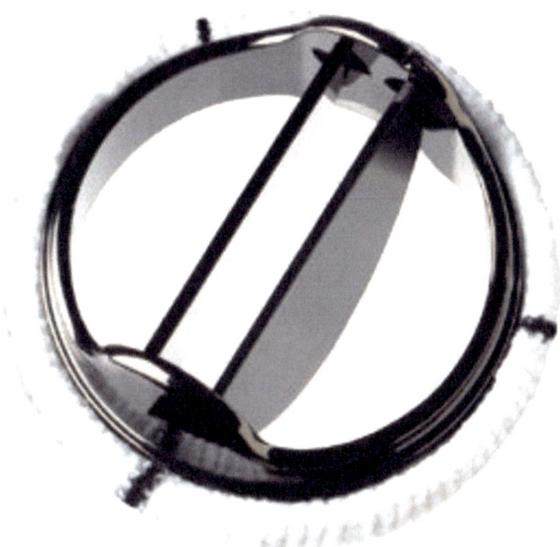

Fig. 6. Metallic valve

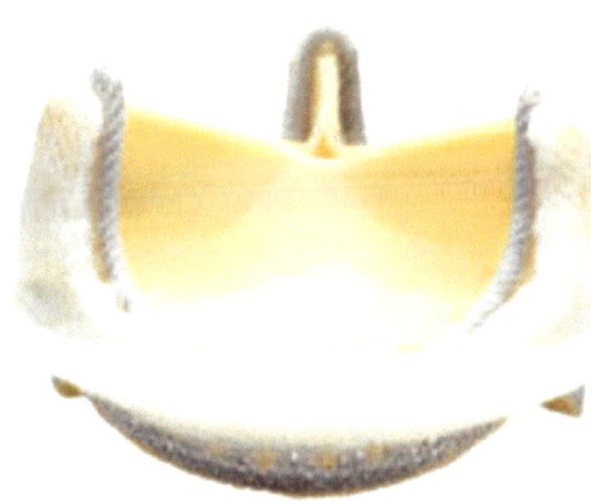

Fig. 7. Bioprosthetic valve

Metallic valves are made of different compound such as titanium and have different types. They would not degenerate over time but their disadvantage is that blood can clot on their surface and cause their dysfunction or systemic embolization. Valve dysfunction can be fatal if severe , by causing cardiac dysfunction. These dysfunctions are managed either surgically or medically depending on their severity and the size of the clot. To prevent these complications AVR patients should receive oral anticoagulation for their life time in order to prevent clot formation on the valve. Precise monitoring is needed for the patients who use these medications because overdosing may cause abnormal and occasionally fatal bleedings.

Under dosing can culminate in clot formation and the aforementioned complications. The most prevalent drug is warfarin which prevents clot formation by inhibiting activation of clotting factors in the liver. The medical follow up of the patients receiving warfarin is by serial checking of International Normalization Ratio (INR) and Prothrombin Time (PT). The optimal INR is about 2.5 in most AVR patients (Butchart 1991)(Cannegieter 1994).
Bioprosthetic valves on the other hand degenerate over time and even may need reoperation, but they do not need constant anticoagulation to prevent clot formation. So the risks associated with anticoagulation such as bleeding is less than metallic valves.
The selection of specific valve is then determined in every patients considering these properties. In a young man who is going to have the valve for many years replacing the valve with a bioprosthetic will expose him to the risk of reoperation because of valve degeneration, so the metallic valve is preferred. On the other hand in an old lady who is high risk for bleeding the bioprosthetic is preferred.

5. References

Anderson R, 2006.The surgical anatomy of aortic valve, Multimedia manual of cardio thoracic surgery doi:10.1510/mmcts.2006.002527

Anderson RH. 2000. Clinical anatomy of the aortic root. *Heart* 2000; 84:670–673

Antunes MJ. 2005. The aortic valve: an everlasting mystery to surgeons. *Eur J Cardiothorac Surg* 2005; 28:855–856.

Baumgartner H, Hung J, Bermejo J, Chambers JB, Evangelista A, Griffin BP, Iung B, Otto CM, Pellikka PA, Quinones M; 2009 American Society of Echocardiography; European Association of Echocardiography. Echocardiographic assessment of valve stenosis: EAE/ASE recommendations for clinical practice. *J Am Soc Echocardiogr*. 2009; 22:1Y23.

Bonow O, Carabello B, Chatterjee K ,De Leon A, et al., MDACC/AHA 2006 Guidelines for the Management of Patients With Valvular Heart Disease A Report of the American College of Cardiology/American Heart Association Task Force on Practice Guidelines (Writing Committee to Revise the 1998 Guidelines for the Management of Patients With Valvular Heart Disease) *JACC*:2006; 05.021:e1-e148 ISSN 0735-1097

Bonow RO, Rosing DR, Maron BJ, et al.1984 Reversal of left ventricular dysfunction after aortic valve replacement for chronic aortic regurgitation: influence of duration of preoperative left ventricular dysfunction. *CIRCULATION* 1984; 70:570 –9. ISSN: 1524-4539

Bonow RO, Dodd JT, Maron BJ, et al. 1988Long-term serial changes in left ventricular function and reversal of ventricular dilatation after valve replacement for chronic aortic regurgitation. *CIRCULATION* 1988; 78:1108 –20. ISSN: 1524-4539

Bonow RO, Rosing DR, McIntosh CL, et al.1983 The natural history of asymptomatic patients with aortic regurgitation and normal left ventricular function. *CIRCULATION* 1983; 68:509 –17. ISSN: 1524-4539

Butchart EG, Lewis PA, Bethel JA, Breckenridge IM.1991 Adjusting anticoagulation to prosthesis thrombogenicity and patient risk factors: recommendations for the Medtronic Hall valve. *CIRCULATION* 1991; 84:III61–9.

Cannegieter SC, Rosendaal FR, Briet E. 1994 Thromboembolic and bleeding complications in patients with mechanical heart valve prostheses. *CIRCULATION* 1994; 89:635– 41. ISSN: 1524-4539

Chan KL, Teo K, Dumesnil JG, Ni A, Tam J.2010 Effect of Lipid lowering with rosuvastatin on progression of aortic stenosis: results of the aortic stenosis progression observation: measuring effects of rosuvastatin (ASTRONOMER) trial. *CIRCULATION*. 2010; 121:306Y314 ISSN: 1524-4539

Frank S, Johnson A, Ross J Jr. 1973 Natural history of valvular aortic stenosis. *Br Heart J* 1973;35:41- 6.

Grossman W, Jones D, McLaurin LP. 1975 Wall stress and patterns of hypertrophy in the human left ventricle. *J Clin Invest* 1975; 56:56–64.

Hiratzka LF, Bakris GL, Beckman JA, Bersin RM, Carr VF, Casey DE Jr, Eagle KA, Hermann LK, Isselbacher EM, Kazerooni EA, Kouchoukos NT, Lytle BW, Milewicz DM, Reich DL, Sen S, Shinn JA, Svensson LG, Williams DM; American College of Cardiology Foundation/American Heart Association Task Force on Practice Guidelines; American Association for Thoracic Surgery; American College of Radiology; American Stroke Association; Society of Cardiovascular Anesthesiologists; Society for Cardiovascular Angiography and Interventions; Society of Interventional Radiology; Society of Thoracic Surgeons; Society for Vascular Medicine. 2010 ACCF/AHA/AATS/ACR/ASA/SCA/SCAI/SIR/STS/SVM 2010 Guidelines for the diagnosis and management of patients with thoracic aortic disease. A Report of the American College of Cardiology Foundation/American Heart Association Task Force on Practice Guidelines, American Association for Thoracic Surgery, American College of Radiology, American Stroke Association, Society of Cardiovascular Anesthesiologists, Society for Cardiovascular Angiography and Interventions, Society of Interventional Radiology, Society of Thoracic Surgeons and Society for Vascular Medicine. *J Am Coll Cardiol*. 2010; 55:e27Ye129.

Kurtz E; Otto, M 2010. Aortic Stenosis Clinical Aspects of Diagnosis and Management, With 10 Illustrative Case Reports From a 25-Year Experience Medicine 6,8: November 2010 ISSN: 0025-7974

Marcus ML, Doty DB, Hiratzka LF, Wright CB, Eastham CL 1982. Decreased coronary reserve: a mechanism for angina pectoris in patients with aortic stenosis and normal coronary arteries. *N Engl J Med* 1982; 307:1362- 6

Moaref A, Shahrzad Sh, and Aslani A, 2009 Acquired AortoVentricular Tunnel: A Rare Complication of Infective Endocarditis *ECHOCARDIOGRAPHY* 2009: 26: 1, 82-83

Nitenberg A, Foult JM, Antony I, Blanchet F, Rahali M.1988 Coronary flow and resistance reserve in patients with chronic aortic regurgitation, angina pectoris and normal coronary arteries. *J Am Coll Cardiol* 1988; 11:478–86.

Pretre R, Kadner A, Dave H, Bettex D, Genoni M. 2006 Tricuspidisation of the aortic valve with creation of a crown-like annulus is able to restore a normal valve function in bicuspid aortic valves. *Eur J Cardiothorac Surg* 2006; 29:1001–1006.

Ricci DR. 1982 Afterload mismatch and preload reserve in chronic aortic regurgitation. *CIRCULATION* 1982; 66:826 -34 ISSN: 1524-4539

Roberts WC. 1970 The congenitally bicuspid aortic valve. A study of 85 autopsy cases. *Am J Cardiol*. 1970; 26:72Y83.

Rosenhek R, Rader F, Loho N, et al. 2004 Statins but not angiotensin converting enzyme inhibitors delay progression of aortic stenosis. *CIRCULATION* 2004; 110:1291–5. ISSN: 1524-4539

Ross J Jr., McCullagh WH.1972 Nature of enhanced performance of the dilated left ventricle in the dog during chronic volume overloading. *Circ Res* 1972; 30:549 –56. ISSN: 1524-4571

Sprigings DC, Fortar JC. 1995 How should we manage symptomatic aortic stenosis in the patient who is 80 or older? *Br Heart J* 1995; 74:481– 4.

Thubrikar MJ, Labrosse MR, Zehr KJ, Robicsek F,Gong GG, Fowler BL. 2005 Aortic root dilatation may alter the dimensions of the valve leaflets. *EUR J CRDIOTHOR SURG.* 2005; 28:850–855

Tornos MP, Olona M, Permanyer-Miralda G, et al.1995 Clinical outcome of severe asymptomatic chronic aortic regurgitation: a long-term prospective follow-up study. *Am Heart J* 1995; 130: 333–9

Webb JG, Chandavimol M, Thompson CR, Ricci DR, Carere RG, Munt BI, Buller CE, Pasupati S, Lichtenstein S.2006 Percutaneous aortic valve implantation retrograde from the femoral artery. *CIRCULATION.* 2006; 113:842Y850. ISSN: 1524-4539

Part 3

Infective Endocarditis

4

Aortic Valve Endocarditis

Lazar Velicki, Stamenko Šušak, Nada Čemerlić-Ađić and Aleksandar Redžek
Institute of Cardiovascular Diseases Vojvodina
Serbia

1. Introduction

Infective endocarditis (IE) is an endovascular infection of cardiovascular structures - usually valves - but also large intra-thoracic vessels and intra-cardiac foreign bodies. It is typically caused by bacteria or fungi. In contrast, sterile thrombotic lesions are termed non-bacterial thrombotic endocarditis (NBTE). IE is generally characterised by lesions of vegetations composed of platelets, fibrin, microorganisms, and inflammatory cells, as well as leaflet disruption to a various degree. Endocarditis may also produce a wide variety of systemic signs and symptoms due to sterile and infected emboli, as well as various immunological phenomena. IE is a fatal disease if left untreated (Horstkotte et al., 2004).
Characterising aspects of IE were first described by Jean François Fernel in his book Medicini in 1554. Lazaire Riviere followed suit with gross autopsy findings of the disease in 1723 after which, in 1852, Kirkes described emboli arising from heart valves in cerebral, renal, splenic and other arteries. Although several reports of IE have been published since - some from well-known physicians like Morgagni and Virchow, it was not until 1885 that IE was comprehensively documented when Sir William Osler accumulated various works and presented them to the public in the form of the comprehensive analysis of this disease (Millar & Moore, 2004).
Despite substantial improvements in diagnosis and treatment of native valve IE, disease incidence is on an increase currently averaging 3.3 new cases each year per 100,000 population in the United Kingdom, similar figures in the United States, and 1.4 to 4 new cases over the same population in European countries (Bashore et al., 2006). Native valve IE continues to be associated with high morbidity and mortality rate. Even though IE was previously associated with poor dentition and rheumatic heart disease, many factors have altered its epidemiology but have maintained its incidence: an aging population with degenerative valvular disease, injection drug use, increasing number of valve replacements, and medical interventions i.e. invasive vascular procedures (Wang & Bashore, 2009). Several variants to valve endocarditis have also been recognized: nosocomial IE, intravenous drug abuse IE, and prosthetic valve endocarditis (PVE). Nosocomial infective endocarditis is defined as acute IE, occurring 48 to 72 hours or more post-admission to hospital, or endocarditis directly related to a hospital-based procedure performed during a prior hospital visit within eight weeks of admission (Haddad et al., 2004). Intravenous drug abuse IE most commonly affects tricuspid valve and is associated with no previous structural damage of the valve. PVE accounts for 10-20% of cases. Incidence of PVE is reported to be most often between 0.2 and 0.8% for each year of life with an implanted valve (Dominik &

Zacek, 2010). Two forms of PVE can be distinguished: early PVE that occurs within 60 days of valve implantation, and late PVE occurring 60 days or more after valve implantation. It is more common after aortic than after mitral valve replacement and affects mechanical and bioprosthetic valves equally (Baddour & Wilson, 2005).

IE may give rise to numerous extracardiac, cardiac, and valvular findings, including infected thrombi (vegetations), sequel of local tissue destruction, and systemic manifestations including vasculitis, emboli, and ischemic events (Kwan-Leung & Embli, 2006). The classic clinical presentation of IE may be characterized as acute or subacute-chronic. Acute IE develops abruptly and progresses rapidly irrespective of person's health or debilitation level. A source of infection or portal of entry is often evident. When bacteria are virulent or bacterial exposure is massive, acute IE can affect normal valves. It is usually presented with signs of hemodynamic deterioration due to valve destruction caused by more aggressive forms of pathogens. The course of subacute IE is more subtle yet harder to diagnose, and may extend over many months. Often no source of infection or portal of entry is evident.

Nowadays, echocardiography offers a highly accurate diagnostic mechanism aimed at early detection and recognition of this disease and its complications also in the absence of positive blood cultures. Trans-esophageal echo (TEE) is preferred over trans-thoracic echo (TTE) because of its high sensitivity and greater ability to visualize local spread of infection at an early stage. Valve incompetence with left ventricular decompensation and congestive heart failure is the usual hemodynamic complication. Surgically demanding cases are those that affect periannular tissue and lead to significantly increased mortality and the rate of recurrent infection (Knosalla et al., 2000). Local spread of infection occurs in about 10 to 40% of native valve IE (Kang et al., 2009). Potential complications from a periannular progression of IE include abscess formation, pseudoaneurysm formation of the mitral-aortic interventricular fibrosa and the subsequent development of aorto-cavitary fistula (ACF). It is estimated that 1.5-2.2% of the patients with IE of aortic valve will develop ACF, more frequently those with prosthetic valve IE than those with native valve IE (odds 1.61:1) (Anguera et al., 2005). ACF is the most dangerous complication of periannular tissue involvement with the mortality of up to 40%. Extension of the IE from aortic to the mitral valve is possible and occurs through mitro-aortic fibrous continuity with development of a septic aneurysm in the anterior mitral leaflet with or without perforation.

2. Pathogenesis

Several conditions must be met in order to develop IE. According to the injury-thrombus-infection theory, the trigger event is the endocardium damage. Endothelial injury is the most plausible factor leading to platelet deposition. Injury develops as a result of hemodynamic and mechanical stress to the endocardium. The predilection site of IE is rough part of the valves (the coaptation area) due to high impact pressures following the closure of the leaflets. Also, turbulent blood flow produced by congenital or acquired heart diseases traumatizes the endothelium inducing apoptosis of valve cells and leading to tissue remodelling. As a result, platelet and fibrin deposition occurs. The phase in which sterile thrombotic vegetations are present on the leaflets is referred to as NBTE. The Venturi effect also contributes to the development and location of NBTE, i.e. vegetations are attached to the flow side of the valves (ventricular side of semilunar valves, tips of the leaflets, sewing rings of prosthetic valves) (Bashore et al., 2006). The entry of micro-organisms into the circulatory system leads to bacteremia and ultimately converts NBTE into IE. Naturally this would depend on the bacteria inoculum sufficient to allow invasion of the pre-existing valve thrombus. Clinical manifestation of IE appears to be influenced by several factors both host and pathogen related (susceptibility of the host genetically determined by defence mechanisms and adherence propensity as well as invasiveness of certain pathogens) (Naber et al., 2009).

On gross examination, vegetations are usually grey, pink, or brown and are often friable. They may be single or multiple and may affect more than one valve. Vegetations may be located anywhere on the valve cusp or leaflet or endocardial surface. In fact this is an important distinguishing feature to note, as valve thrombi associated with nonbacterial thrombotic endocarditis (NBTE) and those related to rheumatic fever do not have this variability in location, and are usually along the lines of valve closure (Kwan-Leung & Embli, 2006). Corresponding microscopic finding would depend on the virulence and duration of the induction and is usually characterized with presence of fibrin, neutrophils and clumps of organisms with foci of calcification or organized thrombi to a certain extent.

2.1 Microbiology

The common causes of native valve IE include members of the normal bacterial flora of the skin, oropharynx and the gastrointestinal and genitourinary tract (Kwan-Leung & Embli, 2006). The most common microorganisms that cause IE include: *Streptococci, Staphylococcus aureus, Enterococcus* species, HACEK organisms (*Hemophilus parainfluenzae, Hemophilus aphrophilus, Actinobacillus actinomycetemcomitans, Cardiobacterium hominis, Eikenella* species, and *Kingella* species) and fungi (Bayer et al., 1998). *S. aureus* is more often associated with the native valve IE than PVE, whereas coagulase negative *Staphyloococci* are more commonly seen in PVE. Furthermore, *Enterococcus spp.* usually leads to subacute form of IE. Anaerobic bacteria are rarely associated with IE and account 2-16% of all cases (Brook, 2008). *Candida* and *Aspergillus* species cause the majority of fungal IE (Bayer et al., 1998). Intravenous drug abusers, prosthetic-valve recipients, and patients with long-term central venous catheters are at highest risk for fungal IE. Fungal infected thrombi are usually quite large and friable leading to valve orifice obstruction.

Procedure	Rate	Micro-organisms
Endoscopy	0-20%	Coagulase negative Staphylococi, Streptococci, diphteroids
Colonoscopy	0-20%	Escherichila coli, Bacteroides species
Barium enema	0-20%	Enterococci, aerobic and anaerobic gram-negative rods
Dental extractions	30-100%	Streptococcus viridans
Transurethral resection of the prostate	20-45%	Coliforms, Enterococci, Staphylococcus aureus
Transesophageal echocardiography	0-25%	Streptococcus viridans, anaerobic organisms, Streptococci

Table 1. Rate of subsequent bacteraemia following certain procedures

Microorganisms have surface adhesions that mediate the adherence to vegetation and avidly bind to valvular and peri-annular tissue with irreversible adhesion (Mocchegiani & Nataloni, 2009). They then produce a biofilm that inhibits host's defence mechanisms and to protect themselves against antimicrobial treatment. This makes antibiotic sterilization extremely difficult. Causative microorganisms vary by site of infection, source of bacteremia, and host risk factors as shown in Table 1 (Towns & Reller, 2003).

Blood culture negative endocarditis (BCNE) is by definition IE in which standard culture methods are inadequate to allow detection of the causative agents. The incidence of BCNE have historically ranged from 2.5% to 31% depending on the study population (Kwan-Leung & Embli, 2006). The most common pathogens that cause BCNE are: *Coxiella burnetti, Bartonella spp.* and *Trophyrema whipplei.* IE associated with these microorganisms most often occurs in patients with some form of immunodeficiency, valvular disease and a history of contact with domestic animals.

3. Clinical presentation and diagnosis

The diagnosis of IE is based upon clinical suspicion derived from signs and symptoms and most importantly the demonstration of associated bacteremia. Clinical presentation of IE may vary significantly with regards to causative pathogen, immunological status of the host, intermittent use of antibiotics, structural heart disease, and presence of foreign objects (heart valves, pacemakers etc.). The diagnosis of IE is straightforward in those patients with classic manifestations: bacteremia or fungemia, evidence of active valvulitis, peripheral emboli, and immunologic vascular phenomena (Bayer et al., 1998). In other patients however the classic peripheral stigmata may be few or absent. All this imposes the necessity for highly sensitive diagnostic algorithm that will be both sensitive for disease detection and specific for its exclusion across all the forms of the disease (Baddour et al., 2005).

Initial signs and symptoms of subacute IE may be vague and ambiguous: low grade fever, fatigability and malaise, night sweats, and weight loss. Clinical manifestation may be prolonged until the development of a heart murmur with or without signs of valvular insufficiency. From this point on, diagnosis can be readily established. However, majority of the patients already have detectable heart murmurs and with a coinciding clinical presentation, IE should be suspected. Peripheral lesions of subacute IE include: petechiae (oral mucosa, conjunctivae, the dorsa of the hands and feet, chest and abdominal wall), subungal haemorrhages (splinter haemorrhages), Osler nods, clubbing fingers, Roth spots (round or oval haemorrhagic retinal lesions), Janeway lesions (irregular erythematous and painless macules on palms and soles). In current times of widespread use of antibiotics, incidence of classic presentation of the peripheral lesions reduced substantially. Some of the peripheral manifestations develop as a result of immunological activities, while others result from embolization. About 35% of patients may develop central nervous system effects such as transient ischemic attacks, stroke, toxic encephalopathy, and brain abscess (Baddour et al., 2005). Renal embolization may lead to hematuria while splenic emboli may cause left upper quadrant pain.

Acute IE is characterized by a more rapid and progressive course of the disease. The invasiveness and aggressiveness of the pathogen causes prompt reaction in the host including hyperpyrexia, profuse sweating, fatigue, and malaise. Signs and symptoms of heart failure develop very often and heart murmur is present in almost every case.

Definite IE	
Pathological criteria	
	Microorganisms demonstrated by culture or histological examination of a vegetation, a vegetation that has embolized, or an intracardiac abscess specimen; or Pathological lesions; vegetation or intracardiac abscess confirmed by histological examination showing active endocarditis
Clinical criteria	
	2 major criteria; or 1 major criterion and 3 minor criteria; or 5 minor criteria
Possible IE	
	1 major criterion and 1 minor criterion; or 3 minor criteria
Rejected	
	Firm alternative diagnosis explaining evidence of IE; or Resolution of IE syndrome with antibiotic therapy for 4 days; or No pathological evidence of IE at surgery or autopsy, after antibiotic therapy for 4 days; or Does not meet criteria for possible IE as above

Table 2. Definition of IE according to the modified Duke criteria (Li et al., 2000)

Major blood culture criteria include
Two blood cultures positive for organisms typically found in patients with IE (i.e., *S viridans, Streptococcus bovis,* a HACEK group organism, community-acquired *S aureus,* or *Enterococci* in the absence of a primary focus)
Blood cultures persistently positive for one of the above organisms from cultures drawn more than 12 hours apart
Three or more separate blood cultures drawn at least 1 hour apart
Single positive blood culture for *Coxiella burnetii* or anti-phase 1 IgG antibody titer > 1:800
Major echocardiographic criteria include
Echocardiogram positive for IE, documented by an oscillating intracardiac mass on a valve or on supporting structures, in the path of regurgitant jets, or on implanted material in the absence of an alternative anatomical explanation
Myocardial abscess
Development of partial dehiscence of a prosthetic valve
New-onset of valvular regurgitation
Minor criteria include
predisposing heart condition
fever
temperature > 38°
vascular phenomena or immunologic phenomena
microbiological evidence that does not meet a major criteria

Table 3. Definition of terms used in the modified Duke criteria for IE diagnosis (Li et al., 2000)

With regard to recurrence of IE, two types are described: relapse - repeat episodes of IE caused by the same microorganism < 6 months after the initial episode; and reinfection - infection with a different microorganism or repeat episode of IE caused by the same microorganism > 6 months after the initial episode.
IE diagnostic criteria published in the previous studies were refined by Durack and colleagues from Duke University Medical Center in 1994. These criteria, which have come to be known as the Duke criteria, incorporated echocardiographic evidence of endocardial involvement (Table 2, Table 3) (Durack et al., 1994; Li et al., 2000). The criteria had improved test performance characteristics over the prior set and have been validated subsequently by many other studies (Wang & Bashore, 2009).
European society of cardiology published diagnostic criteria that should raise suspicion of IE (Table 4) (Horstkotte et al., 2004). These overlap the Duke criteria to an extent, but are also notably different.

High clinical suspicion (urgent indication for echocardiographic screening and possibly hospital admission)
new valve lesion/(regurgitant) murmur
embolic event(s) of unknown origin (esp. cerebral and renal infarction)
sepsis of unknown origin
haematuria, glomerulonephritis, and suspected renal infarction
fever plus one or more of these:
prosthetic material inside the heart; other high predispositions for IE; newly developed ventricular arrhythmias or conduction disturbances; first manifestation of CHF; positive BCs (if the organism identified is typical for NVE/PVE); cutaneous (Osler, Janeway) or ophthalmic (Roth) manifestations; multifocal/rapid changing pulmonic infiltrations (right heart IE); peripheral abscesses (renal, splenic, spine) of unknown origin; predisposition and recent diagnostic/therapeutic interventions known to result in significant
Low clinical suspicion
fever plus none of the above
IE – Infective endocarditis; CHF – Congestive heart failure; BC – Blood cultures; NVE – Native valve endocarditis; PVE – Prosthetic valve endocarditis

Table 4. Criteria that should raise suspicion of IE (Horstkotte et al., 2004)

Although differential diagnosis may seem abundant, after careful clinical management it can be reduced to: non-infectious endocarditis (marantic endocarditis - paraneoplastic syndrome associated with some malignancies and Libman-Sacks endocarditis - associated with systemic lupus erythematosis), and cardiac tumors (atrial myxoma and valve fibroelastoma) (Velicki et al., 2010).

3.1 Echocardiography

Echocardiography plays a crucial role in the diagnosis and management of IE. Diagnosis should be based on the isolation of the microorganism through the blood cultures. In certain cases blood cultures would yield inadequate (non-diagnostic) results due to changing nature of valvular infection necessitating reliance on echocardiography as an indirect diagnostic method. Echocardiography is useful not only for assessing the structural and functional valvular status, but also for the local spread of infection (annular abscess or ACF), as well as predicting the potential for embolization. Echocardiography should be performed in all cases of suspected IE (Baddour et al., 2005).

In most cases TTE would be sufficient in evaluation of aortic valve endocarditis. TEE may be indicated in case of PVE suspicion, evaluation of local spread of infection (better visualization of abscess cavities and ACF), as well as predicting embolization potential based on the vegetation size, consistency, location, number and mobility. Both TTE and TEE can produce false-negative and false-positive results on rare occasions (too small vegetations or already dislodged vegetations, valvular abnormalities not related to a current infection, respectively). Echocardiography should therefore be only one step in a diagnostic chain. More recent studies have shown that in majority of clinical situations of suspected IE, an initial strategy of TEE is more cost-effective than a staged procedure with TTE and is therefore an optimal strategy over empiric antibiotic therapy alone (Habib et al., 2009). At the same time it is important to outline specific definitions of the echocardiographic findings to adequately evaluate local endocarditis presentation (Table 5) (Sachdev et al., 2003).

Finding	Description
Vegetation	Irregularly shaped, discrete echogenic mass, adherent to but distinct from endocardial surface or intra-cardiac device Oscillation of mass (supportive, not mandatory)
Abscess	Thickened area or mass within the myocardium or valve annulus, or evidence of flow into region (supportive, not mandatory)
Aneurysm	Echolucent space with thin surrounding tissue
Fistula	Blood flow between two distinct cardiac blood spaces or chambers through abnormal path/channel
Leaflet perforation	Defect in body of valve leaflet with flow through defect
Valve dehiscence	Prosthetic valve with abnormal rocking motion/excursion in at least one direction

Table 5. Echocardiographic findings in IE and corresponding definitions (Sachdev et al., 2003)

3.2 Periannular extension

Periannular extension of infection is one of the most fearful complications in patients with IE. Perivalvular extension in the setting of native valve IE develops from bacterial necrosis of local tissue and results in high rates of heart failure and death despite surgical therapy (Anguera et al., 2006). Local spread of infection occurs in about 10 to 40% of native aortic valve endocarditis (Kang et al., 2009).

Periannular abscess formation and aortocavitary fistulous tract formation in IE represent a further step in aortic annular erosion and the extension of infection beyond the leaflets and the aortic ring. In the early stage, perivalvular abscess is largely composed of inflammatory infiltrate, but at later stages necrosis and cavitation usually develop leading to destruction of perivalvular tissue. Perivalvular abscess is not a static complication but is progressive and can evolve into serious perivalvular complications including perivalvular leak, fistula and pseudoaneurysm (Kwan-Leung & Embli, 2006). It is estimated that 1.5-2.2% of patients with IE of aortic valve will develop ACF, and even more frequently those with PVE as opposed to those with native valve endocarditis (odds 1.61:1) (Anguera et al., 2005). Due to the central position of the aortic valve, infection of the valve may form fistulas with practically any surrounding chamber (Susak et al., 2009). Because PVE usually begins as periannulitis, it is not surprising that infected prosthetic valves have these complications with a higher frequency than native valves. ACF is the most dangerous complication of periannular tissue involvement with the mortality of up to 40% (Kang et al., 2009). It is estimated that around 60% of patients with ACF develop heart failure before surgery and the extent of the heart failure is more severe than in patients with nonruputred abscesses (Anguera et al., 2006). Extension of the IE from aortic to the mitral valve occurs through mitro-aortic fibrous continuity with development of a septic aneurysm in the anterior mitral leaflet with or without perforation. Myocardial ischemic sequelae may develop as a result of debris embolization from aortic root abscess, or due to extraluminal compression from an enlarged aortic root abscess. Coronary arteries can become directly affected by local extension through the coronary ostia or by creation of mycotic aneurysms.

In the published data, one of the most convincing and consistently reliable variables predictive of periannular complications has been the appearance of an AV block and signs of pericarditis or pericardial effusion (Graupner et al., 2002). Most of these patients will undergo surgery because of classic surgical indications independent of the echocardiographic detection of periannular complications.

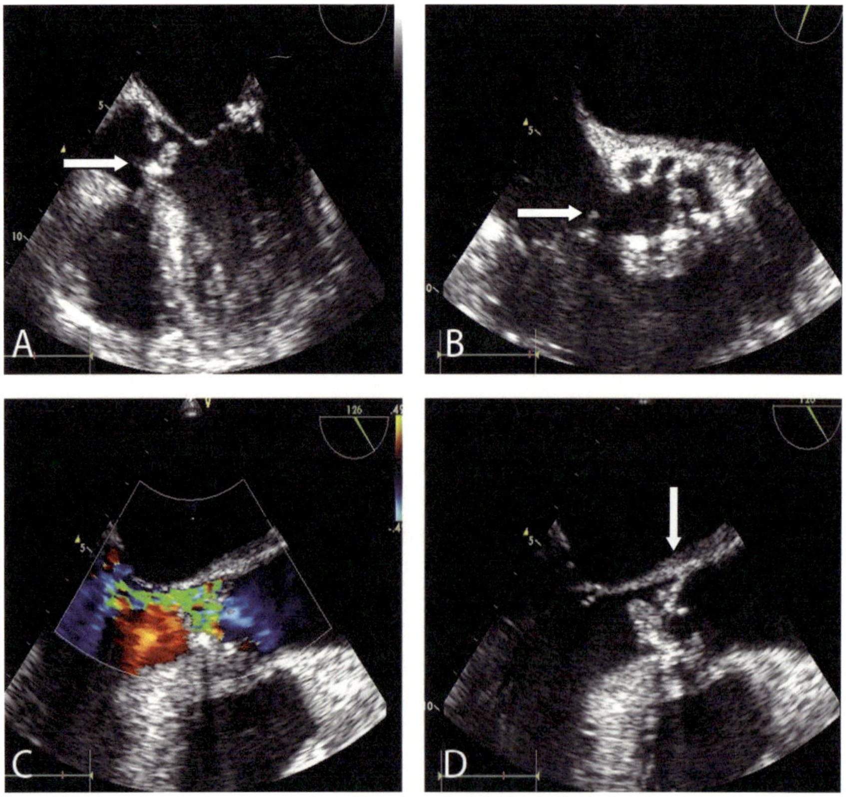

Fig. 1. TEE showing: (A) possible fistula, (B) perforation of the right coronary leaflet, (C) Color flow imaging of the aortic valve showing severe aortic regurgitation due to leaflet perforation, (D) vegetations on the aortic side of the leaflets

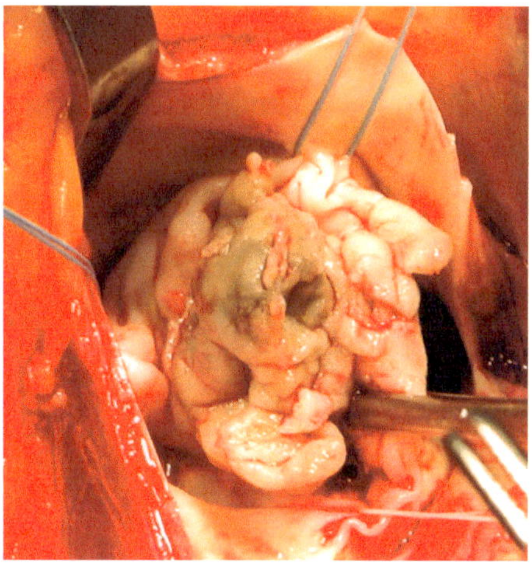

Fig. 2. IE superimposed on severe aortic stenosis with development of small friable vegetations and leaflet abscess

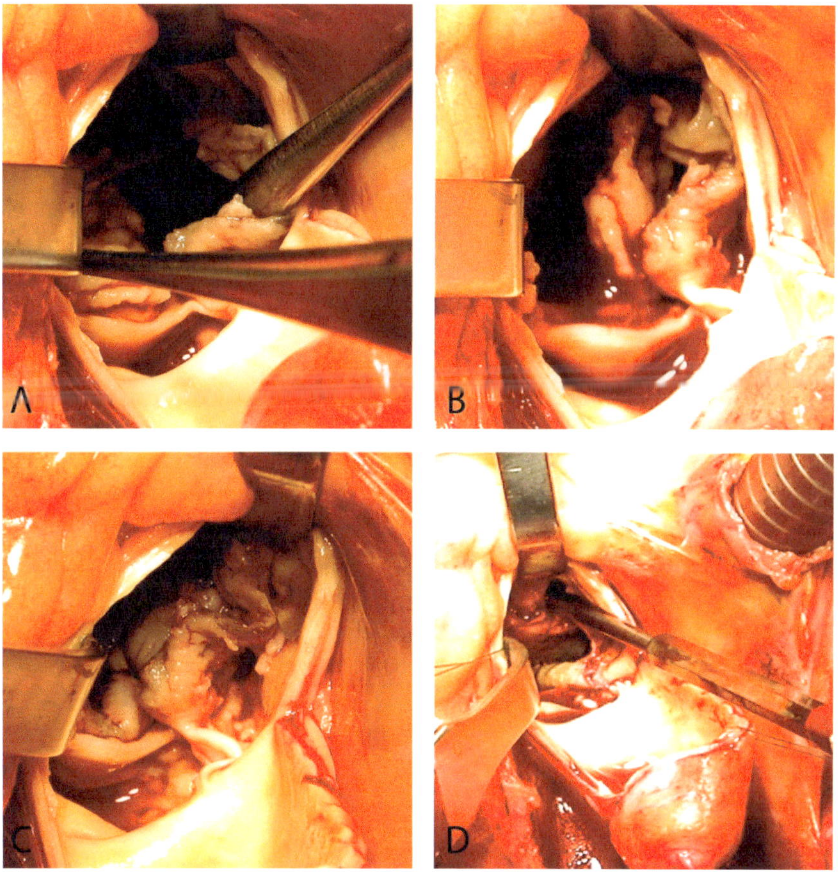

Fig. 3. Complete destruction of the right coronary leaflet (A and B), small vegetations on all leaflets (A, B, C) and ACF to the right ventricle with probe in it (D)

3.3 Prosthetic valve endocarditis

PVE is defined as infection occurring in a prosthetic heart valve and has an overall incidence of 0.32% to 1.2% per patient year and cumulative risk of 5% at 10 years (Mahesh et al., 2005). Rates range from 1% to 3% within the first year however the highest rate of infection occurs in the first three postoperative months. By six months, rates stabilize to 0.4% annually (Kwan-Leung & Embli, 2006). Despite advances in diagnosis, medical and surgical therapy over the past few decades, PVE still carries a substantial risk of morbidity, with overall mortality ranging from 20% to 80% of affected patients (Musci et al., 2010). Important factors in the pathogenesis include type of prosthesis, previous native valve endocarditis, male gender, and long cardiopulmonary bypass time. A number of studies have reported a higher incidence of PVE after mechanical valve replacement in comparison with the biologic valve replacement during the initial few months after implantation. Early PVE may develop when pathogens reach the valve prosthesis by way of direct contamination intraoperatively or via hematogenous spread over the initial days and weeks after surgery. The pathogens have direct access to the prosthesis-annulus interface and to perivalvular tissue along suture pathways because the valve sewing ring, cardiac annulus, and anchoring sutures are not endothelialized early after valve implantation. These structures are coated with host proteins such as fibronectin and fibrinogen to which some organisms can adhere to and initiate infection. On the other hand, as the sewing ring, sutures, and adjacent tissues become endothelialized in months after valve replacement, sites for adherence of microorganisms and access to host tissues adjacent to the prosthesis are altered. The pathogenesis of late PVE has been postulated to resemble native valve endocarditis. This temporal classification is based on marked differences in microbiologic causes of early and late PVEs. Early PVE accounts for approximately 30% of all PVE cases and is predominantly caused by *S. aureus*, gram-negative bacilli, and coagulase negative *Staphylococci*. There are also differences in infection localization with regard to type of prosthesis used to replace aortic valve. Infections in mechanical valves generally involve the sewing ring or adherent thrombi, and can lead to paraprosthetic leaks, ring abscesses, and invasive infection, necessitating operative intervention. Bioprostheses are less susceptible to early infection, which is often restricted to the leaflets, making cure with antibiotics more likely but increasing the chances of late failure due to degeneration of the cusps (Mahesh et al., 2005).

Severe heart failure, staphylococcal infection and complicated PVE are designated as markers of both in-hospital and late mortality, while severe heart failure and *S. aureus* infection were the only independent predictors of in-hospital death (Habib et al., 2008). Data from the International Collaboration on Endocarditis showed that in-hospital death, which occurred in 22.8% of the study patients, was predicted by older age, health-care-associated infection, *S. Aureus* infection and complications of PVE, including heart failure, stroke, intra-cardiac abscess and persistent bacteraemia (Wang et al., 2007).

Because the presence of a prosthetic heart valve is a predisposing factor to the development of endocarditis, antibiotic prophylaxis and therapy at the time of health-care-related procedures has been a mainstay of care of the patient with a prosthetic valve (Wang & Bashore, 2009). For this reason, antibiotic prophylaxis is recommended only for patients with prosthetic heart valves prior to dental procedures (highest rate of possible bacteremia as demonstrated in Table 1.), but not before gastrointestinal or genitourinary procedures (Wilson et al., 2008). However, ESC guidelines do recommend antibiotic prophylaxis in the case of gastrointestinal or genitourinary procedures (Horstkotte et al., 2004).

Patients with suspected PVE should be aggressively treated with broad spectrum antibiotics that are effective against wide range of microorganisms especially *staphylococci* and *streptococci*. In further course of the disease, antibiotic regiment should be optimised based on sensitivity of isolated cultures. This therapy should reduce the risk of systemic embolization by shrinking the size of vegetations. Patient should be carefully monitored and further diagnostic procedures should be performed. TEE is of greatest value because it can provide information of existence and extension of infective process to a surrounding tissue. Negative echocardiography finding does not necessarily exclude PVE. After the diagnosis of PVE, repeat-TEE may be highly sensitive and useful to diagnose complications such as prosthetic valve dysfunction (regurgitation or stenosis), resultant changes in ventricular function or dilation, periannular extension of infection (intra-cardiac abscess or fistula formation), or involvement of other valves (Wang & Bashore, 2009). Surgical consultation should be promptly scheduled given that periannular complications occur in more than 50% of patients and may lead to complete aortic root destruction. Radical surgical debridement with a margin of healthy tissue to eradicate intracardiac foci of infection remains the primary aim of surgery for PVE, enabling secure fixation of the new prosthesis, avoiding recurrent or residual infection, periprosthetic leak or dehiscence, or subannular aneurysm formation (Mahesh et al., 2005).

4. Clinical management

The diagnosis of IE remains challenging and continues to be dependent on a constellation of infectious symptoms and signs in association with bacteremia, auscultatory evidence of valvular involvement, and signs of large and/or small-vessel peripheral arterial embolization (Kwan-Leung & Embli, 2006). With availability of technologically sophisticated imaging modalities, establishing IE diagnosis should not be very hard in theory. Recognition is the first step in proper management of IE. Rapid diagnosis, early risk stratification, institution of appropriate bactericidal therapy, and prompt recognition and treatment of complications are the key elements toward a good outcome (Wang & Bashore, 2009).

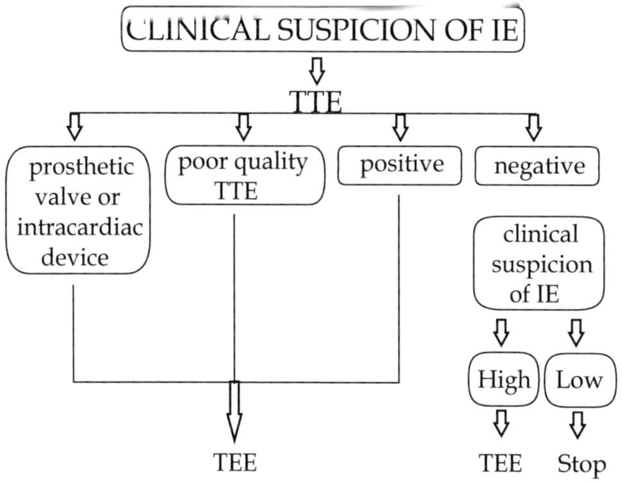

Fig. 4. Indications for initial echocardiography assessment. If initial TEE is negative but suspicion for IE remains, repeat TEE within 7-10 days (Habib et al., 2009)

Diagnosis should be established in regards to clinical presentation and IE diagnostic criteria presented in Table 2., Table 3. and Table 4. Blood cultures remains the single most important investigation in a patient suspected of having IE (*gold standard test*). If appropriate samples are obtained, one could expect to yield growth of the causative organism in over 90% of cases of IE (Kwan-Leung & Embli, 2006). At a minimum, 3 sets of blood cultures should be drawn at least 1h apart prior to antibiotic administration irrespective of body temperature. In most cases, the results of blood cultures would be available within 3 days from the moment they were obtained.

Broad-spectrum parenteral antibiotic therapy should be commenced immediately upon suspicion of IE but after the acquisition of blood cultures. Antibiotic therapy should not be delayed (i.e. should be started even if the blood cultures are not drawn) only when dealing with septic patients with suspected IE. Therapy should be adjusted according to blood culture findings. It should continue for 4-6 weeks so as to eradicate all the pathogens from phagocytic cells and inaccessible vegetations. The precise antibiotic regiment for specific pathogens is presented in detail within the European Society of Cardiology recommendations (Horstkotte et al., 2004). The patient should be evaluated for the signs of immunodepression, malnutrition, or other systemic diseases as these conditions may impair the treatment course and promote development of complications. Additionally, renal function should also be carefully monitored, and due consideration given to probiotic supplements.

Further clinical investigation should be performed using echocardiography and other diagnostic procedures guided by the clinical presentation. As stated earlier, TEE is preferred over TTE because of higher sensitivity and specificity, but TTE may serve as an initial screening test. If echocardiography remains negative but suspicion remains, echocardiography should be repeated within one week. A repeatedly negative study will near-exclude the diagnosis.

Upon completion of the antibiotic regiment, or in the onset of complications or severe hemodynamic deterioration, the patient should be presented to cardiac surgeon to evaluate necessity for the operative intervention and its timing. Table 6 summarizes conditions considered as indications for surgical intervention.

4.1 Surgical therapy

Despite many advances in diagnosis and antibiotic therapy of IE, eradication of the septic focus and abolition of the accompanying systemic manifestations usually require some kind of surgical intervention. Surgically demanding cases are those of active IE affecting entire aortic root with development of local periannular complications. Main challenge with acute IE is to address the two coexisting aspects of the disease: the infectious process necessitating removal of all infected tissues to prevent recurrence, and altered valvular anatomy and function to be corrected and restored (Kwan-Leung & Embli, 2006). With regard to the complex pathology, the mortality and morbidity rates associated with surgical therapy remain relatively high - between 3.8 and 22% (d'Udekem et al., 1997). For the purpose of unifying criteria, hospital mortality is considered to be related to the operation when death occurs in the operating room or during the first 30 days after surgery, but also when the patient dies in hospital beyond 30 days without being discharged (Edmunds et al., 1996). There are many factors that may influence surgical mortality in IE giving cause to a risk stratification scoring system.

Indication	Evidence
Emergency indication for cardiac surgery (same day)	
Acute AR with early closure of mitral valve	A
Rupture of a sinus Valsalva aneurysm into a right heart chamber	A
Rupture into the pericardium	A
Urgent indication for cardiac surgery (within 1–2 days)	
Valvular obstruction	A
Unstable prosthesis	A
Acute AR or MR with heart failure, NYHA III–IV	A
Septal perforation	A
Evidence of annular or aortic abscess, sinus or aortic true or false aneurysm, fistula formation, or new onset conduction disturbances	A
Major embolism + mobile vegetation >10mm + appropriate antibiotic treatment < 7–10 days	B
Mobile vegetation > 15mm + appropriate antibiotic therapy < 7–10 days	C
No effective antimicrobial treatment available	A
Elective indication for cardiac surgery (earlier is usually better)	
Staphylococcal prosthetic valve infective endocarditis	B
Early prosthetic valve infective endocarditis (≤2 months after surgery)	B
Evidence of progressive paravalvar prosthetic leak	A
Evidence of valve dysfunction and persistent infection after 7–10 days of appropriate antibiotic treatment, as indicated by presence of fever or bacteremia, provided there are no noncardiac causes for infection	A
Fungal infective endocarditis caused by a mould	A
Fungal infective endocarditis caused by a yeast	B
Infection with difficult-to-treat organisms	B
Vegetation growing larger during antibiotic treatment > 7 days	C

A: Strong evidence or general agreement that cardiac surgery is useful and effective; B: Inconclusive or conflicting evidence or a divergence of opinion about the usefulness or efficacy of cardiac surgery but with weight of evidence & opinion of the majority being in favour; C: Inconclusive or conflicting evidence or divergence of opinion; lack of clear consensus on the basis of evidence or opinion of the majority.
AR - aortic regurgitation; MR - mitral regurgitation; NYHA - New York Heart Association functional class.

Table 6. Indications for surgical intervention in patients with IE (adapted from Delahaye et al., 2004)

As shown in Table 6., indication for surgical intervention is usually based on development of heart failure that cannot be managed otherwise, signs of uncontrolled infection despite aggressive medical therapy, and manifestation or increased risk of embolization. These surgical indications stand for both native valve endocarditis and PVE. Prior to establishing an indication, surgeon must become aware of all the compromising factors that may affect the outcome of the surgery: phase of the infective process (acute or active phase is associated

with higher mortality), structural and functional status of afflicted valve, comorbidites). In patients with high risk of coronary heart disease, preoperative coronarography should be performed to assess the necessity of coronary artery bypass grafting in the same act.
Knowing that cardiac surgery is an integral part of IE treatment strategy, it is advisable that cardiac surgery team should be included in patient evaluation following IE diagnosis. This will both enable the surgical team to become fully familiar with the patient case as the surgery is eventually called for, but also work with the medical team to determine the need and optimum timing for surgery (Kwan-Leung & Embli, 2006).

4.1.1 Timing of surgery

Surgical treatment is used in approximately half of patients with IE because of severe complications (Habib et al., 2009). The right timing of an operation is absolutely essential for success. The patient status has to be optimized to the maximum capacity in order to achieve maximal benefit from the operation. Operating too soon carries a higher risk of a failure due to unstable patient condition, specific cardiac tissue condition (friability) which may lead to embolization and peri-prosthetic leakage, and greater possibility of recurrence. On the other hand, waiting too long for the operative treatment may lead to a life-threating systemic infection (septic state) with development of multiple organ dysfunction syndrome, or extensive structural destruction of the heart valves and surrounding tissues. Surgical timing strategies have evolved significantly over the previous years, owing to the developments in the medical management and diagnostic tools, but despite this advent, when-to-operate still remains a controversial issue.
In some cases surgery needs to be performed on an emergency (within 24 hours) or urgent (within a few days) basis irrespective of the duration of antibiotic treatment. In other cases surgery can be postponed to allow 1 or 2 weeks of antibiotic treatment under careful clinical and echocardiographic observation before an elective surgical procedure is carried out. Early surgical treatment is justified in patients with high-risk features that make unlikely the possibility of cure with antibiotic treatment, unless they also have co-morbid conditions or complications that make the prospect of recovery remote.
According to European Society of Cardiology Guidelines (Habib et al., 2009), unless severe co-morbidity exists, early surgery is recommended in the following cases: the presence of heart failure, or presence of locally uncontrolled infection in the cases of native valve IE. The decision to operate-on early to prevent embolism is always difficult and specific for every patient. Governing factors include size and mobility of the vegetation, previous embolism, type of microorganism, and duration of antibiotic therapy.

4.1.2 Types of surgical management

During the preoperative evaluation and clinical management a surgeon is presented with a variety of information to evaluate and make an indication for surgical intervention. Exactly what type of intervention is going to be needed will be unclear until the moment the aortic root is open inside the operative theatre. No matter how accurate the pre-operative diagnostics, intra-operative finding will ultimately guide the ongoing operation.
The basic principles of operative treatment are: to remove all destroyed tissue, to resolve local complications if any, and to anatomically reconstruct the valve if it's possible or to replace it entirely. It is evident that the exclusive involvement of the leaflets makes it easier to perform surgical intervention with limited technical difficulty. The problem arises when infection spreads beyond the native annulus.

Aortic valve replacement (AVR) is the cornerstone operation in setting of aortic valve IE. When repair is an option it is preferred over the replacement, although feasibility of aortic valve repair is reduced with prevalence of extensive tissue destruction in an aortic IE setting (Kwan-Leung & Embli, 2006). Vegetectomy, a novel technique, has also been introduced in common practice (Chen et al., 2009). This repair technique may be considered in cases of limited vegetation presence and without severe leaflet involvement or extension into periannular tissue. Vegetations should not be large in size nor abundantly present because the consequent vegetectomy would impair the coaptation process of the valve. Antiobiotic therapy before the operation should be aggressive to eliminate the presence of pathogens and to reduce the chance of recurrence.

Several recent studies evaluated outcome after replacement devices were used, that is, biological or mechanical valves. The results were generally favourable and have noted no significant difference in mortality between the two valve types. The choice of valve type is to surgeon's preference and according to generally accepted indications for AVR. Mechanical valves are charcterized as reliable and durable but require lifelong anticoagulation (taken orally). Bioprosthesis are limited by their durability of 10-15 years but do not require oral anticoagulation therapy. Surgeon needs to be aware of all factors that may influence the choice of valve such as patient age, germinative period, risk of haemorrhage or thrombosis following oral antiocoagulation therapy compliance and so forth. There is no significant difference in either short-term or long-term survival between mechanical and bioprosthetic valves.

In the case of severe aortic root involvement with severe damage of aortic valve and surrounding tissue, a composite graft incorporating a prosthetic valve and a vascular tube graft can be used. If more than 50% of the aortic annulus has been destroyed, homograft (allograft) root replacement may be the treatment of choice. These are the most serious conditions that can be seen in aortic root as a consequence of IE. Aortic homograft represent the ideal tissue to reconstruct the complicated aortic root as they allow for a radical treatment by eliminating abscesses, closing fistulae, the associated treatment of the sinotubular junction and ascending aorta, and the implantation of a biological device that does not require anticoagulation and is resistant to infection (Mestres et al., 1993). Although no conclusive data is available comparing homografts and prosthetic valves with respect to durability and risk of recurrent IE, current data from surgical series indicate satisfactory results with the use of homografts (Riberi et al., 1997). Another indication for use of homograft is PVE which represents a difficult operation with need of extensive removal of necrotic tissue and debris (Sabik et al., 2002). A recent study compared 5-year survival rate for different valve implant types. It demonstrated that the survival is comparable for mechanical valves and homografts, but is significantly lower for bioprosthesis (Nguyen et al., 2010). Another research group also investigated relationship between mechanical valves and homografts in native valve endocarditis establishing advantage of mechanical prosthesis over homografts (Klieverik et al., 2009).

Stentless aortic valves may also be used for AVR in the case of IE (Perrotta & Lentini, 2010). Stentless Aortic Valve Conduit in patients with native or prosthetic aortic valve endocarditis appears to demonstrate good results, similar to those of cryopreserved homografts. Study comparing two groups of patients treated with stentless valves and homografts, demonstrating an equal reinfection rate of 4% and lower mortality for the stentless group (12% vs. 16%, respectively). The reinfection rate is found to be lower for the homograft and stentless groups than for the patients treated with standard prostheses, respectively, 5.8%,

3.7% and 33%. The stentless valve offers a reinfection rate and postoperative echocardiographic data comparable to those achieved with homografts (Siniawski et al., 2003).

Study	Conduit/ prosthesis	No. of pts	Peri-annular aortic root abscess (%)	Op. mortality (%)	Freedom from recurrent infection (follow-up duration)	Freedom from reop. (follow-up)	Survival rate (%) (follow-up)
Yankah et al. (2005)	Homograft in NVE	161	100	9.3	91% (10 years)	82.9% (17 years)	87 (11 years)
Sabik et al. (2002)	Homograft in PVE	103	78	3.9	95% (10 years)	-	73 (5 years) 56 (10 years)
Siniawski et al. (2005)	Shelhigh noreact stentless prosthesis	75	100	12 (60 days)	96% (17±10 months)	-	
	Homograft	68	100	16 (60 days)	96% (17±10 months)		
Kon et al. (2002)	Stentless porcine aortic root bioprosthesis	104	-	3.9	96.9% (8 years)	100 (8 years)	59.8 (8 years)
Schmidtke et al. (2007)	Ross procedure	296	-	0.3	0 (47.3 ± 28.6 months)	-	99.7 (47.3 ± 28.6 months)
Avierinos et al. (2007)	Homograft	54	63	9	44 ± 10% (10 years survival-free from the combined endpoint, including recurrence IE, prosthesis dysfunctions and long-term cardiovascular mortality)		
	Convent. prosthesis	73	-	-			

Table 7. Comparision of multiple conduits for periannular extension of aortic valve endocarditis (reproduced with permission from Kang et al., 2009)

Another suggested procedure that may be used in the setting of IE is the Ross procedure (Joyce et al., 1994). The Ross procedure consists of autotransplantation of the pulmonary valve. Studies reporting reproducible results following the Ross procedure in the treatment of IE have not yet been published in quantity that would allow comparison with other available approaches. In the setting of PVE, the Ross procedure should be introduced for further improvement of surgical results (Ishikawa et al., 2009).

Short-term and long-term results following operation due to IE are generally satisfactory. There is however a statistical difference in survival among patients with native valve IE and PVE. One year survival in native valve endocarditis is reported to be from 91% to 93%, while in PVE 79,7%. Five year survival in native valve IE ranges between 54% and 93%, and for PVE it is 64,2%. Ten year survival for native valve IE is reported to be from 54% to 67,5%, and for PVE from 33.5% to 58% (Kwan-Leung & Embli, 2006).

5. References

Anguera, I., Miro, J. M., Evangelista, A., Cabell, C. H., San Roman, J. A., Vilacosta, I., Almirante, B., Ripoll, T., Farinas, M. C., Anguita, M., Navas, E., Gonzalez-Juanatey, C., Garcia-Bolao, I., Munoz, P., de, A. A., Sarria, C., Rufi, G., Miralles, F., Pare, C., Fowler, V. G., Jr., Mestres, C. A., de, L. E., Guma, J. R., Moreno, A. & Corey, G. R. (2006). Periannular complications in infective endocarditis involving native aortic valves. *Am. J. Cardiol.*, Vol.98, No.9, pp. 1254-1260, ISSN 0002-9149.

Anguera, I., Miro, J. M., Vilacosta, I., Almirante, B., Anguita, M., Munoz, P., Roman, J. A., de, A. A., Ripoll, T., Navas, E., Gonzalez-Juanatey, C., Cabell, C. H., Sarria, C., Garcia-Bolao, I., Farinas, M. C., Leta, R., Rufi, G., Miralles, F., Pare, C., Evangelista, A., Fowler, V. G., Jr., Mestres, C. A., de, L. E. & Guma, J. R. (2005). Aorto-cavitary fistulous tract formation in infective endocarditis: clinical and echocardiographic features of 76 cases and risk factors for mortality. *Eur. Heart J.*, Vol.26, No.3, pp. 288-297, ISSN 0195-668X.

Baddour, L. M., Wilson, W. R., Bayer, A. S., Fowler, V. G., Jr., Bolger, A. F., Levison, M. E., Ferrieri, P., Gerber, M. A., Tani, L. Y., Gewitz, M. H., Tong, D. C., Steckelberg, J. M., Baltimore, R. S., Shulman, S. T., Burns, J. C., Falace, D. A., Newburger, J. W., Pallasch, T. J., Takahashi, M. & Taubert, K. A. (2005). Infective endocarditis: diagnosis, antimicrobial therapy, and management of complications: a statement for healthcare professionals from the Committee on Rheumatic Fever, Endocarditis, and Kawasaki Disease, Council on Cardiovascular Disease in the Young, and the Councils on Clinical Cardiology, Stroke, and Cardiovascular Surgery and Anesthesia, American Heart Association: endorsed by the Infectious Diseases Society of America. *Circulation*, Vol.111, No.23, pp. e394-e434, ISNN 0009-7322.

Baddour, L.M. & Wilson, L.M. (2005). Infections of prosthetic valves and other cardiovascular devices: intravascular devices, In: *Mandell, Douglas and Bennett's Principles and Practice of Infectious Diseases 5th edition*, Mandell, G.L., Bennett, J.E. & Dolin, R., pp. 1022-1044,.Elsevier, ISBN 978-0443075933, Philadelphia, USA.

Bashore, T. M., Cabell, C. & Fowler, V., Jr. (2006). Update on infective endocarditis. *Curr. Probl. Cardiol.*, Vol.31, No.4, pp. 274-352, ISSN 0146-2806.

Bayer, A. S., Bolger, A. F., Taubert, K. A., Wilson, W., Steckelberg, J., Karchmer, A. W., Levison, M., Chambers, H. F., Dajani, A. S., Gewitz, M. H., Newburger, J. W., Gerber, M. A., Shulman, S. T., Pallasch, T. J., Gage, T. W. & Ferrieri, P. 1998. Diagnosis and management of infective endocarditis and its complications. *Circulation,* Vol.98, No.25, pp. 2936-2948, ISSN 0009-7322.

Brook, I. (2008). Infective endocarditis caused by anaerobic bacteria. *Arch. Cardiovasc. Dis.*, Vol.101, No.10, pp. 665-676, ISSN 1875-2136.

Chen, X., Chen, X., Gu, F. & Xie, D. (2009). An alternative surgical approach for aortic infective endocarditis: vegetectomy. *Eur. J. Cardiothorac. Surg.*, Vol.35, No.6, pp. 1096-1098, ISSN 1010-7940.

David, T. E., Gavra, G., Feindel, C. M., Regesta, T., Armstrong, S. & Maganti, M. D. (2007). Surgical treatment of active infective endocarditis: a continued challenge. *J. Thorac. Cardiovasc. Surg.*, Vol.133, No.1, pp. 144-149, ISSN 0022-5233.

Delahaye, F., Celard, M., Roth, O. & de, G. G. (2004). Indications and optimal timing for surgery in infective endocarditis. *Heart*, Vol.90, No.6, pp. 618-620, ISSN 1366-5278.

Dominik, J. & Zacek, P. (2010). *Heart Valve Surgery*, Springer, ISBN 978-3-642-12205-7, Berlin, Germany.

d'Udekem, Y., David, T. E., Feindel, C. M., Armstrong, S. & Sun, Z. (1997). Long-term results of surgery for active infective endocarditis. *Eur. J. Cardiothorac. Surg.*, Vol.11, No.1, pp. 46-52, ISSN 1010-7940.

Durack, D. T., Lukes, A. S. & Bright, D. K. (1994). New criteria for diagnosis of infective endocarditis: utilization of specific echocardiographic findings. Duke Endocarditis Service. *Am. J. Med.*, Vol.96, No.3, pp. 200-209, ISSN 0002-9343.

Edmunds, L. H., Jr., Clark, R. E., Cohn, L. H., Grunkemeier, G. L., Miller, D. C. & Weisel, R. D. (1996). Guidelines for reporting morbidity and mortality after cardiac valvular operations. Ad Hoc Liaison Committee for Standardizing Definitions of Prosthetic Heart Valve Morbidity of The American Association for Thoracic Surgery and The Society of Thoracic Surgeons. *J. Thorac. Cardiovasc. Surg.*, Vol.112, No.3, pp. 708-711, ISSN 0022-5223.

Graupner, C., Vilacosta, I., SanRoman, J., Ronderos, R., Sarria, C., Fernandez, C., Mujica, R., Sanz, O., Sanmartin, J. V. & Pinto, A. G. (2002). Periannular extension of infective endocarditis. *J. Am. Coll. Cardiol.*, Vol.39, No.7, pp. 1204-1211, ISSN 0735-1097.

Habib, G., Hoen, B., Tornos, P., Thuny, F., Prendergast, B., Vilacosta, I., Moreillon, P., de Jesus, A. M., Thilen, U., Lekakis, J., Lengyel, M., Muller, L., Naber, C. K., Nihoyannopoulos, P., Moritz, A. & Zamorano, J. L. (2009). Guidelines on the prevention, diagnosis, and treatment of infective endocarditis (new version 2009): the Task Force on the Prevention, Diagnosis, and Treatment of Infective Endocarditis of the European Society of Cardiology (ESC). Endorsed by the European Society of Clinical Microbiology and Infectious Diseases (ESCMID) and the International Society of Chemotherapy (ISC) for Infection and Cancer. *Eur. Heart J.*, Vol.30, No.19, pp. 2369-2413, ISSN 0195-668X.

Habib, G., Thuny, F. & Avierinos, J. F. (2008). Prosthetic valve endocarditis: current approach and therapeutic options. *Prog. Cardiovasc. Dis.*, Vol.50, No.4, pp. 274-281, ISSN 0033-0620.

Haddad, S. H., Arabi, Y. M., Memish, Z. A. & Al-Shimemeri, A. A. (2004). Nosocomial infective endocarditis in critically ill patients: a report of three cases and review of the literature. *Int. J. Infect. Dis.*, Vol.8, No.4, pp. 210-216, ISSN 1201-9712.

Horstkotte, D., Follath, F., Gutschik, E., Lengyel, M., Oto, A., Pavie, A., Soler-Soler, J., Thiene, G., von, G. A., Priori, S. G., Garcia, M. A., Blanc, J. J., Budaj, A., Cowie, M., Dean, V., Deckers, J., Fernandez, B. E., Lekakis, J., Lindahl, B., Mazzotta, G., Morais, J., Oto, A., Smiseth, O. A., Lekakis, J., Vahanian, A., Delahaye, F., Parkhomenko, A., Filipatos, G., Aldershvile, J. & Vardas, P. (2004). Guidelines on prevention, diagnosis and treatment of infective endocarditis executive summary; the task force on infective endocarditis of the European society of cardiology. *Eur. Heart J.*, Vol.25, No.3, pp. 267-276, ISSN 0195-668X.

Ishikawa, S., Kawasaki, A., Neya, K., Abe, K., Suzuki, H., Koizumi, S., Shibuya, H., Horikawa, M. & Ueda, K. (2009). Surgical treatments for infective endocarditis involving valve annulus. *Ann. Thorac. Cardiovasc. Surg.*, Vol.15, No.6, pp. 378-381, ISSN 1341-1098.

Joyce, F., Tingleff, J., Aagaard, J. & Pettersson, G. (1994). The Ross operation in the treatment of native and prosthetic aortic valve endocarditis. *J. Heart Valve Dis.*, Vol.3, No.4, pp. 371-376, ISSN 0966-8519.

Kang, N., Wan, S., Ng, C. S. & Underwood, M. J. (2009). Periannular extension of infective endocarditis. *Ann. Thorac. Cardiovasc. Surg.*, Vol.15, No.2, pp. 74-81, ISSN 1341-1098.

Klieverik, L. M., Yacoub, M. H., Edwards, S., Bekkers, J. A., Roos-Hesselink, J. W., Kappetein, A. P., Takkenberg, J. J. & Bogers, A. J. (2009). Surgical treatment of active native aortic valve endocarditis with allografts and mechanical prostheses. *Ann. Thorac. Surg.*, Vol.88, No.6, pp. 1814-1821, ISSN 0003-4975.

Knosalla, C., Weng, Y., Yankah, A. C., Siniawski, H., Hofmeister, J., Hammerschmidt, R., Loebe, M. & Hetzer, R. (2000). Surgical treatment of active infective aortic valve endocarditis with associated periannular abscess--11 year results. *Eur. Heart J.*, Vol.21, No.6, pp. 490-497, ISSN 0195-668X.

Kwan-Leung, C. & Embli, J.M. (2006). *Endocarditis: diagnosis and management*, Springer, ISBN 978-1-84625-452-6, London, UK.

Li, J. S., Sexton, D. J., Mick, N., Nettles, R., Fowler, V. G., Jr., Ryan, T., Bashore, T. & Corey, G. R. (2000). Proposed modifications to the Duke criteria for the diagnosis of infective endocarditis. *Clin. Infect. Dis.*, Vol.30, No.4, pp. 633-638, ISSN 1058-4838.

Mahesh, B., Angelini, G., Caputo, M., Jin, X. Y. & Bryan, A. (2005). Prosthetic valve endocarditis. *Ann. Thorac. Surg.*, Vol.80, No.3, pp. 1151-1158, ISSN 0003-4975.

Mestres, C. A., Ginel, A., Cartana, R. & Pomar, J. L. (1993). Cryopreserved homografts in aortic and mitral prosthetic endocarditis: expanding the use of biological tissues in complex cardiac infections. *J. Heart Valve Dis.*, Vol.2, No.6, pp. 679-683, ISSN 0966-8519.

Millar, B. C. & Moore, J. E. (2004). Emerging issues in infective endocarditis. *Emerg. Infect. Dis.*, Vol.10, No.6, pp. 1110-1116, ISSN 1080-6040.

Mocchegiani, R. & Nataloni, M. (2009). Complications of infective endocarditis. *Cardiovasc. Hematol. Disord. Drug Targets*, Vol.9, No.4, pp. 240-248, ISSN 1568-0061.

Musci, M., Hubler, M., Amiri, A., Stein, J., Kosky, S., Meyer, R., Weng, Y. & Hetzer, R. (2010). Surgical treatment for active infective prosthetic valve endocarditis: 22-year single-centre experience. *Eur. J. Cardiothorac. Surg.*, Vol.38, No.5, pp. 528-538, ISSN 1010-7940.

Naber, C. K., Baddour, L. M., Giamarellos-Bourboulis, E. J., Gould, I. M., Herrmann, M., Hoen, B., Karchmer, A. W., Kobayashi, Y., Kozlov, R. S., Lew, D., Miro, J. M., Moellering, R. C., Jr., Moreillon, P., Peters, G., Rubinstein, E., Seifert, H. & Corey, G. R. (2009). Clinical consensus conference: survey on Gram-positive bloodstream infections with a focus on Staphylococcus aureus. *Clin. Infect. Dis.*, Vol.48, No.Suppl 4, pp. S260-S270, ISSN 1058-4838.

Nguyen, D. T., Delahaye, F., Obadia, J. F., Duval, X., Selton-Suty, C., Carteaux, J. P., Hoen, B. & Alla, F. (2010). Aortic valve replacement for active infective endocarditis: 5-year survival comparison of bioprostheses, homografts and mechanical prostheses. *Eur. J. Cardiothorac. Surg.*, Vol.37, No.5, pp. 1025-1032, ISSN 1010-7940.

Perrotta, S. & Lentini, S. (2010). In patients with severe active aortic valve endocarditis, is a stentless valve as good as the homograft? *Interact. Cardiovasc. Thorac. Surg.*, Vol.11, No.3, pp. 309-313, ISSN 1569-9293.

Riberi, A., Caus, T., Mesana, T., Goudard, A., Mouly, A., Habib, G. & Monties, J. R. (1997). Aortic valve or root replacement with cryopreserved homograft for active infectious endocarditis. *Cardiovasc. Surg.*, Vol.5, No.6, pp. 579-583, ISSN 0967-2109.

Sabik, J. F., Lytle, B. W., Blackstone, E. H., Marullo, A. G., Pettersson, G. B. & Cosgrove, D. M. (2002). Aortic root replacement with cryopreserved allograft for prosthetic valve endocarditis. *Ann. Thorac. Surg.*, Vol.74, No.3, pp. 650-659, ISSN 0003-4975.

Sachdev, M., Peterson, G. E. & Jollis, J. G. (2003). Imaging techniques for diagnosis of infective endocarditis. *Cardiol. Clin.*, Vol.21, No.2, pp. 185-195, ISSN 0733-8651.

Siniawski, H., Lehmkuhl, H., Weng, Y., Pasic, M., Yankah, C., Hoffmann, M., Behnke, I. & Hetzer, R. (2003). Stentless aortic valves as an alternative to homografts for valve replacement in active infective endocarditis complicated by ring abscess. *Ann. Thorac. Surg.*, Vol.75, No.3, pp. 803-808, ISSN 0003-4975.

Susak, S., Torbica, V., Velicki, L. & Golubovic, M. (2009). Rare type of quadricuspid aortic valve requiring surgical replacement. *Thorac. Cardiovasc. Surg.*, Vol.57, No.6, pp. 364-366, ISSN 0171-6425.

Towns, M. L. & Reller, L. B. (2003). Diagnostic methods. Current best practices and guidelines for isolation of bacteria and fungi in infective endocarditis. *Cardiol. Clin.*, Vol.21, No.2, pp. 197-205, ISSN 0733-8651.

Velicki, L., Nicin, S., Mihajlovic, B., Kovacevic, P., Susak, S. & Fabri, M. (2010). Cardiac myxoma: clinical presentation, surgical treatment and outcome. *J. BUON.*, Vol.15, No.1, pp. 51-55, ISSN 1107-0625.

Wang, A. & Bashore, T. (2009). *Valvular Heart Disease,* Humana Press, ISBN 978-1-58829-982-6, New York, USA

Wang, A., Athan, E., Pappas, P. A., Fowler, V. G., Jr., Olaison, L., Pare, C., Almirante, B., Munoz, P., Rizzi, M., Naber, C., Logar, M., Tattevin, P., Iarussi, D. L., Selton-Suty, C., Jones, S. B., Casabe, J., Morris, A., Corey, G. R. & Cabell, C. H. (2007). Contemporary clinical profile and outcome of prosthetic valve endocarditis. *JAMA,* Vol.297, No.12, pp. 1354-1361, ISSN 0098-7484.

Wilson, W., Taubert, K. A., Gewitz, M., Lockhart, P. B., Baddour, L. M., Levison, M., Bolger, A., Cabell, C. H., Takahashi, M., Baltimore, R. S., Newburger, J. W., Strom, B. L., Tani, L. Y., Gerber, M., Bonow, R. O., Pallasch, T., Shulman, S. T., Rowley, A. H., Burns, J. C., Ferrieri, P., Gardner, T., Goff, D. & Durack, D. T. (2008). Prevention of infective endocarditis: guidelines from the American Heart Association: a guideline from the American Heart Association Rheumatic Fever, Endocarditis and Kawasaki Disease Committee, Council on Cardiovascular Disease in the Young, and the Council on Clinical Cardiology, Council on Cardiovascular Surgery and Anesthesia, and the Quality of Care and Outcomes Research Interdisciplinary Working Group. *J. Am. Dent. Assoc.,* Vol.139, Suppl, pp. 3S-24S, ISSN 0002-8177.

5

Native and Prosthetic Aortic Valve Endocarditis

Ioan Tilea[1], Brindusa Tilea[2], Cristina Maria Tatar[1] and Mihaela Ispas[3]
[1]*Internal Medicine Clinic, Division of Cardiology, University of Medicine and Pharmacy Tirgu Mures,*
[2]*Infectious Disease Clinic, University of Medicine and Pharmacy Tirgu Mures,*
[3]*Cardiology Clinic, Institute of Cardiovascular Diseases and Transplantation Tirgu Mures, Romania*

1. Introduction

1.1 Definitions

Infective endocarditis (IE) is an endovascular, microbial infection of intracardiac structures facing the blood, including infections of the large intrathoracic vessels and of intracardiac foreign bodies. The early characteristic lesion is a variably sized vegetation, although destruction, ulceration, or abscess formation may be seen earlier by echocardiography (Habib et al, 2009).

Prosthetic valve endocarditis (PVE) is classified as early or late, depending on when infection is diagnosed: early PVE (within 12 months after surgery) and late PVE (12 months or more after surgery).

Nosocomial IE is defined as an infection occurring > 72 h after admission to the hospital or IE acquired in association with a significant invasive procedure performed during a recent hospitalization ≤ 8 weeks before the onset of symptoms.

Persistent infection is defined as a repeat episode of IE caused by the same microorganism developing < 1 year after the first episode (Hill et al, 2007).

1.2 Historical perspective

The hypothesis of the role of parasites (microorganisms) microscopically observed in vegetations and in the cardiac valves of patients with endocarditis was first put forth by Winge in Sweden in 1869. Winge's work led Klebs and Rosenbach in Germany to establish, between 1878 and 1881, an animal model of experimental endocarditis in which the aortic valves of rabbits were perforated with a metallic probe (loaded with septic material) introduced through the carotid artery. Ten years after Winge's work, Pasteur emphasized the importance of bacteriologic "blood cultures". During the period 1881-1886, Netter and Grancher (Pasteur's associates) introduced a method for drawing aseptic blood samples from patients with clinical endocarditis and doing bacteriologic blood cultures. In Vienna in 1885-1886, Orth, Weichselbaum, and Wyssokowitsch further developed Rosenbach's procedure of inducing experimental endocarditis by injecting material from a bacterial culture into a rabbit's ear vein. The development of an experimental model of endocarditis by investigators in the latter part of the nineteenth century provided anatomopathological and bacteriologic data that in turn led to a better understanding of IE (Contrepois, 1995).

1.3 Epidemiology

The epidemiological profile of IE has changed substantially over the last few years. In industrialized countries, the typical pattern of IE is now an elderly patient with a degenerative heart valve disease or with a prosthetic valve or an intracardiac device such as a pacemaker or defibrillator leads. Major changes have occurred in the mode of acquisition of IE and in its microbiological profile (Thuny et al, 2010). Significant geographical variations have been shown. The highest increase in the rate of staphylococcal IE has been reported in the USA, where chronic hemodialysis, diabetes mellitus, and intravascular devices are the three major factors associated with the development of *Staphylococcus aureus* (*S. aureus*) endocarditis. In other countries, the main predisposing factor for *S. aureus* IE may be intravenous drug abuse (Habib et al, 2009).

1.4 Incidence

The incidence of IE ranges from one country to another within 3–10 episodes/100,000 person-years. This may reflect methodological differences between surveys rather than true variation. Of note, in these surveys, the incidence of IE was very low in young patients but increased dramatically with age—the peak incidence was 14.5 episodes/100,000 person-years in patients between 70 and 80 years old.

In all epidemiological studies of IE, the male:female ratio is 2:1, although why there is a higher proportion of men is poorly understood. Furthermore, female patients may have a worse prognosis and undergo valve surgery less frequently than their male counterparts (Habib et al, 2009).

Patients with prosthetic aortic valves are reported to have an incidence of PVE of 0.3 to 1.2 episodes per 100 patients/year, and approximately 1.4% of patients undergoing aortic valve replacement develop PVE during the first postoperative year.

1.5 Types of infective endocarditis

IE should be regarded as a set of clinical situations that are sometimes very different from each other. In an attempt to avoid overlap, the following four categories of IE must be separated according to the site of infection and the presence or absence of intracardiac foreign material: left-sided native valve IE, left-sided prosthetic valve IE, right-sided IE, and device-related IE (the latter includes IE developing on pacemaker or defibrillator leads with or without associated valve involvement).

With regard to acquisition, the following situations can be identified: community-acquired IE, healthcare-associated IE (nosocomial and non-nosocomial), and IE in intravenous drug abusers (IVDAs) (Habib et al, 2009).

1.6 Microbiology

The microbiology of IE of the aortic valve depends on whether the valve is native or prosthetic, and whether the infection is hospital- or community-acquired.

According to microbiological findings, the following categories are proposed:

1. IE with positive blood cultures.
   This is the most important category, representing 85% of all IE. Causative microorganisms are most often staphylococci, streptococci, and enterococci (Murdoch et al, 2009).
   a. IE due to streptococci and enterococci.
      Oral (formerly *viridans*) streptococci form a mixed group of microorganisms, which includes species such as *S. sanguis, S. mitis, S. salivarius, S. mutans,* and *Gemella*

morbillorum. Microorganisms of this group are almost always susceptible to penicillin. Members of the *S. milleri* or *S. anginosus* group (*S. anginosus, S. intermedius,* and *S. constellatus*) must be distinguished since they tend to form abscesses and cause hematogenously disseminated infections, that often require a longer duration of antibiotic treatment. Likewise, nutritionally variant "defective" streptococci, recently reclassified into other species (*Abiotrophia* and *Granulicatella*), should also be distinguished since they are often tolerant to penicillin [minimal bactericidal concentration (MBC) much higher than the minimal inhibitory concentration (MIC)]. Group D streptococci form the *Streptococcus bovis/ Streptococcus equinus* complex, including commensal species of the human intestinal tract, and were until recently gathered under the name of *Streptococcus bovis*. They, like oral streptococci, are usually sensitive to penicillin. Among enterococci, *E. faecalis, E. faecium*, and, to a lesser extent, *E. durans*, are the three species that cause IE.

b. Staphylococcal IE.
Traditionally, native valve staphylococcal IE is due to *S. aureus*, which is most often susceptible to oxacillin, at least in community-acquired IE. In contrast, staphylococcal prosthetic valve IE is more frequently due to coagulase-negative staphylococci (CNS) with oxacillin resistance. However, in a recent study of 1779 cases of IE collected prospectively in 16 countries, *S. aureus* was the most frequent cause, not only of IE, but also of prosthetic valve IE (Fowler et al, 2005). Conversely, CNS can also cause native valve IE (Chu et al, 2004, 2008) especially *S. lugdunensis*, which frequently has an aggressive clinical course.

2. IE with negative blood cultures because of prior antibiotic treatment.
This situation arises in patients who received antibiotics for unexplained fever before any blood cultures were done and in whom the diagnosis of IE was not considered; usually the diagnosis is eventually considered in the face of relapsing febrile episodes following antibiotic discontinuation. Blood cultures may remain negative for many days after antibiotic cesation, and causative organisms are most often oral streptococci or CNS.
3. IE frequently associated with negative blood cultures.
They are usually due to fastidious organisms such as nutritionally variant streptococci, fastidious Gram-negative bacilli of the HACEK group (*H. parainfluenzae, H. aphrophilus, H. paraphrophilus, H. influenzae, Actinobacillus actinomycetemcomitans, Cardiobacterium hominis, Eikenella corrodens, Kingella kingae,* and *K. denitrificans*), *Brucella*, and fungi.
4. IE associated with constantly negative blood cultures.
They are caused by intracellular bacteria such as *Coxiella burnetii, Bartonella, Chlamydia,* and, as recently demonstrated, *Tropheryma whipplei*, the agent of Whipple's disease (Richardson et al, 2003). Overall, these account for up to 5% of all IE. Diagnosis in such cases relies on serological testing, cell culture, or gene amplification (Habib et al, 2009).

1.7 Pathophysiology

Healthy valve endothelium is resistant to colonization and infection by circulating bacteria. However, mechanical disruption of the endothelium results in the exposure of underlying extracellular matrix proteins, the production of tissue factor, and the deposition of fibrin and platelets as a normal healing process. Such nonbacterial thrombotic endocarditis (NBTE) facilitates bacterial adherence and infection (Prendergast, 2006).

Endothelial damage may result from mechanical lesions induced by turbulent blood flow, electrodes or catheters, inflammation, as in rheumatic carditis, or, in the elderly, degenerative changes associated with inflammation, micro-ulcers, and microthrombi.
Endothelial inflammation without valve lesions may also promote IE. Local inflammation triggers endothelial cells to express integrins of the b1 family (very late antigen). Integrins are transmembrane proteins that can connect extracellular determinants to the cellular cytoskeleton. Integrins of the b1 family bind circulating fibronectin to the endothelial surface while *S. aureus* and some other IE pathogens carry fibronectin-binding proteins on their surface. Hence, when activated endothelial cells bind fibronectin, they provide an adhesive surface for circulating staphylococci. Once adherent, *S. aureus* trigger their active internalization into valve endothelial cells, where they can either persist and escape host defenses and antibiotics, or multiply and spread to distant organs. Thus, there are at least two scenarios for primary valve infection: one involving a physically damaged endothelium, favoring infection by most types of organism, and one occurring on physically undamaged endothelium, promoting IE due to *S. aureus* and other potential intracellular pathogens.
The role of bacteremia has been studied in animals with catheter-induced NBTE. Both the magnitude of bacteremia and the ability of the pathogen to attach to damaged valves are important. Of note, bacteremia does not occur only after invasive procedures, but also as a consequence of chewing and tooth brushing. Such spontaneous bacteremia is low-grade and of short duration.
Classical IE pathogens (*S. aureus*, *Streptococcus spp.*, and *Enterococcus spp.*) share the ability to adhere to damaged valves, trigger local procoagulant activity, and nurture infected vegetations in which they can survive. They are equipped with numerous surface determinants that mediate adherence to host matrix molecules present on damaged valves (e.g. fibrinogen, fibronectin, platelet proteins) and trigger platelet activation. Following colonization, adherent bacteria must escape host defenses.
Gram-positive bacteria are resistant to complement. However, they may be the target of platelet microbicidal proteins (PMPs), which are produced by activated platelets and kill microbes by disturbing their plasma membrane. Bacteria recovered from patients with IE are consistently resistant to PMP-induced killing, whereas similar bacteria recovered from patients with other types of infection are susceptible. Thus, escaping PMP-induced killing is a typical characteristic of IE-causing pathogens (Habib et al, 2009).

2. Diagnosis

The diagnosis of IE remains a continuous challenge. It must be suspected in the presence of a new regurgitant heart murmur, embolic events of unknown origin, sepsis of unknown cause, and fever. IE should be suspected if fever is associated with intracardiac prosthetic material, a previous history of IE, previous valvular or congenital heart disease, and other predisposition or conditions for IE (immunocompromised state, evidence of congestive heart failure, conduction disturbance, vascular or immunologic phenomena, unexplained focal or non-specific neurological symptoms and signs, etc.). Echocardiography (transthoracic, transesophageal) and microbiological diagnosis confirm the diagnosis.
When diagnosing IE, molecular biology techniques such as PCR are rapid and reliably detect fastidious and nonculturable agents in patients, but they have inherent limitations, such as they cannot be reliably applied to whole blood samples, they risk contamination,

they yield false-negatives because of PCR inhibitors in clinical samples, they are unable to provide information about bacterial sensitivity to antimicrobial agents, and they are persistently positive despite clinical remission.

The variability in the clinical presentation of IE requires a diagnostic strategy that is both sensitive for disease detection and specific for its exclusion across all forms of the disease. In 1994, a diagnostic schema, termed the Duke criteria, was proposed. It stratified patients with suspected IE into 3 categories: "definite" cases, identified either clinically or pathologically (IE proved at surgery or autopsy); "possible" cases (not meeting the criteria for definite IE); and "rejected" cases (no pathological evidence of IE at autopsy or surgery, rapid resolution of the clinical syndrome with either no treatment or short-term antibiotic therapy, or a firm alternative diagnosis) (Durack et al, 1994; Baddour et al, 2005).

The revised Duke Clinical Diagnostic Criteria for IE were published in 2000, and included the following changes: the category "possible IE" was defined as having at least 1 major criterion and 1 minor criterion or 3 minor criteria; the minor criterion "echocardiogram consistent with IE but not meeting major criterion" was eliminated, given the widespread use of transesophageal echocardiography (TEE); bacteremia because of *S. aureus* was considered a major criterion, regardless of whether the infection was nosocomially acquired or whether a removable source of infection was present; and positive Q-fever serology was changed to a major criterion (Li et al, 2000).

Major Criteria
Two positive blood cultures for organisms typical of endocarditis
Three positive blood cultures for organisms consistent with endocarditis
Serologic evidence of *Coxiella burnetii*
Echocardiographic evidence of endocardial involvement: oscillating intracardiac mass on a heart valve, on supporting structures, in the path of regurgitant jets, or on implanted material without another anatomic explanation, cardiac abscess, new dehiscence of prosthetic valve, new valvular regurgitation
Minor Criteria
Predisposing heart disorder, intravenous drug abuse, fever ≥ 38°C
Vascular phenomena: arterial embolism, septic pulmonary embolism, mycotic aneurysm, intracranial hemorrhage, conjunctival petechiae, Janeway lesions
Immunologic phenomena: glomerulonephritis, Osler's nodes, Roth's spots, rheumatoid factor
Microbiologic evidence of infection consistent with but not meeting major criteria
Serologic evidence of infection with organisms consistent with endocarditis
For definite clinical diagnosis: 2 major criteria or 1 major criterion and 3 minor criteria or 5 minor criteria
For possible clinical diagnosis: 1 major criterion and 1 minor criterion or 3 minor criteria.
For rejection of diagnosis: Firm alternative diagnosis explaining the findings of IE, resolution of symptoms and signs after antimicrobial therapy for ≤ 4 days, no pathologic evidence of infective endocarditis found during surgery or autopsy, or failure to meet the clinical criteria for possible endocarditis

Table 1. Revised Duke Clinical Diagnostic Criteria for IE (Adapted from Li et al, 2000)

2.1 Clinical features

Symptoms and signs of IE are nonspecific: fever (94%), malaise (81%), fatigue (66%), loss of appetite (52%), dyspnoea (50%), cough (45%), sweating (37%), chills (37%), weight loss (35%), myalgia/arthralgia (25%), back pain (9%), vascular phenomena (53%), and splenomegaly (31%). Cardiac symptoms or signs (that is, new or altered cardiac murmur, heart failure) are recorded in half of the patients. In 36% of the episodes, neurological signs are present. They are more common in patients over 55 years old. Intracranial hemorrhages occur in 2%. Splenomegaly is found less often in patients over 55 years old than in younger patients. Most patients developed hematuria (79%) or anaemia (91%). Patients with anemia are more prone to malaise and loss of appetite. Anaemia occurs more often in patients with vegetations (Netzer et al, 2000).

2.2 Microbiological diagnosis

2.2.1 Blood cultures

Positive blood cultures remain the cornerstones of diagnosis and provide live bacteria for susceptibility testing. Three sets (including at least one aerobic and one anaerobic), each containing 10 ml of blood obtained from a peripheral vein using a meticulously sterile technique, is virtually always sufficient to identify the usual microorganisms—the diagnostic yield of repeated sampling thereafter is low. Sampling from central venous catheters should be avoided in view of the high risk of contaminants (false-positives, typically staphylococcal) and misleading findings (Habib et al, 2009). Although infective endocarditis secondary to anaerobic infection is uncommon, cultures should be sent for both aerobic and anaerobic incubation. No evidence suggests that cultures should be taken coincident with peaks of temperature, as bacteremia is constant (Beynon et al, 2006).

2.2.2 Culture-negative infective endocarditis and atypical organisms

Blood-culture negative IE (BCNIE) occurs in 2.5-31% of all cases of IE, often delaying diagnosis and the initiation of treatment, with profound impact on clinical outcome. BCNIE arises most commonly as a consequence of prior antibiotic administration, underlying the need for withdrawing antibiotics and repeating blood cultures in this situation. An increasingly common scenario is infection by fastidious organisms (including *Legionella*, *Coxiella*, the HACEK group and fungi such as *Candida*, *Histoplasma*, and *Aspergillus* species) with limited proliferation under conventional culture conditions, or requiring specialized tools for identification. These organisms may be particularly common in IE and affect patients with prosthetic valves, indwelling venous lines, pacemakers, renal failure, and immunocompromised states.

2.2.3 Histological/immunological techniques

Pathological examination of resected valvular tissue or embolic fragments remains the gold standard for diagnosing IE and may also guide antimicrobial treatment if the causative agent can be identified using special stains or immunohistological techniques. Electron microscopy is highly sensitive and may help characterize new microorganisms, but it is time consuming and expensive. *Coxiella burnetii* and *Bartonella* species may be easily detected using serological testing with indirect immunofluorescence or an enzyme-linked immunosorbent assay (ELISA), and recent data (Watkin et al, 2006) demonstrate similar utility for staphylococci. An immunological analysis of urine may allow the detection of microorganism degradation products, and ELISA detection of *Legionella* species has been described (Helbig et al, 2001). Incorporating these methods into accepted diagnostic criteria awaits prospective validation.

2.2.4 Molecular biology techniques

The polymerase chain reaction (PCR) allows rapid and reliable detection of fastidious and nonculturable agents in patients with IE.

PCR uses nucleic acid target or signal amplification, alone or in combination with sequence analysis. The technique is particularly useful when negative cultures are caused by previous administration of antibiotics (as the technique is culture independent) or the presence of a fastidious organism and to identify the culprit organism in polymicrobial infection (Beynon et al, 2006).

2.3 Echocardiography

Echocardiography plays a key role in IE, concerning its diagnosis, the diagnosis of its complications, its follow-up under therapy and prognostic assessment. Echocardiography is particularly useful for the initial assessment of embolic risk and in decision-making in IE.

Transesophageal echocardiography (TEE) plays a major role both before surgery and during surgery (intraoperative echocardiography).

Echocardiographic results must be taken into consideration for both the decision to operate or not and the choice of the optimal timing for surgery. In all cases, however, the results of echocardiographic studies may be interpreted taking into account the clinical features of the patient (Habib et al, 2010).

2.3.1 Transthoracic echocardiography

Transthoracic echocardiography (TTE) is the initial technique of choice for investigating IE. In low-risk patients, a normal transthoracic echocardiogram provides confirmation that endocarditis is unlikely and suggests that investigations should be directed elsewhere (Beynon et al, 2006). If the clinical suspicion is high, TEE should be used.

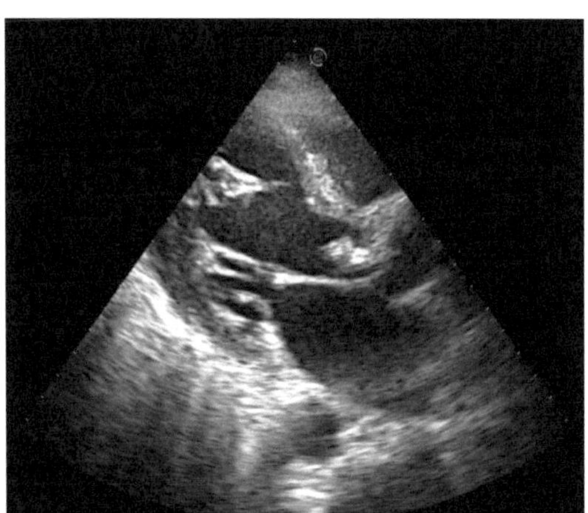

Fig. 1. Parasternal long axis view from TTE of a native aortic valve vegetation with aortic valve rupture

The sensitivity of TTE ranges from 40% to 63%. There is no better technique for noninvasive visualization of vegetations than echocardiography. Overall, the TTE detection rate for vegetations in patients with a clinical suspicion of endocarditis averages around 50%. The diagnostic yield of the technique in detecting vegetations is influenced by several factors: image quality; echogenicity and vegetation size; vegetation location; presence of previous valvular disease or valvular prosthesis; experience and skill of the examiner; and pretest probability of endocarditis (Evangelista & Gonzalez-Alujas, 2004).

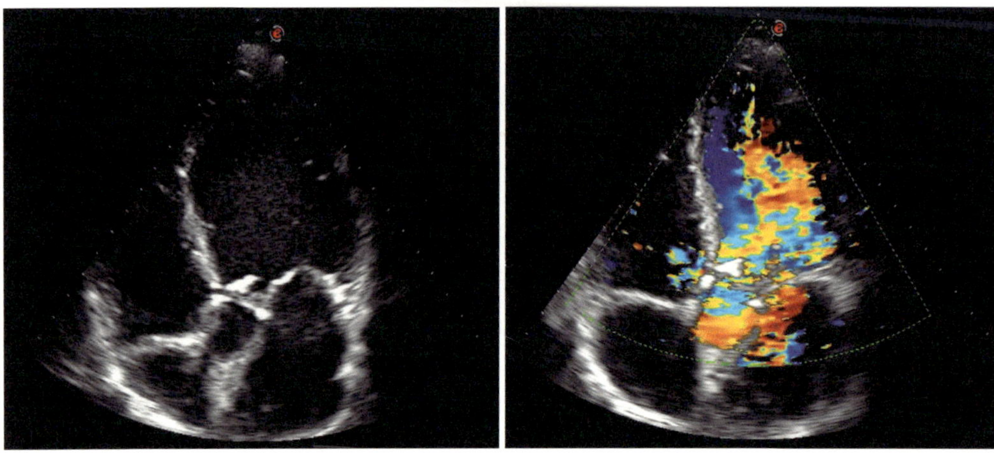

Fig. 2. Native aortic valve vegetation (left TTE and right color Doppler ultrasound)

2.3.2 Transesophageal echocardiography

In most cases, TTE is sufficient. TEE is indicated when mechanical prosthetic valves are present, to detect right-sided lesions and to visualize myocardial abscesses. TEE may be considered an invasive procedure, but it is only modestly uncomfortable to the patient, can be rapidly done, and is low-risk. It is more sensitive than conventional TTE for detecting valvular vegetations. Furthermore, it may detect an unsuspected paravalvular abscess, and it correlates well with surgical and pathologic findings. The sensitivity of TEE ranges from 90% to 100%.

In high-risk groups, TEE, with its higher sensitivity and specificity, may be needed if the TTE is normal and suspicion of IE remains high. TEE is also used to investigate potential complications of IE (Beynon et al, 2006). TEE is particularly useful in patients with prosthetic valves and for evaluating myocardial invasion. Negative TEE has a negative predictive value of over 92% for IE (Mylonakis & Calderwood, 2001).

2.4 Other imaging technologies

Other advances in imaging technology have had minimal impact in routine clinical practice. Using harmonic imaging has improved study quality, while three-dimensional echocardiography and other alternative modes of imaging— computed tomography (CT), magnetic resonance imaging (MRI), positron emission tomography (PET), and radionuclide scanning— have yet to be evaluated in IE. Multislice CT has recently been shown to give better results than does TEE when evaluating IE-associated valvular abnormalities, particularly when assessing the perivalvular extent of abscesses and pseudoaneurysms (Habib et al, 2009).

2.5 Other tests

Blood and urine studies: Complete blood count (CBC), electrolytes, creatinine, blood urea nitrogen (BUN), glucose, and coagulation panel. Erythrocyte sedimentation rate (ESR), while not specific, is elevated in more than 90% of cases. Proteinuria and microscopic hematuria are present in approximately 50% of cases.

Chest X-ray: This has a limited value, although it may demonstrate signs of congestive heart failure. Multiple embolic pyogenic abscesses may be visualized.

Electrocardiography: This may help detect the 10% of patients who develop a conduction delay during IE by documenting an increased P-R interval. Nonspecific changes are common. A first-degree atrioventricular (AV) block and new interventricular conduction delays may signal septal involvement in aortic valve disease; both are poor prognostic signs.

Coronary angiography: This is recommended pre-surgery according to the ESC Guidelines on the Management of Valvular Heart Disease in men over 40 years, in post-menopausal women, and in patients with at least one cardiovascular risk factor or a history of coronary artery disease. Exceptions arise when there are large aortic vegetations that may be dislodged during catheterization, or when emergency surgery is necessary. In these situations, high-resolution CT may be used to rule out significant coronary artery disease.

3. Treatment

The major goals of therapy for IE are to eradicate the infectious agent from the thrombus and to address the complications of valvular infection. The latter includes both the intracardiac and extracardiac consequences of IE. Some of the effects of IE require surgical intervention.

3.1 Medical treatment

Successful treatment of IE relies on microbe eradication by antimicrobial drugs. Surgery contributes by removing infected material and draining abscesses. Host defenses are of little help. This explains why bactericidal regimens are more effective than bacteriostatic therapy, both in animal experiments and in humans.

Aminoglycosides synergize with cell wall inhibitors (i.e. b-lactams and glycopeptides) for bactericidal activity and are useful for shortening the duration of therapy (e.g. oral streptococci) and eradicate problematic organisms (e.g. *Enterococcus spp.*).

One major hindrance to drug-induced killing is bacterial antibiotic tolerance. Tolerant microbes are not resistant, i.e. they are still susceptible to growth inhibition by the drug, but escape drug-induced killing and may resume growth after treatment discontinuation.

Slow-growing and dormant microbes display phenotypic tolerance towards most antimicrobials (except rifampin to some extent). They are present in vegetations and biofilms, e.g. in PVE, and justify the need for prolonged therapy (6 weeks) to sterilize infected heart valves fully.

Some bacteria carry mutations rendering them tolerant during both active growth and stationary (dormant) phases. Bactericidal drug combinations are preferred to monotherapy against tolerant organisms.

Drug treatment for PVE should last longer (at least 6 weeks) than that for native-valve endocarditis (NVE) (2–6 weeks), but is otherwise similar, except for staphylococcal PVE, for which the regimen should include rifampin whenever the strain is susceptible.

In NVE needing a valve to be replaced by a prosthesis during antibiotic therapy, the postoperative antibiotic regimen should be that recommended for NVE, not for PVE. In both NVE and PVE, the duration of treatment is based on the first day of effective antibiotic therapy, not on the day of surgery.
After surgery, a new full course of treatment should start only if valve cultures are positive, and the choice of antibiotic should be based on the susceptibility of the latest recovered bacterial isolate (Habib et al, 2009).

3.1.1 Empirical therapy

IE treatment should be promptly started. The initial choice of empirical treatment depends on several considerations:

- whether the patient has received prior antibiotic therapy or not
- whether the infection affects a native valve or a prosthesis and, if so, when surgery occurred (early vs. late PVE)
- knowledge of local epidemiology, especially for antibiotic resistance and specific genuine culture-negative pathogens.

NVE and late PVE regimens should cover staphylococci, streptococci, HACEK species, and *Bartonella spp.* Early PVE regimens should cover methicillin-resistant staphylococci and, ideally, non-HACEK Gram-negative pathogens (Habib et al, 2009).

Antibiotic	Dosage and route	Duration (weeks)	Level of evidence	Comments
Native valves				
Ampicillin-sulbactam,	12 g/day i.v. in 4 doses	4-6	II C	Patients with BCNIE should be treated in consultation with an infectious disease specialist.
or Amoxicillin-clavulanate, with	12 g/day i.v. in 4 doses	4-6	II C	
Gentamicin	3 mg/kg/day i.v. or i.m. in 2 or 3 doses	4-6		
Vancomycin with	30 mg/kg/day i.v. in 2 doses	4-6	II C	For patients unable to tolerate β-lactams
Gentamicin with	3 mg/kg/day i.v. or i.m. in 2 or 3 doses	4-6		Ciprofloxacin is not uniformly active on *Bartonella spp.* Adding doxycycline is an option if *Bartonella spp.* is likely.
Ciprofloxacin	1000 mg/day orally in 2 doses or 800 mg/day i.v. in 2 doses	4-6		
Prosthetic valves (early, < 12 months post-surgery)				
Vancomycin with	30 mg/kg/day i.v. in 2 doses	6	II C	If no clinical response, surgery and maybe extending the antibiotic spectrum to Gram-negative pathogens must be considered.
Gentamicin with	3 mg/kg/day i.v. or i.m. in 2 or 3 doses	2		
Rifampin	1200 mg/day orally in 2 doses			
Prosthetic valves (late, ≥ 12 months post-surgery)				
Same as for native valves				

Table 2. Proposed antibiotic regimens for initial empirical treatment of IE (before or without pathogen identification) (Adapted from Habib et al, 2009)

3.1.2 Penicillin-susceptible oral streptococci and group D streptococci

The cure rate is expected to be > 95%. In uncomplicated cases, short-term (2-week) therapy can be administered by combining penicillin or ceftriaxone with gentamicin or netilmicin. Ceftriaxone alone or combined with gentamicin or netilmicin given once a day is particularly convenient for outpatient therapy. Patients allergic to b-lactams should receive vancomycin. Teicoplanin has been proposed as an alternative and requires loading doses (6 mg/kg/12 h for 3 days) followed by 6–10 mg/kg/day. Loading is critical because the drug is highly bound to serum proteins and penetrates slowly into vegetations.

3.1.3 Penicillin-resistant oral streptococci and group D streptococci

Such resistant streptococci are increasing. Antibiotic therapy for penicillin-resistant and penicillin-susceptible oral streptococci is qualitatively similar. However, in penicillin-resistant cases, aminoglycoside treatment may be prolonged to 3–4 weeks, and short-term therapy regimens are not recommended. Little experience exists with highly resistant isolates (MIC > 4 mg/L)—vancomycin might be preferred in such circumstances.

3.1.4 *Streptococcus pneumoniae*, b-hemolytic streptococci (groups A, B, C, and G)

IE due to *S. pneumoniae* has become rare since the introduction of antibiotics. It is associated with meningitis in up to 30% of cases, which requires special consideration in penicillin-resistant cases. Treatment is similar to that of oral streptococci, except for the use of short-term (2-week) therapy, which has not been formally investigated. In cases with meningitis, penicillin must be avoided because it poorly penetrates the cerebrospinal fluid, and should be replaced with ceftriaxone or cefotaxime alone or cefotaxime combined with vancomycin.
IE due to group A, B, C, or G streptococci—including the *S. milleri* group (*S. constellatus, S. anginosus,* and *S. intermedius*)—is relatively rare. Group A streptococci are uniformly susceptible to b-lactams, whereas other serogroups may display resistance. IE due to group B streptococci was once associated with the peripartum period, but now occurs in adults, especially the elderly. Group B, C, and G streptococci and *S. milleri* produce abscesses and thus may require adjunctive surgery. The mortality of group B PVE is very high, and cardiac surgery is recommended. Antibiotic treatment is similar to that of oral streptococci, except that short-term therapy is not recommended.

3.1.5 Nutritionally variant streptococci

Nutritionally variant streptococci produce IE with a protracted course, which is associated with higher rates of complications and treatment failure (up to 40%), possibly due to delayed diagnosis and treatment. Antibiotic recommendations include penicillin, ceftriaxone, or vancomycin for 6 weeks, combined with an aminoglycoside for at least the first 2 weeks.

3.1.6 *S. aureus* and coagulase-negative staphylococci

S. aureus is usually responsible for acute and destructive IE, whereas CNS produce more protracted valve infections (except *S. lugdunensis* and some cases of *S. capitis*). *S. aureus* PVE carries a very high risk of mortality (> 45%) and often requires early valve replacement. Other differences in comparison with NVE include the overall duration of therapy, prolonged additional use of aminoglycosides, and the addition of rifampin. Although the level of evidence is poor, adding rifampin in the treatment of staphylococcal PVE is standard practice, although treatment may be associated with microbial resistance, hepatotoxicity, and drug interactions.

Antibiotic	Dosage and route	Duration (weeks)	Level of evidence
Native valves			
Methicillin-susceptible staphylococci			
Flucloxacillin or Oxacillin with Gentamicin	12 g/day i.v. in 4-6 doses 3 mg/kg/day i.v. or i.m. in 2 or 3 doses Pediatric doses: Oxacillin or flucloxacillin 200 mg/kg/day i.v. in 4-6 equally divided doses. Gentamicin 3 mg/kg/day i.v. or. i.m. in 3 equally divided doses.	4– 6 3– 5 days	I B
Penicillin-allergic patients or methicillin-resistant staphylococci			
Vancomycin with Gentamicin	30 mg/kg/day i.v. in 2 doses 3 mg/kg/day i.v. or i.m. in 2 or 3 doses Pediatric doses: Vancomycin 40 mg/kg/day i.v. in 2-3 equally divided doses.	4– 6 3– 5 days	I B
Prosthetic valves			
Methicillin-susceptible staphylococci:			
Flucloxacillin, or Oxacillin with Rifampin and Gentamicin	12 g/day i.v. in 4-6 doses 1200 mg/day i.v. orally in 2 doses 3 mg/kg/day i.v. in 2 or 3 doses Pediatric doses: Oxacillin and flucloxacillin as above. Rifampin 20 mg/kg/day i.v. or orally in 3 equally divided doses.	≥ 6 ≥ 6 2	I B
Penicillin-allergic patients and methicillin-resistant staphylococci:			
Vancomycin with Rifampin and Gentamicin	30 mg/kg/day i.v. in 2 doses 1200 mg/day i.v. or orally in 2 doses 3 mg/kg/day i.v. or i.m. in 2 or 3 doses Pediatric doses: As above.	≥ 6 ≥ 6 2	I B

Table 3. Antibiotic treatment of IE due to *Staphylococcus spp.* (Habib et al, 2009)

3.1.7 Methicillin-resistant and vancomycin-resistant staphylococci

MRSA produce low-affinity plasma-binding protein (PBP) 2A, which confers cross-resistance to most b-lactams. They are usually resistant to multiple antibiotics, leaving only vancomycin to treat severe infections. However, vancomycin-intermediate *S. aureus* (VISA) (MIC 4–16 mg/L) and hetero-VISA (MIC ≤ 2 mg/L, but with subpopulations growing at higher concentrations) have emerged worldwide, and are associated with IE treatment failures (Howden et al, 2006). Moreover, some highly vancomycin-resistant *S. aureus* have been isolated from infected patients in recent years, requiring new approaches to treatment. New lipopeptide daptomycin (6 mg/kg/day i.v.) was recently approved for *S. aureus* bacteremia and right-sided IE (Fowler et al, 2006). Observational studies suggest that daptomycin might also be considered in left-sided IE and may overcome methicillin and vancomycin resistance (Levine & Lamp, 2007). Importantly, daptomycin needs to be administered in appropriate doses to avoid further resistance. Other choices include newer b-lactams with relatively good PBP2A affinity, quinupristin-dalfopristin with or without b-lactams, b-lactams plus oxazolidinones, and b-lactams plus vancomycin. Such cases warrant collaborative management with an infectious diseases specialist.

3.1.8 *Enterococcus spp.*

Enterococcal IE is primarily caused by *E. faecalis* (90% of cases) and, more rarely, by *E. faecium* or other species. They pose two major problems. First, enterococci are highly tolerant to antibiotic-induced killing, and eradication requires prolonged administration (up to 6 weeks) of synergistic bactericidal combinations of cell-wall inhibitors with aminoglycosides. Secondly, they may be resistant to multiple drugs, including aminoglycosides, b-lactams (via PBP5 modification and sometimes b-lactamases), and vancomycin. Fully penicillin-susceptible strains (penicillin MIC ≤ 8 mg/L) are treated with penicillin or ampicillin (or amoxicillin) combined with gentamicin. Ampicillin (or amoxicillin) might be preferred since MICs are 2–4 times lower. Prolonged courses of gentamicin require regular monitoring of serum drug levels and renal and vestibular function. One study reported success with short-course administration of aminoglycosides (2–3 weeks) in 74 (81%) of 91 episodes of enterococcal IE (Olaison & Schadewitz, 2002). This option might be considered in cases where prolonged treatment is limited by toxicity.

High-level gentamicin resistance is frequent in both *E. faecalis* and *E. faecium*. An aminoglycoside MIC > 500 mg/L is associated with the loss of bactericidal synergism with cell-wall inhibitors, and aminoglycosides should not be used in such conditions. Streptomycin may remain active in such cases and is a useful alternative. An additional recently described (Gavalda et al, 2007) option against gentamicin-resistant *E. faecalis* is the combination of ampicillin and ceftriaxone, which synergize by inhibiting complementary PBPs. Otherwise, more prolonged courses of b-lactams or vancomycin should be considered. B-Lactam and vancomycin resistance are observed primarily in *E. faecium*. Since dual resistance is rare, b-lactam might be used against vancomycin-resistant strains, and vice versa. Varying results have been reported with quinupristin–dalfopristin, linezolid, daptomycin, and tigecycline. Again, these situations require the expertise of an infectious diseases specialist.

3.1.9 Gram-negative bacteria

HACEK-related species: HACEK Gram-negative bacilli are fastidious organisms needing specialized investigations. Because they grow slowly, standard MIC tests may be difficult to

Pathogens	Proposed therapy	Treatment outcome
Brucella spp.	Doxycycline (200 mg/24 h) plus cotrimoxazole (960 mg/12 h) plus rifampin (300-600 mg/24 h) for ≥ 3 months orally (Adding streptomycin (15 mg/kg/24 h in two doses) for the first few weeks is optional)	Treatment success defined as an antibody titer < 1:60
Coxiella burnetii **(agent of Q fever)**	Doxycycline (200 mg/24 h) plus hydroxychloroquine (200-600 mg/24 h) orally or Doxycycline (200 mg/24 h) plus quinolone (ofloxacin, 400 mg/24 h) orally (>18 months treatment) Doxycycline plus hydroxychloroquine (with monitoring of serum hydroxychloroquine levels) is superior to doxycycline alone and to doxycycline + fluoroquinolone	Treatment success defined as anti-phase I IgG titer < 1:200, and IgM titers < 1:50
Bartonella spp.	Ceftriaxone (2 g/24 h) or ampicillin (or amoxicillin) (12 g/24 h) i.v. or Doxycycline (200 mg/24 h) orally for 6 weeks plus Gentamicin (3 mg/24 h) or netilmicin i.v. (for 3 weeks)	Treatment success expected in ≥ 90%
Legionella spp.	Erythromycin (3g/24h) i.v. for 2 weeks, then orally for 4 weeks plus Rifampin (300-1200 mg/24h) or Ciprofloxacin (1.5 g/24 h) orally for 6 weeks	Optimal treatment unknown. Because of high susceptibility, quinolones should probably be included.
Mycoplasma spp.	Newer fluoroquinolones (> 6 months treatment) Newer fluoroquinolones are more potent than ciprofloxacin against intracellular pathogens such as *Mycoplasma spp.*, *Legionella spp.*, and *Chlamydia spp.*	Optimal treatment unknown.
Tropheryma whipplei **(agent of Whipple's disease**	Cotrimoxazole Penicillin (1.2 MU/24 h) and streptomycin (1 g/24 h) i.v. for 2 weeks, then Cotrimoxazole orally for 1 year or Doxycycline (200 mg/24 h) plus Hydroxychloroquine (200-600 mg/24 h) orally for ≥ 18 months	Long-term treatment, optimal duration unknown.

Table 4. Antibiotic treatment of BCNIE. (Adapted from Brouqui & Raoult, 2001)

interpret. Some HACEK group bacilli produce b-lactamases, and ampicillin is therefore no longer the first-line option. Conversely, they are susceptible to ceftriaxone, other third-generation cephalosporins, and quinolones—the standard treatment is ceftriaxone 2 g/day for 4 weeks. If they do not produce b-lactamase, intravenous ampicillin (12 g/day i.v. in four or six doses) plus gentamicin (3 mg/kg/day in two or three doses) for 4 weeks is an option. Ciprofloxacin (2 x 400 mg/day i.v. or 1000 mg/day orally) is a less well-validated option (Das et al, 1997).

Non-HACEK species: Recommended treatment is early surgery plus long-term (≥ 6 weeks) therapy with bactericidal combinations of b-lactams and aminoglycosides, sometimes with additional quinolones or cotrimoxazole. *In vitro* bactericidal tests and monitoring serum antibiotic concentrations may be helpful. Because of their rarity and severity, these conditions should be managed with the input of an infectious diseases specialist (Habib et al, 2009).

3.1.10 Blood culture-negative IE

Due to the lack of large series, the optimal duration of the treatment of IE due to these pathogens is unknown. The presented durations are based on selected case reports.

Treating Whipple IE remains highly empirical. Successes have been reported with long-term (> 1 year) cotrimoxazole therapy. γ-Interferon is protective in intracellular infections and has been proposed as adjuvant therapy in Whipple's disease.

3.1.11 Fungi

Fungi are most frequently observed in PVE and in IE affecting IVDAs and immunocompromised patients. *Candida* and *Aspergillus spp.* predominate, the latter resulting in BCNIE. Mortality is very high (> 50%), and treatment necessitates dual antifungal administration and valve replacement. Most cases are treated with various forms of amphotericin B with or without azoles, although recent case reports describe successful therapy with the new echinocandin caspofungin (Garzoni et al, 2007; Lye et al, 2005). Suppressive treatment with oral azoles is often maintained long term and sometimes for life.

3.2 Surgical treatment

Surgery has an established role in the management of IE across a wide range of patients, a role that appears poised to increase as the complexity of patients with this difficult condition rises and the benefits of earlier surgery emerge.

Contemporary data in Europe indicate that surgical treatment is used in approximately half of patients with IE because of severe complications. Reasons to consider early surgery in the active phase, i.e. while the patient is still receiving antibiotic treatment, are to avoid progressive heart failure (HF) and irreversible structural damage caused by severe infection and to prevent systemic embolisms. On the other hand, surgical therapy during the active phase of the disease is associated with significant risk.

Surgery performed very early may improve survival in patients with the most severely complicated IE. However, a greater risk of relapses and postoperative valvular dysfunctions should be expected with very early surgery (Thuny et al, 2009).

3.2.1 Indications for surgery in IE

- **Congestive HF**: Congestive HF caused by severe aortic regurgitation or, more rarely, by valve obstruction caused by vegetations, severe acute aortic regurgitation with echocardiographic signs of elevated left ventricular end-diastolic pressure or significant pulmonary hypertension, congestive HF as a result of prosthetic dehiscence or obstruction;

- **Periannular extension**: Most patients with abscess formation or fistulous tract formation;
- **Systemic embolism**: Recurrent emboli despite appropriate antibiotic therapy, large vegetations (> 10 mm) after 1 or more clinical or silent embolic events after the initiation of antibiotic therapy, large vegetations and other predictors of a complicated course, very large vegetations (> 15 mm) without embolic complications, especially if valve-sparing surgery is likely (remains controversial);
- **Cerebrovascular complications**: Silent neurological complication or transient ischemic attack and other surgical indications, ischemic stroke and other surgical indications, provided that cerebral hemorrhage has been excluded and neurological complications are not severe (e.g. coma);
- **Persistent sepsis:** Fever or positive blood cultures persisting for > 5 to 7 days despite an appropriate antibiotic regimen, assuming that vegetations or other lesions requiring surgery persist and that extracardiac sources of sepsis have been excluded;
- **Relapsing IE:** Especially when caused by organisms other than sensitive streptococci or in patients with prosthetic valves;
- **Difficult organisms:** *S. aureus* IE involving a prosthetic valve and most cases involving a left-sided native valve, IE caused by other aggressive organisms (*Brucella*, *Staphylococcus lugdunensis*), IE caused by multiresistant organisms (e.g. methicillin-resistant *S. aureus* or vancomycin-resistant enterococci) and rare infections caused by Gram-negative bacteria, *Pseudomonas aeruginosa* IE, fungal IE, Q fever IE, and other relative indications for intervention;
- **PVE**: Virtually all cases of early PVE, virtually all cases of PVE caused by *S. aureus*, late PVE with HF caused by prosthetic dehiscence or obstruction (Prendergast & Tornos, 2010).

The three main indications for early surgery in IE are: HF, uncontrolled infection, and prevention of embolic events.

3.2.2 Timing of surgery

- **Emergency surgery (within 24 hours):** NVE or PVE and severe congestive HF or cardiogenic shock caused by: acute valvular regurgitation, severe prosthetic dysfunction (dehiscence or obstruction), fistula into a cardiac chamber or the pericardial space
- **Urgent surgery (within days):** NVE with persistent congestive HF, signs of poor hemodynamic tolerance, or abscess; PVE with persistent congestive heart failure, signs of poor hemodynamic tolerance, or abscess; PVE caused by staphylococci or Gram-negative organisms, large vegetation (> 10 mm) with an embolic event, large vegetation (> 10 mm) with other predictors of a complicated course, very large vegetation (> 15 mm), especially if conservative surgery is available, large abscess or periannular involvement with uncontrolled infection;
- **Early elective surgery (during the in-hospital stay):** Severe aortic regurgitation with congestive HF and good response to medical therapy, PVE with valvular dehiscence or congestive heart failure and good response to medical therapy, presence of abscess or periannular extension, persistent infection when extracardiac focus has been excluded, fungal or other infections resistant to medical cure (Prendergast & Tornos, 2010).

3.2.3 Surgical approach and techniques

The two primary objectives of surgery are the total removal of infected tissue and the reconstruction of cardiac morphology, including repair or replacement of the affected valve. The mode of surgery (replacement versus repair) or type of prosthesis used (mechanical versus biological) has no influence on operative mortality, although repair techniques, when applicable, offer long-term advantages, including a reduced risk of late complications (notably, recurrent IE) and obviate the need for lifelong anticoagulation medication. Homografts offer a reduced risk of recurrent infection in aortic IE, although their use remains controversial owing to a higher risk of late complications. Cardiac transplantation may be considered in extreme cases with recurrent PVE (Pavie, 2006).

Where infection is confined to the valve cusps or leaflets, any method of repairing or replacing the valve may be used. However, valve repair is favored whenever possible. Perforations in a single valve cusp or leaflet may be repaired with an autologous glutaraldehyde-treated or bovine pericardial patch.

In complex cases with locally uncontrolled infection, total excision of infected and devitalized tissue should be followed by valve replacement and repair of associated defects to secure valve fixation. Mechanical and biological prostheses have similar operative mortality (Edwards et al, 1998). The use of foreign material should be kept to a minimum. Small abscesses can be closed directly. Radical resection of the abscess is essential. The general consensus is that an aortic valve homograft is the ideal conduit for an aortic root abscess, but that it is not a substitute for radical extirpation of the abscess and all inflamed tissue (David et al, 2007).

In aortic IE, replacing the aortic valve with a mechanical or biological prosthesis is the technique of choice. Using cryopreserved or sterilized homografts has been suggested to reduce the risk of persistent or recurrent infection (Lopes et al, 2007). However, mechanical prostheses and xenografts compare favorably, and with improved durability. Homografts or stentless xenografts may be preferred in PVE or in cases where there is extensive aortic root destruction with aorto-ventricular discontinuity (Sabik et al, 2002). A tailored tubular Dacron graft to concomitantly reconstruct the left ventricular outflow tract and replace the aortic root is a useful and safe operative technique for patients with destroyed aorto-ventricular junction.

A monoblock aorto-mitral homograft has been suggested as a surgical option for extensive bivalvular IE (Obadia et al, 2006).

3.2.4 Operative mortality and morbidity

Perioperative mortality and morbidity vary according to the type of infective agent, the extent of destruction of cardiac structures, the degree of left ventricular dysfunction, and the patient's hemodynamic condition at the time of surgery. Currently, operative mortality in IE lies between 5% and 15%.

The outcomes of PVE are worse than those of NVE. The main reason the operative mortality for PVE is higher than that for NVE is the complexity of the operation and the fact that it is often associated with a paravalvular abscess (David et al, 2006).

When surgery must be done within the first week of antimicrobial therapy, a recent study showed that in-hospital mortality is 15%, with risks of recurrence and non-infective postoperative valvular dysfunction of 12% and 7%, respectively (Thuny et al, 2008).

In less complex cases, where disease is limited to the valve structures alone allowing complete excision of the infected tissue, mortality should be similar to routine valve surgery.

The cause of death is often multifactorial, but the main reasons are multiorgan failure, HF, intractable sepsis, coagulopathy, and stroke.

3.2.5 Postoperative complications

Immediate postoperative complications are relatively common. Among the most frequent are severe coagulopathy requiring treatment with clotting factors, re-exploration of the chest for bleeding or tamponade, acute renal failure requiring hemodialysis, stroke, low cardiac output syndrome, pneumonia, and atrioventricular block following radical resection of an aortic root abscess with a need for pacemaker implantation. A preoperative ECG demonstrating left bundle branch block predicts the need for a postoperative permanent pacemaker.

3.3 Prophylaxis for IE

The European Society of Cardiology Guideline proposes limiting antibiotic prophylaxis to patients with the highest risk of IE undergoing the highest risk dental procedures. Patients with the highest risk of IE are patients with a prosthetic valve or a prosthetic material used for cardiac valve repair, patients with previous IE, patients with congenital heart disease, in particular those with complex cyanotic heart disease and those who have postoperative palliative shunts, conduits, or other prostheses. Procedures at risk involve the manipulation of the gingival or periapical region of teeth or perforation of the oral mucosa, including scaling and root canal procedures. Good oral hygiene and regular dental review are very important for reducing the risk of IE. Aseptic measures are mandatory during venous catheter manipulation and during any invasive procedures in order to reduce the rate of healthcare-associated IE (Habib et al, 2009).

The American Heart Association Guideline includes cardiac transplant recipients who develop cardiac valvulopathy on the list of patients with the highest risk of IE. It also recommends prophylaxis for procedures on respiratory tract or infected skin, skin structures, or musculoskeletal tissue only for patients with underlying cardiac conditions associated with the highest risk of adverse outcome from IE (Wilson et al, 2007).

An antibiotic for prophylaxis should be given in a single dose 30-60 minutes before the procedure. Amoxicillin is the preferred choice for oral therapy because it is well absorbed in the GI tract and provides high and sustained serum concentrations. For individuals who are allergic to penicillin or amoxicillin, the use of cephalexin or another first-generation oral cephalosporin, clindamycin, azithromycin, or clarithromycin is recommended. Because of possible cross-reactions, a cephalosporin should not be given to patients with a history of anaphylaxis, angioedema, or urticaria after treatment with any form of penicillin, including ampicillin or amoxicillin (Habib et al, 2009; Wilson et al, 2007).

4. Complications of IE

4.1 Heart failure

HF is the most frequent complication of IE and represents the most frequent indication for surgery in IE. HF is observed in 50–60% of cases overall and is more often present when IE affects the aortic (29%) rather than the mitral (20%) valve (Baddour et al, 2005). HF can be caused by severe aortic regurgitation, intracardiac fistulae, or, more rarely, by valve obstruction, when a large vegetation partially obstructs the valve orifice.

Clinical presentation of HF may include severe dyspnea, pulmonary edema, and cardiogenic shock. In addition to clinical findings, TTE is crucially important for the initial evaluation and follow-up. Echocardiography is also of more general value for hemodynamic assessment of valvular dysfunction, measurement of pulmonary artery pressure, and assessment and monitoring of left ventricular systolic function and left and right heart filling pressures. Brain natriuretic peptide (NT-proBNP) is potentially useful for diagnosing and monitoring HF in IE.

HF may progress from mild to severe during treatment, and two-thirds of these cases occur during the active phase of the disease. Moderate-to-severe HF is the most important predictor of in-hospital and 6-month mortality (Baddour et al, 2005).

4.2 Uncontrolled infection

Uncontrolled infection is the second most frequent cause for surgery and encompasses persisting infection (> 7–10 days), infection due to resistant organisms, and locally uncontrolled infection.

Uncontrolled infection is most frequently related to perivalvular extension (the most frequent cause, associated with a poor prognosis and a high likelihood of the need for surgery) or difficult-to-treat organisms, such as fungi, multiresistant organisms, e.g. MRSA or vancomycin-resistant enterococci, and also in the rare infections caused by Gram-negative bacteria.

Signs of locally uncontrolled infection include increasing vegetation size, abscess formation, false aneurysms, or the creation of fistulae. Persistent fever is also usually present.

Unless severe comorbidity exists, the presence of locally uncontrolled infection indicates early surgery in patients with NVE (Habib et al, 2009).

4.3 Systemic embolism

Embolic events are a frequent and life-threatening complication of IE related to the migration of cardiac vegetations. It has been reported to occur in 13% to 49% of cases. The brain and spleen are the most frequent sites of embolisms in aortic IE.

Embolisms after adequate antimicrobial treatment are frequent, and most embolisms occur within the first two weeks of therapy. Embolisms before antimicrobial therapy are a risk factor for embolisms after antimicrobial therapy has begun. Controlling infection is important for preventing embolisms. The benefits of surgery to prevent embolisms are greatest during the first week of antibiotic therapy, when embolic risk peaks.

Several factors are associated with increased risk of embolisms: the size and mobility of vegetations, the location of the vegetation, an increase or decrease in the size of the vegetation under antibiotic therapy, particular microorganisms (staphylococci, *Streptococcus bovis, Candida spp.*), previous embolisms, multivalvular IE, and biological markers.

The risk of embolization seems to increase with increasing vegetation size, and this is particularly significant in staphylococcal endocarditis (Vilacosta et al, 2002).

4.4 Neurological complications

Neurologic events develop in 20–40% of all patients with IE.

Neurologic complications of IE most commonly occur as a result of embolization from endocardial vegetation, with the resultant occlusion of cerebral arteries. An ischemic or hemorrhagic stroke or a transient ischemic attack (TIA) can then develop. The dissemination of infected embolic material into cerebral or meningeal vessels may also lead to meningitis

or brain abscesses. More nonspecific neurologic manifestations associated with IE include headache, seizures, and toxic encephalopathy. Cerebral hemorrhage is the most dramatic, though fortunately rare, neurologic complication of IE. It can be caused by a rupture of a mycotic aneurysm even months to years after the IE has been cured.
Neurologic manifestations of IE occur mainly before antimicrobial treatment has begun, thus reinforcing the belief that rapidly diagnosing and initiating antimicrobial therapy may still be the most effective means of preventing neurologic complications (Heiro et al, 2000).
After a first neurological event, most patients still have an indication for surgery that is generally not contraindicated.

4.5 Infectious aneurysms

Infectious (mycotic) aneurysms (IAs) result from septic arterial embolisms to the intraluminal space or vasa vasorum, or from the subsequent spread of infection through the intimal vessels. An intracranial location is most frequent, and the reported frequency of 2–4% (Corr et al, 1995) is probably an underestimate since some IAs are clinically silent.
The most important sequelae of these aneurysms is bleeding, which can occur days, weeks, months, or, rarely, years after successful therapy for the underlying IE. Cerebral mycotic aneurysms tend to occur in the more distal portions of the middle cerebral artery near the surface of the brain involving the secondary and tertiary branches. This characteristic pattern helps to separate them clinically from berry aneurysms, which tend to occur near the base of the brain and the circle of Willis.

4.6 Acute renal failure

Acute renal failure is a common complication of IE, which occurs in 30% of patients and predicts a poor prognosis. Causes of acute renal failure are often multifactorial and include the following: immune complex and vasculitic glomerulonephritis, renal infarction, hemodynamic impairment in cases with HF or severe sepsis, or, after cardiac surgery, antibiotic toxicity, notably related to aminoglycosides, vancomycin, and even high-dose penicillin, nephrotoxicity of contrast agents used for imaging (Majumdar et al, 2000).
Hemodialysis may be required in some patients, but acute renal failure is often reversible.

4.7 Rheumatic complications

Musculoskeletal symptoms (arthralgia, myalgia, back pain) are frequent during IE, and rheumatic complications may be the first manifestations of the disease. Peripheral arthritis occurs in 14% and spondylodiscitis in 3–15% of cases.
Vertebral osteomyelitis is a known but rare complication of IE, occurring most frequently in patients with *S. aureus* infection. Acute septic arthritis involving 2 or more joints should raise a suspicion of IE (Speechly-Dick & Swanton, 1994).

4.8 Splenic abscess

Although splenic emboli are common, splenic abscess is rare. Persistent or recurrent fever and bacteremia suggest the diagnosis, and these patients should be evaluated using abdominal CT, MRI, or ultrasound. Treatment consists of appropriate antibiotic regimens. A splenectomy may be considered for splenic rupture or large abscesses that respond poorly to antibiotics alone, and should be done before valvular surgery, unless the latter is urgent. Percutaneous drainage is an alternative for high-risk surgical candidates. (Chou et al, 1992)

4.9 Myocarditis, pericarditis

Cardiac failure may also be due to myocarditis, which is frequently associated with abscess formation. Regional myocardial infarction may be caused by coronary embolisms or compression. Ventricular arrhythmias may indicate myocardial involvement and imply a poor prognosis. Myocardial involvement is best assessed using TTE.

Pericarditis may be associated with an abscess, myocarditis, or bacteremia, often as a result of *S. aureus* infection. Purulent pericarditis is rare and may necessitate surgical drainage. Rarely, ruptured pseudoaneurysms or fistulae may communicate with the pericardium, with dramatic and often fatal consequences (Sexton & Spelman, 2002).

5. Outcome and long-term prognosis

The prognosis of aortic valve endocarditis depends largely on when the disease is diagnosed, which microorganism is involved, and how promptly it is treated.

Patients with PVE have a more serious prognosis than patients with NVE.

Late complications occurring after the initial infection contribute to the poor prognosis of IE. Following in-hospital treatment, the main complications include a recurrence of infection, HF, a need for valve surgery, and death.

The risk of recurrence among survivors of IE varies between 2.7% and 22.5%. There are two types of recurrence: relapse and reinfection. The term "relapse" refers to a repeat episode of IE caused by the same microorganism as the previous episode. In contrast, "reinfection" is used primarily to describe infection with a different microorganism (Chu et al, 2005). Relapses are most often due to an insufficient duration of the original treatment, a suboptimal choice of initial antibiotics, and a persistent focus of infection (e.g. a periprosthetic abscess).

Progressive HF can occur as a consequence of valve destruction, even when the infection is healed. After the completion of treatment, recommendations for surgery follow conventional guidelines.

Following the in-hospital phase, principal factors that determine long-term mortality are age, comorbidity, and HF, particularly when surgery has not been done, which suggests that long-term mortality is related to the underlying conditions rather than to the IE itself.

A high early surgery rate is related to good long-term results and does not increase in-hospital mortality. Medical treatment, however, also offers favorable long-term results in cases of responsive IE where poor prognostic factors are absent (Bishara et al, 2001).

The IE prognosis is not uniform. Mortality is high during the initial phase, but after one year, the risk of dying is low, although still above that of the general population. Part of the risk is probably the direct consequence of IE, but part is due to the course of the underlying heart disease (Delahaye et al, 1995).

6. Conclusions

IE is a changing disease with predisposing risk factors, etiology, manifestations, and therapeutics in continuous evolution.

Although modern antibiotic and surgical treatments have substantially improved outcomes in recent decades, IE remains a life-threatening disease. As mortality during the active phase of the infection has declined, long-term morbidity and mortality caused by late sequelae such as congestive HF, valve incompetence, and predisposition to recurrent IE are becoming more important. Moreover, the focus has shifted away from infections of native valves to endocarditis of prosthetic valves in the elderly and to endocarditis in users of injected drugs. Effective therapy has become progressively more difficult to achieve because of the proliferation of implanted biomechanical devices and the rise in the number of resistant organisms.

Endocarditis has evolved into several variations, keeping it near the top of the list of diseases that must not be misdiagnosed or overlooked.

7. Acknowledgement

This paper is supported by the Sectoral Operational Programme Human Resources Development, financed from the European Social Fund and by the Romanian Government under the contract number POSDRU 89/1.5/S/64109

8. References

Baddour LM, Wilson WR, Bayer AS, Fowler VG Jr, Bolger AF, Levison ME, Ferrieri P, Gerber MA, Tani LY, Gewitz MH, Tong DC, Steckelberg JM, Baltimore RS, Shulman ST, Burns JC, Falace DA, Newburger JW, Pallasch TJ, Takahashi M & Taubert KA (2005). Infective endocarditis: diagnosis, antimicrobial therapy, and management of complications: a statement for healthcare professionals from the Committee on Rheumatic Fever, Endocarditis, and Kawasaki Disease, Council on Cardiovascular Disease in the Young, and the Councils on Clinical Cardiology, Stroke, and Cardiovascular Surgery and Anesthesia, American Heart Association: endorsed by the Infectious Diseases Society of America. *Circulation*; 111:e394–e434.

Beynon RP, Bahl VK & Prendergast BD (2006). *Infective endocarditis*, BMJ; 333:334–9

Bishara J, Leibovici L, Gartman-Israel D, Sagie A, Kazakov A, Miroshnik E, Ashkenazi S & Pitlik S (2001). Long-term outcome of infective endocarditis: the impact of early surgical intervention. *Clin Infect Dis*; 33:1636–1643.

Brouqui P & Raoult D (2001). Endocarditis due to rare and fastidious bacteria. *Clin Microbiol Rev*; 14:177–207.

Contrepois A (1995). Notes on the Early History of Infective Endocarditis and the Development of an Experimental Model *Clin Infect Dis.*; 20(2): 461-466

Corr P, Wright M & Handler LC (1995). Endocarditis-related cerebral aneurysms: radiologic changes with treatment. *AJNR Am J Neuroradiol*; 16:745–748.

Chou YH, Hsu CC, Tiu CM & Chang T (1992). Splenic abscess: sonographic diagnosis and percutaneous drainage or aspiration. *Gastrointest Radiol*; 17:262–266.

Chu VH Jr., Cabell CH, Abrutyn E, Corey GR, Hoen B, Miro JM, Olaison L, Stryjewski ME, Pappas P, Anstrom KJ, Eykyn S, Habib G, Benito N & Fowler VG Jr. (2004). Native valve endocarditis due to coagulase-negative staphylococci: report of 99 episodes from the International Collaboration on Endocarditis Merged Database. *Clin Infect Dis*; 39:1527–1530.

Chu VH, Sexton DJ, Cabell CH, Reller LB, Pappas PA, Singh RK, Fowler VG Jr, Corey GR, Aksoy O & Woods CW (2005). Repeat infective endocarditis: differentiating relapse from reinfection. *Clin Infect Dis*; 41:406–409.

Chu VH Jr., Woods CW, Miro JM, Hoen B, Cabell CH, Pappas PA, Federspiel J, Athan E, Stryjewski ME, Nacinovich F, Marco F, Levine DP, Elliott TS, Fortes CQ, Tornos P, Gordon DL, Utili R, Delahaye F, Corey GR & Fowler VG Jr. (2008). Emergence of coagulase-negative staphylococci as a cause of native valve endocarditis. *Clin Infect Dis*; 46:232–242.

David TE, Gavra G, Feindel CM, Regesta T, Armstrong S & Maganti MD (2007) Surgical treatment of active infective endocarditis: a continued challenge. *J Thorac Cardiovasc Surg*; 133:144–149.

David TE, Regesta T, Gavra G, Armstrong S & Maganti MD (2007). Surgical treatment of paravalvular abscess: long-term results. *Eur J Cardiothorac Surg*; 31:43–48.

Das M, Badley AD, Cockerill FR, Steckelberg JM & Wilson WR (1997). Infective endocarditis caused by HACEK microorganisms. *Annu Rev Med*; 48:25–33.

Delahaye F, Ecochard R, De Gevigney G, Barjhoux C, Malquarti V, Saradarian W & Delaye J (1995). The long term prognosis of infective endocarditis, *Eur Heart J* 16 (suppl B): 48-53.

Durack DT, Lukes AS & Bright DK (1994). New criteria for diagnosis of infective endocarditis: utilization of specific echocardiographic findings. *Am J Med*; 96:200-9.

Edwards MB, Ratnatunga CP, Dore CJ & Taylor KM (1998). Thirty-day mortality and longterm survival following surgery for prosthetic endocarditis: a study from the UK heart valve registry. *Eur J Cardiothorac Surg*; 14:156–164.

Evangelista A & Gonzalez-Alujas MT (2004). Echocardiography in infective endocarditis. *Heart*; 90:614–617.

Fowler VG Jr, Boucher HW, Corey GR, Abrutyn E, Karchmer AW, Rupp ME, Levine DP, Chambers HF, Tally FP, Vigliani GA, Cabell CH, Link AS, DeMeyer I, Filler SG, Zervos M, Cook P, Parsonnet J, Bernstein JM, Price CS, Forrest GN, Fatkenheuer G, Gareca M, Rehm SJ, Brodt HR, Tice A, Cosgrove SE (2006). Daptomycin versus standard therapy for bacteremia and endocarditis caused by Staphylococcus aureus. *N Engl J Med*; 355:653–665.

Fowler VG Jr, Miro JM, Hoen B, Cabell CH, Abrutyn E, Rubinstein E, Corey GR, Spelman D, Bradley SF, Barsic B, Pappas PA, Anstrom KJ, Wray D, Fortes CQ, Anguera I, Athan E, Jones P, van der Meer JT, Elliott TS, Levine DP & Bayer AS (2005). Staphylococcus aureus endocarditis: a consequence of medical progress. *JAMA*; 293:3012-3021.

Garzoni C, Nobre VA & Garbino J. (2007). Candida parapsilosis endocarditis: a comparative review of the literature. *Eur J Clin Microbiol Infect Dis*; 26:915–926.

Gavalda J, Len O, Miro JM, Munoz P, Montejo M, Alarcon A, de la Torre-Cisneros J, Pena C, Martinez-Lacasa X, Sarria C, Bou G, Aguado JM, Navas E, Romeu J, Marco F, Torres C, Tornos P, Planes A, Falco V, Almirante B & Pahissa A (2007). Brief communication: treatment of Enterococcus faecalis endocarditis with ampicillin plus ceftriaxone. *Ann Intern Med*; 146:574–579.

Habib G, Badano L, Tribouilloy C, Vilacosta I, Zamorano JL, Galderisi M, et al. (2010). Recommendations for the practice of echocardiography in infective endocarditis. *Eur J Echocardiogr*; 11:202-19.

Habib G, Hoen B, Tornos P, Thuny F, Prendergast B, Vilacosta I, Moreillon P, de Jesus Antunes M, Thilen U, Lekakis J, Lengyel M, Mueller L, Naber CK, Nihoyannopoulos P, Moritz A & Zamorano GL (2009). Guidelines on the prevention, diagnosis, and treatment of infective endocarditis (new version 2009). *Eur Heart J*; doi:10.1093/eurheartj/ehp285.

Heiro M, Nikoskelainen J, Engblom E, Kotilainen E, Marttila R & Kotilainen P (2000). Neurologic manifestations of infective endocarditis: a 17-year experience in a teaching hospital in Finland. *Arch Intern Med*; 160:2781–2787.

Helbig JH, Uldum SA, Luck PC & Harrison TG (2001). Detection of Legionella pneumophila antigen in urine samples by the BinaxNOW immunochromatographic assay and comparison with both Binax legionella urinary enzyme immunoassay (EIA) and Biotest Legionella Urin Antigen EIA. *J Med Microbiol*; 50:509–516.

Hill EE, Herijgers P, Claus P, Vanderschueren S, Herregods MC & Peetermans WE (2007). Infective endocarditis: changing epidemiology and predictors of 6-month mortality: a prospective cohort study. *Eur Heart J*; 28:196–203.

Horstkotte D, Follath F, Gutschik E, Lengyel M, Oto A, Pavie A, Soler-Soler J, Thiene G, von Graevenitz A, Priori SG, Garcia MA, Blanc JJ, Budaj A, Cowie M, Dean V, Deckers J, Fernandez Burgos E, Lekakis J, Lindahl B, Mazzotta G, Morais J, Oto A, Smiseth OA, Lekakis J, Vahanian A, Delahaye F, Parkhomenko A, Filipatos G, Aldershvile J & Vardas P (2004). Guidelines on prevention, diagnosis and treatment of infective endocarditis executive summary; the task force on infective endocarditis of the European society of cardiology. *Eur Heart J*; 25:267–276.

Howden BP, Johnson PD, Ward PB, Stinear TP & Davies JK (2006). Isolates with low-level vancomycin resistance associated with persistent methicillin-resistant Staphylococcus aureus bacteremia. *Antimicrob Agents Chemother*; 50:3039–3047.

Levine DP & Lamp KC (2007). Daptomycin in the treatment of patients with infective endocarditis: experience from a registry. *Am J Med*; 120:S28–S33.

Li JS, Sexton DJ, Mick N, Nettles R, Fowler VG Jr, Ryan T, Bashore T & Corey GR. (2000) Proposed modifications to the Duke criteria for the diagnosis of infective endocarditis. *Clin Infect Dis*; 30: 633–638.

Lopes S, Calvinho P, de Oliveira F & Antunes M (2007). Allograft aortic root replacement in complex prosthetic endocarditis. *Eur J Cardiothorac Surg*; 32:126–130; discussion 131–132.

Lye DC, Hughes A, O'Brien D & Athan E (2005). Candida glabrata prosthetic valve endocarditis treated successfully with fluconazole plus caspofungin without surgery: a case report and literature review. *Eur J Clin Microbiol Infect Dis*; 24:753–755.

Majumdar A, Chowdhary S, Ferreira MA, Hammond LA, Howie AJ, Lipkin GW & Littler WA (2000). Renal pathological findings in infective endocarditis. *Nephrol Dial Transplant*; 15:1782–1787.

Murdoch DR, Corey GR, Hoen B, Miro JM, Fowler VG Jr, Bayer AS, Karchmer AW, Olaison L, Pappas PA, Moreillon P, Chambers ST, Chu VH, Falco V, Holland DJ, Jones P, Klein JL, Raymond NJ, Read KM, Tripodi MF, Utili R, Wang A, Woods CW &

Cabell CH (2009). Clinical presentation, etiology, and outcome of infective endocarditis in the 21st century: the International Collaboration on Endocarditis-Prospective Cohort Study. *Arch Intern Med*; 169: 463–473.

Mylonakis E & Calderwood SB (2001). Infective endocarditis in adults. *N Engl J Med*; 345:1318–1330.

Netzer R O-M, Zollinger E, Seiler C & Cerny A (2000). Infective endocarditis: clinical spectrum, presentation and outcome. An analysis of 212 cases 1980–1995, *Heart*; 84:25–30

Obadia JF, Henaine R, Bergerot C, Ginon I, Nataf P, Chavanis N, Robin J, Andre-Fouet X, Ninet J & Raisky O (2006). Monobloc aorto-mitral homograft or mechanical valve replacement: a new surgical option for extensive bivalvular endocarditis. *J Thorac Cardiovasc Surg*; 131:243–245.

Olaison L & Schadewitz K (2002). Enterococcal endocarditis in Sweden, 1995–1999: can shorter therapy with aminoglycosides be used? *Clin Infect Dis*; 34:159–166.

Pavie A (2006). Heart transplantation for end-stage valvular disease: indications and results. *Curr Opin Cardiol*; 21:100–105.

Prendergast BD (2006). The changing face of infective endocarditis. *Heart*; 92: 879–885.

Prendergast BD & Tornos P (2010). Surgery for Infective Endocarditis. Who and When? *Circulation*; 121:1141-1152

Richardson DC, Burrows LL, Korithoski B, Salit IE, Butany J, David TE & Conly JM (2003). Tropheryma whippelii as a cause of afebrile culture-negative endocarditis: the evolving spectrum of Whipple's disease. *J Infect*; 47:170–173.

Sabik JF, Lytle BW, Blackstone EH, Marullo AG, Pettersson GB & Cosgrove DM (2002). Aortic root replacement with cryopreserved allograft for prosthetic valve endocarditis. *Ann Thorac Surg*; 74:650–659; discussion 659.

Sexton DJ & Spelman D (2002). Current best practices and guidelines. Assessment and management of complications in infective endocarditis. *Infect Dis Clin North Am*; 16:507–521.

Speechly-Dick ME & Swanton RH (1994). Osteomyelitis and infective endocarditis. *Postgrad Med J*; 70:885–890

Thuny F, Beurtheret S, Gariboldi V, Mancini J, Avierinos JF, Riberi A, Casalta JP, Gouriet F, Tafanelli L, Giorgi R, Collart F, Raoult D & Habib G (2008). Outcome after surgical treatment performed within the first week of antimicrobial therapy during infective endocarditis: a prospective study. *Arch Cardiovasc Dis*; 101:687–695.

Thuny F, Beurtheret S, Mancini J, Gariboldi V, Casalta JP, Riberi A, Giorgi R, Gouriet F, Tafanelli L, Avierinos JF, Renard S, Collart F, Raoult D & Habib G. The timing of surgery influences mortality and morbidity in adults with severe complicated infective endocarditis: a propensity analysis. *Eur Heart J*; doi: 10.1093/eurheartj/ehp089

Thuny F, Avierinos JF & Habib G (2010). Changing patterns in epidemiological profiles and prevention strategies in infective endocarditis: from teeth to healthcare-related infection *Eur Heart J*; 31(15): 1826-1827

Vilacosta I, Graupner C, San Roman JA, Sarria C, Ronderos R, Fernandez C, Mancini L, Sanz O, Sanmartin JV, Stoermann W (2002). Risk of embolization after institution of antibiotic therapy for infective endocarditis. *J Am Coll Cardiol*; 39: 1489–1495.

Watkin RW, Lang S, Lambert PA, Littler WA & Elliott TS (2006). The serological diagnosis of staphylococcal infective endocarditis. *J Infect*; 53:301–307.

Wilson W, Taubert KA, Gewitz M, Lockhart PB, Baddour LM, Levison M, et al. (2007). Prevention of infective endocarditis: guidelines from the American Heart Association: a guideline from the American Heart Association Rheumatic Fever, Endocarditis, and Kawasaki Disease Committee, Council on Cardiovascular Disease in the Young, and the Council on Clinical Cardiology, Council on Cardiovascular Surgery and Anesthesia, and the Quality of Care and Outcomes Research Interdisciplinary Working Group. *Circulation*; 116(15):1736-54.

Part 4

Aortic Sclerosis/Aortic Stenosis

6

The Progression of Aortic Sclerosis to Aortic Stenosis

Uzma Jalal Serageldin Raslan and Farouk Mookadam
Department of Cardiovascular Diseases, Mayo Clinic, Scottsdale, AZ, USA

1. Introduction

Aortic stenosis is the most frequent valvular heart disease in the western world and its incidence continues to rise. Until recently, aortic valve sclerosis (AVS) was considered to be a normal degenerative process associated with aging. For this reason, the common and well recognized soft, basal ejection murmur of aortic sclerosis was generally regarded by physicians to be of little or no clinical significance. In the last decade, AVS has been the focus of both clinical and animal research. AVS has emerged as a biomarker for cardiovascular risk, and ultimately leads to aortic stenosis in 16% of adults (Stewart et al., 1997; Cosmi et al., 2002).
Calcific aortic valve disease ranges from aortic sclerosis, defined as focal, irregular thickening of aortic valve leaflets with no hemodynamically significant derangement (i.e., peak velocity of ≤ 2 m/s and no significant aortic regurgitation), to severe calcification (with impaired leaflet motion and an aortic jet velocity of ≥ 2.5 m/s) referred to as aortic stenosis. The paradigm of aortic stenosis has shifted from being considered a degenerative aging process; it is now recognized as a dynamic inflammatory process with features similar to atherosclerotic plaque. These features include endothelial disruption, focal deposition of low density lipoprotein (LDL) cholesterol and lipoprotein A, accumulation of macrophages and T lymphocytes, and calcification (Freeman et al., 2004).

2. Epidemiology and etiology

Aortic valve sclerosis is present in approximately 25% of people 65 to 74 years old and in 50 % of people over 84 years (Lindroos et al., 1993; Stewart et al., 1997; Otto et al., 1999), while aortic stenosis affects 2% of the population over 65 years old, 3 % over 75 years old, and 4% over 85 years old (Stewart, 1997). The severity of aortic sclerosis on a scale of 0-3 has been quantified by echocardiography for echogenicity, thickening, or calcification of the valve leaflet as follows (Chandra et al., 2004):

- 0- Normal (No involvement)
- 1- Mild (Minor involvement of one leaflet)
- 2- Moderate (Minor involvement of two leaflets or extensive involvement of one leaflet)
- 3- Severe (Extensive involvement of two leaflets or involvement of all three leaflets)

In adults, valvular aortic stenosis is due to degenerative calcific changes of a trileaflet valve, rheumatic disease, or secondary calcification of a congenitally bicuspid valve (Roberts, 1970; Selzer, 1987). In developed countries, the most common cause of adult acquired aortic stenosis at present is a chronic inflammatory and fibrotic process of the aortic valve very similar to atherosclerosis. Histologically, the valve consists of 3 layers: [1] the ventricularis (on the ventricular side of the leaflet), composed of elastin rich fibers; [2] the fibrosa (on the aortic side of leaflet), composed of fibroblasts and collagen fibres; and [3] the spongiosa (at the base of leaflet, between the fibrosa and ventricularis), a layer of loose connective tissue composed of fibroblasts, mesenchymal cells, and mucopolysaccharide- rich matrix. Progressive fibrosis and calcification can occur on a bileaflet or a trileaflet valve; it occurs earlier in life in the bicuspid valve. The most common cause of aortic stenosis in patients 65 years old and over is called "senile calcific aortic stenosis". With aging, the protein collagen of the valve leaflets is destroyed, and calcium is deposited on the leaflets. Turbulence across the valve increases, which causes scarring, thickening, and stenosis of the valve once valve leaflet mobility is reduced by calcification.

Rheumatic fever is the cause of aortic stenosis in developing countries. Rheumatic involvement of the aortic valve is characterized by commissural fusion between the aortic valve leaflets. When rheumatic fever is the cause of aortic stenosis, the mitral valve is also affected in most patients (Campbell, 1968).

3. Clinical presentation

The classic triad of symptoms in significant aortic stenosis is angina, syncope, and dyspnea, all of which typically occur with exertion. Occasionally, gastrointestinal bleeding occurs secondary to arteriovenous malformations, platelet dysfunction, and defective coagulation in what is termed as Heyde syndrome (Zigelman et al., 2009; Batur et al., 2003; Sucker, 2007). In older adults, symptoms are often delayed due to an age- associated decrease in activity, and symptom are attributed to other conditions common in the elderly; therefore, special attention should be focused on the elicitation of symptoms.

Angina is the first symptom in one-third of the patients, and it eventually occurs in one-half of patients with aortic stenosis. It is due to a supply and demand mismatch caused by a combination of left ventricular hypertrophy, increased afterload, increased wall strain, and excessive compression of the coronary arteries. Syncope related to aortic stenosis is usually associated with exertion or excitement. These conditions cause vasodilation and lowering of blood pressure. In aortic stenosis, the heart is unable to increase cardiac output due to fixed left ventricular outflow tract (LVOT) obstruction, and is unable to compensate for the drop in blood pressure. This results in decreased cerebral perfusion, thereby causing syncope. Dyspnea is a late- presenting symptom of severe aortic stenosis caused by failure of the left ventricle to compensate for the outflow obstruction.

On physical examination, the hallmark of aortic stenosis is a late peaking crescendo-decrescendo systolic murmur. It is best heard at the upper- right or left- sterna border, radiating to the carotids. Older adults exhibit certain variations of this characteristic pattern. The occurrence of heart failure and chronic lung disease common in this population results in a significant reduction in the intensity of the murmur, while pure aortic sclerosis without stenosis may present with an apical systolic high- pitched murmur (Gallavardin phenomenon) (Hage et al., 2011).

4. Risk factors

Several lines of evidence suggest that, in addition to the pathophysiological similarities to atherosclerosis, aortic stenosis and coronary disease share many risk factors, such as male gender, older age group, tobacco use, diabetes mellitus, hypercholesterolemia, hypertension, hyperparathyroidism, renal disease, decreased bone density, and metabolic syndrome (Figure 1). Increased C-reactive protein (CRP) as a risk factor for aortic stenosis is controversial. Reports from a few studies show a positive association between aortic stenosis and increased CRP; however, a recent prospective trial (Novaro et al., 2007) involving 5621 subjects followed over a period of 5 years, and using echocardiography and CRP measurements, showed that there was no association between CRP and the development of aortic stenosis. In addition, being Caucasian and short in stature were found to have a positive association with development of aortic stenosis.

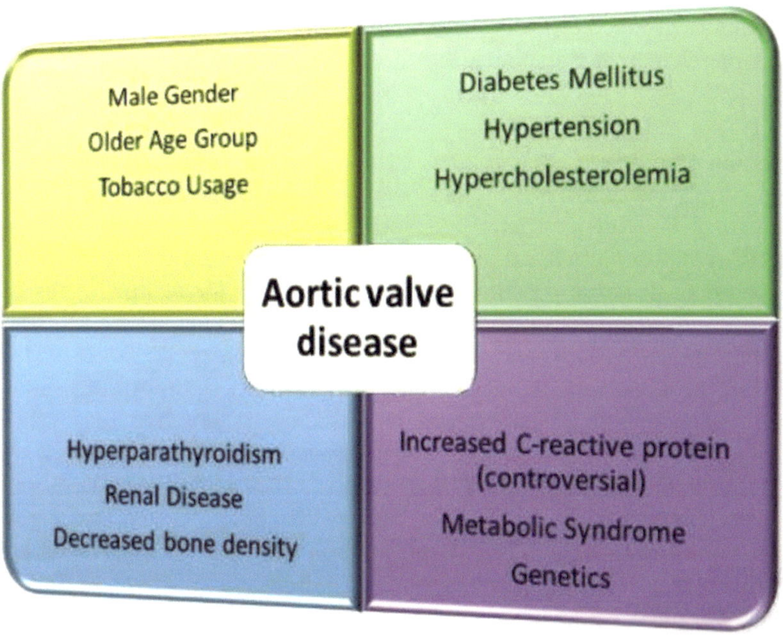

Fig. 1. Schematic view of risk factors involved in aortic valve disease

5. Pathogenesis

5.1 Early lesion

The early sclerotic lesion shows focal subendothelial plaque like lesions on the aortic surface of the leaflet that extends into the adjacent fibrosa layer. The initiating factor for these lesions is the endothelial disruption due to increased mechanical or decreased shear stress. The Mechanical stress of the aortic valve is highest on the aortic side of the leaflet in the flexion area. These lesions show similarities to atherosclerosis, with a prominent accumulation of atherogenic lipoproteins, low density lipoprotein (LDL) oxidation, inflammatory cell infiltrate, and microcalcification (O'Brien et al., 1996; Olsson et al., 1999; Otto et al., 1994).

5.2 Inflammation and lipoproteins

Over the course of time, mechanical stress leads to endothelial dysfunction, which is then perpetuated by inflammatory cell infiltrate consisting of both T-lymphocytes and macrophages. Monocytes infiltrate the endothelium and differentiate into macrophages via adhesion molecules (Ghaisas et al., 2000). After infiltrating into the endothelium, these inflammatory cells upregulate inflammatory cytokines, transforming growth factor, and interleukin, all of which act on valvular fibroblasts and promote cellular proliferation, extracellular matrix remodeling, and local calcification. Focal, extracellular lipid accumulation is seen within each valve leaflet, in small areas in the subendothelial region, with displacement of elastic lamina and extension into adjacent fibrosa (Otto et al., 1994). LDL that is taken into the subendothelial layer undergoes oxidative modification and subsequent macrophage ingestion to become foam cells. Studies have shown that aortic stenosis is associated with high levels of plasma asymmetric dimethylarginine, a marker of endothelial dysfunction (Ngo et al., 2007) and that nitric oxide (NO) is involved in inhibiting valve calcification (Kennedy et al., 2009). Aortic sclerosis has been associated with NO resistance in platelets, which explains the thrombotic risk in patients with aortic sclerosis (Ngo et al., 2009).

5.3 Angiotensin converting enzyme and extracellular matrix

Angiotensin converting enzyme(ACE) has been identified in aortic sclerotic lesions(O'Brien et al., 2002).There is evidence that the majority of this enzyme is extracellular and co-localized with apolipoprotein B, even though some of it may be locally produced. The aortic valve is exposed to pulsatile repetitive pressure and shear stress during systole, whereas cyclical stretch and turbulent shear stress occur during diastole. These are transmitted to valve interstitial cells (VICs) by endothelial cells and the matrix (Sacks et al., 2007), which results in cell proliferation, increased collagen deposition, apoptosis, and enhanced cathepsin S and K expression. Furthermore, increased cyclic stretch increases the expression and activity of matrix metalloproteinase (MMP)-1, 2, and 9, whereas it reduces the expression as well as the activity of cathepsin L and tissue inhibitor of metalloproteinase-1 (TIMP-1) (Balachandran et al., 2009). In patients with aortic stenosis and coronary artery disease, an increase in soluble vascular cell adhesion molecule-1 (VCAM-1) occurs along with a decrease in soluble intercellular adhesion molecule-1 (ICAM-1) and s-E selectin (Linhartova et al., 2009). Increased expression of elastolytic cathepsins S, K, and V and their inhibitor cystatin C is also observed (Helske et al., 2006). The association of calcific aortic valve disease and increase in endothelin-1 and endothelin A receptor support the evidence of inflammation and fibrosis in aortic calcific disease (Peltonen et al., 2009).

5.4 Angiogenesis and osteogenesis

As the disease progresses, active bone formation is seen. Angiogenesis is predominant in the pathogenesis of aortic stenosis and is the hallmark for longitudinal bone growth. Angiogenetic factors such as vascular endothelial growth factor (VEGF) have been shown to be necessary for enchondral bone formation in calcified valves (Gerber et al., 1999).The lipids and inflammatory cells localize within the microscopic calcific areas, which results in macrophage- derived osteopontin, a key element in tissue calcification (Abdel-Azeez et al., 2010).Synthesis of bone sialoprotein, tenacin C and extracellular matrix proteins also ensues(Kaden et al., 2003; Satta et al., 2002; Kaden et al., 2004).There is evidence that native aortic valve disease involves mediators of bone homeostasis like osteoprotegrin (OPG), receptor activator of nuclear factor κ B (RANK), and receptor activator of nuclear factor κ B ligand (RANKL), and that OPG/RANKL ratio was less in stenotic than in sclerotic valves (Steinmetz et al., 2008).

5.5 Genetics

Genetic factors may be important in the development of aortic valve calcification. Genetic polymorphism of interlukin 10, connective tissue growth factor, chemokine receptor 5, apoprotein polymorphism, and estrogen receptors have been shown to influence valvular calcification (Ortlepp et al., 2004). In addition, the B allele of vitamin D receptor has an association with aortic valve stenosis, which confirms the abnormal bone signaling pathway in the pathogenesis of the disease (Ortlepp et al., 2001). Another finding that implies the role of genetics in aortic valve disease is the loss of function mutation of Notch 1 receptor in patients with aortic stenosis (Garg et al., 2005).

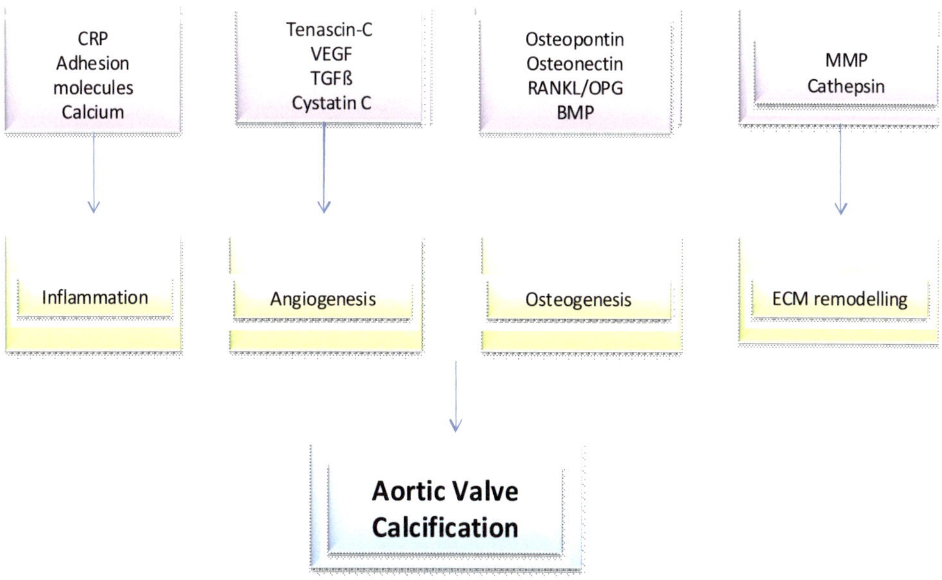

CRP: C-reactive protein; VEGF: Vascular endothelial growth factor; TGF: Transforming growth factor; RANKL: Receptor activator of nuclear factor κ B ligand; OPG: Osteoprotegerin; BMP: Bone morphogenetic protein; MMP: Matrix Metalloproteinase

Fig. 2. Schematic view of mediators in pathogenesis of aortic valve calcification

6. Animal models

Several elegant animal studies have advanced the pathogenetic understanding of aortic valve disease. Rajamannan et al. (2001) compared the aortic valves in rabbits fed on a high cholesterol diet to those fed on a standard diet. The microscopy of the hypercholesterolemia rabbits demonstrated a cholesterol infiltrative pattern along with low- grade apoptosis, neither of which was seen in the control rabbits. Furthermore, Rajamannan et al. (2005a) showed that aortic valves from hypercholesterolemic rabbits had evidence of atherosclerotic streaks, increased CRP, early calcification, and minor levels of nitric oxide synthase (eNOS) compared with controls. The rabbits treated with atorvastatin had less lipid accumulation and higher levels of eNOS. More recently (Rajamannan et al., 2005b), aortic valve calcification was shown to be similar to osteogenesis with a similar spectroscopic appearance and bone matrix markers (osteopontin, bone sialoprotein, osteocalcin) with increase in low-density receptor- related protein (Lrp5) using models fed on a cholesterol

Authur (Year)	Population(N)/ Age (Years)	Outcome Measures	Conclusion
Ngo et al. (2009)	n=253; 51-77	Transthoracic Echo, AVBS score	Association of platelet NO resistance with aortic sclerosis
Linhartova et al. (2009)	n=223;	Coronary angiography, Echo	Association of aortic stenosis with s-VCAM1 in CAD pts
Peltonen et al. (2009)	n=36; 58± 6	Immunohistochemistry, RT-PCR	Upregulation of ET1 & ETA receptor in aortic stenosis
Abdel-Azeez et al. (2010)	n=120	OPN & hsCRP measurement, coronary angio, Echo, lipid profile	OPN is an independent factor of aortic sclerosis
Steinmetz et al. (2008)	n=69	Immunostaining, Morphometry	OPG/RANKL/RANK system is involved in aortic valve calcification
Ortlepp et al. (2001)	n=200	Restricted fragment length polymorphism, PCR	Association of aortic stenosis with Vitamin D receptor genotype
Garg et al. (2005)	n=14	DNA collection, luciferase assay, PCR, Phenotypic evaluation, Genetic linkage analysis	NOTCH 1 mutation causes early defect in aortic valve & calcium deposition

Echo, Echocardiography; Angio, Angiography; RT-PCR, Reverse transcriptase-Polymerase chain reaction; AVBS, Aortic valve ultrasonic back scatter; NO, nitric oxide.

Table 1. Description of human studies

diet and atorvastatin. In addition, intervention with a statin showed a reduction in bone formation, less cellular proliferation, a lower Lrp5/beta catenin protein level, and an increase in endothelial NO synthase concentration (Rajamannan et al., 2005a, 2005b). Recently it was shown (Barrick et al., 2009) that epidermal growth factor receptor (EGFR) signaling contributes to normal valvulogenesis and that reduced EGFR was associated with aortic stenosis in mice models. Another mouse- model study (Matsumoto et al., 2010) showed the beneficial effect of regular exercise training in preventing aortic sclerosis by various pathways, e.g., reducing inflammation and oxidative stress, inhibiting osteogenic pathway, and maintaining endothelial integrity. Various studies suggest that vitamin D and an atherogenic diet induce aortic stenosis only when they act in combination (Drolet et al., 2008), and that an association of aortic valve stenosis and tissue factor was demonstrated (Marechaux et al., 2009).

7. Treatment

Accumulating animal and human studies suggest that aortic sclerosis is an inflammatory disease akin to atherosclerosis in addition to being an important biomarker of atherosclerosis and coronary artery disease. It is a slowly progressive disease that leads to aortic stenosis and, therefore, should be treated aggressively.

Authur (Year)	Model (N)	Intervention	Outcome Measures	Follow Up	Conclusion
Rajamannan et al. (2001)	Rabbits; n=16	Cholesterol	AV dissection	12 weeks	Aortic valve apoptosis
Rajamannan et al. (2005)	Rabbits; n=48	Cholesterol, Atorvastatin	eNOS expression, Western blot, Micro CT	3 months	Hypercholester-olemia produces bone mineralization in AV. Atorvastatin inhibits AVC & increases eNOS concentration
Rajamannan et al. (2005)	Rabbits; n= 54	Cholesterol, Atorvastatin	Micro CT, Calcein inj, Osteopontin expression	24 weeks	Positive bone formation in calcific AV but atorvastatin attenuates it.
Barrick et al. (2009)	Egfr-null mice; n=119	None	Echo, Histology, gene expression, Ventricular pressure	15months	EGFR is required for valvulogenesis & decreased EGFR is seen in AS
Matsumoto et al. (2010)	Mice; n=94	Cholesterol, regular ET, Occasional ET	Histologic analysis, Immunohistochemistry	16 weeks	Regular ET prevents AV sclerosis
Drolet et al. (2008)	Rabbits	Cholesterol, Vitamin D	Transvalvular gradient, AVA, Immunohistological study, Echo	12 weeks	Atherosclerosis & calcifying factors induce AS in combination
Marechauxs et al. (2009)	Rabbits; n= 45	Cholesterol, Vitamin D	Immunohistology, Doppler AV performance, Histology	12 weeks	Association of AV sclerosis with tissue factor

REF, Reference; eNOS, Endothelial nitric oxide synthase; CT, Computed tomography; AV, Aortic valve; AVC, Aortic valve calcification; EGFR, Epidermal growth factor receptor; ET, Exercise training; AVA, Aortic valve area; Echo, Echocardiography; Inj, Injection.

Table 2. Description of animal model

7.1 Pharmacological therapy

Statins are known pleiotropic drugs with an anti-inflammatory and antioxidant effect in addition to their ability to lower lipid levels, stabilize, plaque, and prevent platelet aggregation. This underscores their role in preventing atherosclerotic vascular disease. With cumulative evidence on the similarities between vascular atherosclerosis and aortic valve disease, the hypothesis that statins halt the progression of aortic sclerosis to stenosis was proposed. Statins and ACE-I were considered the first-line candidates for slowing down the

Authur (Year)	Population(N) /Age (Years)	Intervention	Outcome Measures	Study Type	Conclusion
Antonini-Canterin et al. (2008)	n=1046; 70±8	Statins	Echocardiogram	Retro-spective	Statins were effective in aortic sclerosis & mild stenosis.
Shavelle et al. (2002)	n=65; 67-68 (mean)	Statins	Electron beam computed tomogram	Retro-spective	Statins reduce aortic valve calcium accumulation.
Bellamy et al. (2002)	n=156; 77±12	Statins	Doppler echocardiogram	Pro-spective	Statin therapy results in slower progression of AS.
Moura et al. (2007)	n=121; 73±8.9	Rosuvastatin	Echo, serum lipids & inflammatory markers	Pro-spective	Rosuvastatin 20mg is beneficial in slowing AS progression
Cowell et al. (SALTIRE) (2005)	n=155	Atorvastatin 80mg	Doppler Echocardiogram, Helical CT	Double-blinded rando-mized	Statins do not halt the AS progression
Rossebo et al. (SEAS) (2008)	n=1873; 68±10	Simvastatin 10mg, Ezetimbe 40mg	Cardiovascular events, nonfatal MI	Double-blinded rando-mized	Simvastatin and ezetimibe did not reduce the composite outcome of combined aortic-valve events and ischemic events in patients with aortic stenosis
Chan et al. (ASTRON OMER) (2010)	N=269;	Rosuvastatin 40 mg	Echocardiogram	Double-blinded rando-mized	Rosuvastatin did not reduce progression of AS
Hamilton et al. (2011)	Rabbits	Cholesterol, statins	MRI, Excised AV tissue thickness, lipid accumulation	Pro-spective	In advance stages of AS, statin therapy is ineffective

REF, Reference; AS, Aortic stenosis; CT, Computed tomography; MI, Myocardial infarction; MRI, Magnetic resonance imaging

Table 3. Description of statin studies

progression of aortic sclerosis and mild aortic stenosis (Antonini-Canterin et al., 2008; Shavelle et al., 2002; Bellamy et al., 2002), but not for moderate-to-severe stenosis. Moura et al. (2007), in a 1.5-year prospective study, were the first to show the positive effect of statins in slowing the progression of aortic stenosis. Contrary evidence from three prospective randomized trials suggests that statins do not slow the progression of aortic valve disease but lower cholesterol and thus reduce coronary events. The three trials were SALTIRE (The Scottish Aortic Stenosis and Lipid Lowering Trial), SEAS (Simvastatin and Ezetimbe in Aortic Stenosis), and ASTRNOMER (Aortic Stenosis Progression Observation Measuring Effects of Rosuvastatin), which involved 155, 1873 and 269 participants, respectively (Cowell et al., 2005; Rossebo et al., 2008; Chan et al., 2010). In a recent animal experiment with rabbits (Hamilton et al., 2011), it was shown that statin therapy did not regress the disease process in valves with established sclerosis. Thus, medical intervention at an early stage of aortic sclerosis or trivial stenosis may be beneficial, but large outcome- based studies are lacking.

8. Conclusion

Aortic stenosis is the most common valvular pathology in older adults. It is emerging with increasing clarity that aortic valve sclerosis is an active inflammatory process and may be construed as a cardiovascular disease risk biomarker. Physicians should no longer ignore the murmur of aortic sclerosis as innocent; rather, it should be a beacon alerting us of the dangers that lie ahead for patients who harbor this murmur.

It is also evident that aortic sclerosis progresses to aortic stenosis. In fact, this progression is not infrequent. The take- home message from the larger trials and natural history studies seems to be that the target for therapy in established, calcific aortic stenosis may be too late, and that early, aggressive medical intervention be undertaken before the irrevocable process of calcification has occurred. Future studies are needed to fully estimate the benefits of medical therapy as well as the optimal timing for such interventions. Newer therapeutic options targeting the molecular and cellular mechanisms involved in the pathogenesis of aortic valve disease either singularly or in concert are needed.

9. References

Abdel-Azeez, H. A., Al-Zaky, M. (2010). Plasma osteopontin as a predictor of coronary artery disease: association with echocardiographic characteristics of atherosclerosis. J Clin Lab Anal, 24(3): 201-206.

Antonini-Canterin, F., Hirsu, M., Popescu, B. A., et al. (2008). Stage-related effect of statin treatment on the progression of aortic valve sclerosis and stenosis. Am J Cardiol, 102(6): 738-742.

Balachandran, K., Sucosky, P., Jo, H., et al. (2009). Elevated cyclic stretch alters matrix remodeling in aortic valve cusps: implications for degenerative aortic valve disease. Am J Physiol Heart Circ Physiol, 296(3): H756-764.

Barrick, C. J., Roberts, R. B., Rojas, M., et al. (2009). Reduced EGFR causes abnormal valvular differentiation leading to calcific aortic stenosis and left ventricular hypertrophy in C57BL/6J but not 129S1/SvImJ mice. Am J Physiol Heart Circ Physiol, 297(1): H65-75.

Batur, P., Stewart, W. J., Isaacson, J. H. (2003). Increased prevalence of aortic stenosis in patients with arteriovenous malformations of the gastrointestinal tract in Heyde syndrome. Arch Intern Med, 163(15): 1821-1824.

Bellamy, M.F., Pellikka, P.A., Klarich, K.W., et al. (2002). Association of cholesterol levels, hydroxymethylglutaryl coenzyme-A reductase inhibitor treatment, and progression of aortic stenosis in the community. J Am Coll Cardiol, 40(10): 1723-1730.

Campbell, M. (1968). Calcific aortic stenosis and congenital bicuspid aortic valves. Br Heart J, 30(5): 606-616.

Chan, K.L., Teo, K., Dumesnil, J.G., et al. (2010). Effect of Lipid lowering with rosuvastatin on progression of aortic stenosis: results of the aortic stenosis progression observation: measuring effects of rosuvastatin (ASTRONOMER) trial. Circulation, 121(2): 306-314.

Chandra, H. R., Goldstein, J.A., Choudhary, N., et al. (2004). Adverse outcome in aortic sclerosis is associated with coronary artery disease and inflammation. J Am Coll Cardiol, 43(2): 169-175.

Cosmi, J.E., Kort, S., Tunick, P.A., et al. (2002). The risk of the development of aortic stenosis in patients with "benign" aortic valve thickening. Arch Intern Med, 162(20): 2345-2347.

Cowell, S.J., Newby, D.E., Prescott, R.J., et al. (2005). A randomized trial of intensive lipid-lowering therapy in calcific aortic stenosis. N Engl J Med, 352(23): 2389-2397.

Drolet, M.C., Couet, J., Arsenault, M. (2008). Development of aortic valve sclerosis or stenosis in rabbits: role of cholesterol and calcium. J Heart Valve Dis, 17(4): 381-387.

Freeman, R.V., Crittenden, G., Otto, C. (2004). Acquired aortic stenosis. Expert Rev Cardiovasc Ther, 2(1): 107-116.

Garg, V., Muth, A.N., Ransom, J.F., et al. (2005). Mutations in NOTCH1 cause aortic valve disease. Nature, 437(7056): 270-274.

Gerber, H. P., Vu, T. H., Ryan, A. M., et al. (1999). VEGF couples hypertrophic cartilage remodeling, ossification and angiogenesis during endochondral bone formation. Nat Med, 5(6): 623-628.

Ghaisas, N. K., Foley, J. B., O'Briain, D. S., et al. (2000).Adhesion molecules in nonrheumatic aortic valve disease: endothelial expression, serum levels and effects of valve replacement. J Am Coll Cardiol, 36(7): 2257-2262.

Hage, F. G., Adegunsoye, A., Mundkur, M., et al. (2011). The role of echocardiography in the evaluation and management of aortic stenosis in the older adult. Int J Cardiol.

Hamilton, A. M., Boughner, D. R., Drangova, M., et al. (2011). Statin treatment of hypercholesterolemic-induced aortic valve sclerosis. Cardiovasc Pathol, 20(2): 84-92.

Helske, S., Syvaranta, S., Lindstedt, K.A., et al. (2006). Increased expression of elastolytic cathepsins S, K, and V and their inhibitor cystatin C in stenotic aortic valves. Arterioscler Thromb Vasc Biol, 26(8): 1791-1798.

Kaden, J. J., Bickelhaupt, S., Grobholz, R., et al. (2004). Expression of bone sialoprotein and bone morphogenetic protein-2 in calcific aortic stenosis. J Heart Valve Dis, 13(4): 560-566.

Kaden, J. J., Dempfle, C. E., Grobholz, R., et al. (2003). Interleukin-1 beta promotes matrix metalloproteinase expression and cell proliferation in calcific aortic valve stenosis. Atherosclerosis, 170(2): 205-211.

Kennedy, J. A., Hua, X., Mishra, K., et al. (2009). Inhibition of calcifying nodule formation in cultured porcine aortic valve cells by nitric oxide donors. Eur J Pharmacol, 602(1): 28-35.

Lindroos, M., Kupari, M., Heikkila, J., et al. (1993). Prevalence of aortic valve abnormalities in the elderly: an echocardiographic study of a random population sample. J Am Coll Cardiol, 21(5): 1220-1225.
Linhartova, K., Sterbakova, G., Racek, J., et al. (2009). Linking soluble vascular adhesion molecule-1 level to calcific aortic stenosis in patients with coronary artery disease. Exp Clin Cardiol, 14(3): e80-83.
Marechaux, S., Corseaux, D., Vincentelli, A., et al.(2009). Identification of tissue factor in experimental aortic valve sclerosis. Cardiovasc Pathol, 18(2): 67-76.
Matsumoto, Y., Adams, V., Jacob, S., et al. (2010). Regular exercise training prevents aortic valve disease in low-density lipoprotein-receptor-deficient mice. Circulation, 121(6): 759-767.
Moura, L. M., Ramos, S. F., Zamorano, J. L., et al. (2007).Rosuvastatin affecting aortic valve endothelium to slow the progression of aortic stenosis. J Am Coll Cardiol, 49(5): 554-561.
Ngo, D. T., Heresztyn, T., Mishra, K., et al. (2007). Aortic stenosis is associated with elevated plasma levels of asymmetric dimethylarginine (ADMA). Nitric Oxide, 16(2): 197-201.
Ngo, D. T., Sverdlov, A. L., Willoughby, S. R., et al. (2009). Determinants of occurrence of aortic sclerosis in an aging population. JACC Cardiovasc Imaging, 2(8): 919-927.
Novaro, G. M., Katz, R., Aviles, R. J., et al. (2007). Clinical factors, but not C-reactive protein, predict progression of calcific aortic-valve disease: the Cardiovascular Health Study. J Am Coll Cardiol, 50(20): 1992-1998.
O'Brien, K. D., Reichenbach, D. D., Marcovina, S. M., et al. (1996). Apolipoproteins B, (a), and E accumulate in the morphologically early lesion of 'degenerative' valvular aortic stenosis. Arterioscler Thromb Vasc Biol, 16(4): 523-532.
O'Brien, K. D., Shavelle, D. M., Caulfield, M. T., et al. (2002).Association of angiotensin-converting enzyme with low-density lipoprotein in aortic valvular lesions and in human plasma. Circulation, 106(17): 2224-2230.
Olsson, M., Thyberg, J., Nilsson, J. (1999).Presence of oxidized low density lipoprotein in nonrheumatic stenotic aortic valves. Arterioscler Thromb Vasc Biol, 19(5): 1218-1222.
Ortlepp, J. R., Hoffmann, R., Ohme, F., et al. (2001).The vitamin D receptor genotype predisposes to the development of calcific aortic valve stenosis. Heart, 85(6): 635-638.
Ortlepp, J. R., Schmitz, F., Mevissen, V., et al. (2004). The amount of calcium-deficient hexagonal hydroxyapatite in aortic valves is influenced by gender and associated with genetic polymorphisms in patients with severe calcific aortic stenosis. Eur Heart J, 25(6): 514-522.
Otto, C. M., Kuusisto, J., Reichenbach, D. D., et al. (1994). Characterization of the early lesion of 'degenerative' valvular aortic stenosis. Histological and immunohistochemical studies. Circulation, 90(2): 844-853.
Otto, C. M., Lind, B.K., Kitzman, D. W., et al. (1999). Association of aortic-valve sclerosis with cardiovascular mortality and morbidity in the elderly. N Engl J Med, 341(3): 142-147.
Peltonen, T., Taskinen, P., Napankangas, J., et al. (2009).Increase in tissue endothelin-1 and ETA receptor levels in human aortic valve stenosis. Eur Heart J, 30(2): 242-249.

Rajamannan, N. M., Sangiorgi, G., Springett, M., et al. (2001). Experimental hypercholesterolemia induces apoptosis in the aortic valve. J Heart Valve Dis, 10(3): 371-374.

Rajamannan, N.M., Subramaniam, M., Caira, F., et al (2005). Atorvastatin inhibits hypercholesterolemia-induced calcification in the aortic valves via the Lrp5 receptor pathway. Circulation, 112(9 Suppl): I229-234.

Rajamannan, N. M., Subramaniam, M., Stock, S. R., et al. (2005). Atorvastatin inhibits calcification and enhances nitric oxide synthase production in the hypercholesterolaemic aortic valve. Heart, 91(6): 806-810.

Roberts, W. C. (1970). Anatomically isolated aortic valvular disease. The case against its being of rheumatic etiology. Am J Med, 49(2): 151-159.

Rossebo, A. B., Pedersen, T. R., Boman, K., et al. (2008). Intensive lipid lowering with simvastatin and ezetimibe in aortic stenosis. N Engl J Med, 359(13): 1343-1356.

Sacks, M. S., Yoganathan, A. P. (2007). Heart valve function: a biomechanical perspective. Philos Trans R Soc Lond B Biol Sci, 362(1484): 1369-1391.

Satta, J., Melkko, J., Pollanen, R., et al. (2002). Progression of human aortic valve stenosis is associated with tenascin-C expression. J Am Coll Cardiol, 39(1): 96-101.

Selzer, A. (1987). Changing aspects of the natural history of valvular aortic stenosis. N Engl J Med, 317(2): 91-98.

Shavelle, D. M., Takasu, J., Budoff, M. J., et al. (2002). HMG CoA reductase inhibitor (statin) and aortic valve calcium. Lancet, 359(9312): 1125-1126.

Steinmetz, M., Skowasch, D., Wernert, N., et al. (2008). Differential profile of the OPG/RANKL/RANK-system in degenerative aortic native and bioprosthetic valves. J Heart Valve Dis, 17(2): 187-193.

Stewart, B. F., Siscovick, D., Lind, B. K., et al. (1997). Clinical factors associated with calcific aortic valve disease. Cardiovascular Health Study. J Am Coll Cardiol, 29(3): 630-634.

Sucker, C. (2007). The Heyde syndrome: proposal for a unifying concept explaining the association of aortic valve stenosis, gastrointestinal angiodysplasia and bleeding. Int J Cardiol, 115(1): 77-8.

Zigelman, C. Z., Edelstein, P. M. (2009). Aortic valve stenostenosis. Anesthesiol Clin, 27(3): 519-532, table of contents

7

Calcific Aortic Valve Disease

Jesper Hjortnaes and Elena Aikawa
Brigham and Women's Hospital, Harvard Medical School, Boston, Massachusetts, United States of America

1. Introduction

Aortic stenosis due to calcific aortic valve disease (CAVD) is currently the main indication for aortic valve replacement in developed countries (Iung et al, 2003). Due to an aging population and a decline in rheumatic heart disease, CAVD has become the most common heart valve disease in the Western countries, affecting approximately 25% of adults over 65 years, of which 2-3% has clinically significant aortic stenosis (Stewart et al, 1997). Even mild CAVD is associated with adverse outcomes, with a 50% increased risk of cardiovascular death (Lloyd-Jones et al, 2009). There are no known therapies that slow disease progression, and surgical valve replacement is the only effective treatment for aortic stenosis. More than 85,000 aortic valve replacement surgeries are done in the United States, and over 275,000 are performed worldwide. This numbers are expected to triple by 2050 (Takkenberg et al, 2008). These statistics emphasize the burden of aortic valve disease and the necessity of understanding its mechanisms, underscored recently by recommendations set out by The National Heart, Lung and Blood Institute Aortic Stenosis Working Group (http://www.nhlbi.nih.gov/meetings/workshops/cas.htm).

CAVD is a progressive disease that starts with initial changes in the cell biology of the valve leaflets, which develop into atherosclerotic-like lesions and aortic sclerosis, and eventually lead to calcification of the valve, causing left ventricular outflow tract obstruction (Rajamannan et al, 2007, Otto, 2008). Although CAVD progresses with age, it is not an inevitable consequence of aging. CAVD traditionally has been considered a degenerative phenomenon, in which years of mechanical stress on an otherwise normal valve, cause calcium to deposit on the surface of the aortic valve leaflets. The evolving concept, however, is that CAVD is an actively regulated process that cannot be characterized simply as "senile" or "degenerative". The progressive calcification process involves lipid accumulation, increasing angiotensin-converting enzyme activity, inflammation, neovascularization, and extracellular matrix degradation.

Furthermore, the risk factors for CAVD are similar to those for atherosclerosis: age, gender, hypercholesterolemia, diabetes, smoking, renal failure, and hypertension (Stewart et al, 1997). In addition, pathological studies of explanted human stenotic aortic valves have identified lesions similar to those in atherosclerotic plaques, which contain inflammatory cells and calcific deposits (Otto et al, 1994). The involvement of high cholesterol levels is corroborated by studies demonstrating that patients with familial hypercholesterolemia develop aortic valve lesions that calcify with age (Rajamannan et al, 2001). Furthermore, preclinical studies have demonstrated atherosclerotic-like lesions in aortic valve leaflets in

atherosclerosis in rabbits and mice. From the notion that CAVD and atherosclerosis might share a similar mechanism, statins (3-hydroxy-3-methylglutaryl-coenzyme A [HMG-CoA] reductase inhibitors) emerged as a potential therapy for treating CAVD. Indeed, retrospective studies have demonstrated a reduction in disease progression when patients were treated with statins (Aronow et al, 2001, Novaro et al, 2001, Bellamy et al, 2002). In addition, animal studies confirmed that statin treatment inhibits calcificication (Rajamannan et al, 2005, Aikawa et al, 2007). Large prospective clinical trials, however have not shown slowed CAVD progression in patients treated with high doses of statins (Cowell et al, 2005, Rossebo et al, 2008). This may be due to the late implementation of the statins, after aortic valve calcification has progressed to the irreversible stage.
The aortic valve consists of endothelial cells and valvular interstitial cells that maintain the health of the valve and are important in valvular disease. Valvular interstitial cells likely mediate the progression of CAVD (Mohler et al, 1999). Signals in aortic valve biology that trigger activation, differentiation, or pathological change are unclear. However, we know that in CAVD, valvular interstitial cells differentiate to myofibroblasts and osteoblast-like cells, which are eventually responsible for calcium deposition (Mohler et al, 2001). Possible pathological triggers include hemodynamic shear stress, solid tissue stresses, reactive oxygen species (ROS), inflammatory cytokines and growth factors, and physiological imbalances such as the metabolic syndrome, diabetes mellitus, end-stage renal disease, and calcium or phosphate imbalance (Schoen, 2008, New & Aikawa, 2011, Miller et al, 2010). The cellular and molecular factors involved in the development of aortic valve stenosis, however, remain largely obscure. The poor prognosis and increased mortality after the onset of symptoms provide a rationale for the pursuit of a better understanding of the disease process, which can lead to effective therapeutic strategies to prevent CAVD. This chapter discusses our current understanding of the pathophysiology, risk factors, cellular mechanisms, diagnosis, and clinical management of CAVD, and describes areas of future research vital for diagnosing, treating, and potentially preventing this disease.

2. Normal aortic valve physiology and function

Aortic heart valves maintain unidirectional blood flow throughout the cardiac cycle with minimal obstruction, without regurgitation. The aortic valve prevents retrograde flow back into the left ventricle during diastole. Heart valves open and close approximately 40 million times a year, and 3 billion times over an average lifetime. Mechanical forces exerted by the surrounding blood and heart drive the aortic valve's function. The dynamic structure and physiology of aortic heart valves enables them to avoid excess stress concentration and to withstand wear and tear over many years (Breuer et al, 2004). Aortic valve functionality must be seen in conjunction with the aortic root, and be viewed as one apparatus (Schoen, 2008). A variety of pathological processes can lead to aortic valve malfunction, with serious clinical consequences. This malfunction usually is associated with calcific changes of the valve connective tissue, and eventually causes aortic stenosis. Before we elaborate on the pathological mechanisms of CAVD, we will discuss normal aortic valve anatomy and physiology and their relationship to aortic valve function.

2.1 Aortic valve anatomy

The aortic cusps are thin, flexible structures that come together to seal the valve orifice during diastole. The aortic valve is normally composed of three cusps or leaflets. The individual cusps are attached to the aortic wall in a semilunar fashion, ascending to the commissures (where adjacent cusps come together at the aorta) and descending to the basal attachment of each cusp to the aortic wall; this anatomical structure is also called the aortic valve annulus. A portion of the annulus is attached to cardiac muscle, while the other half is continuous with the fibrous leaflets of the mitral valve. The functional unit of the aortic valve includes the cusps and their respective aortic sinus complexes, also called the aortic root. The aortic root is a bulb-shaped structure to which the aortic cusps are attached. Behind the aortic valve cusps are dilated pockets in the aortic root known as the *sinuses of Valsalva*, from which the coronary arteries originate. The nomenclature of the aortic valve cusps and their respective sinuses are based on the position of the coronary artery ostia – the left coronary cusp, the right coronary cusp, and the non-coronary cusp (and their associated sinuses).

In the middle of the free margin of each cusp on the ventricular surface is a pronounced thickening, known as the *nodule of Arantius.* Coaptation of these three nodules ensures complete closure of the valve during diastole. Along the ventricular surface of each cusp, between the free edge and the closing edge, is a crescent shaped region called a *lunula.* These thin areas of leaflet contact the corresponding regions of both adjacent cusps to ensure a competent seal. The remainder of the cusp (noncoapting portion) is known as the *belly.* Native human aortic valves are virtually avascular, and receive nutrients through hemodynamic convection and diffusion. In most cases, the dimensions of the three leaflets are slightly unequal (Roberts, 1970). The dynamic, complex three-dimensional anatomy of the aortic trileaflet cusps and the aortic root allows for stress sharing between leaflets, the sinuses of Valsalva, and the aortic wall (Thubrikar et al, 1986a, Katayama et al, 2008).

2.2 Aortic valve function

The aortic valve functions synergistically with the aortic root to maintain efficient cyclic opening and closing – opening when exposed to forward flow, and then rapidly and completely closing under minimal reverse pressure. Importantly, opening of the valve precedes, rather than responds to, the forward movement of blood from the ventricle (Thubrikar et al, 1979, Higashidate et al, 1995). This illustrates the complex function of the valve, and is one of the reasons for considering movement of the whole root – from the level of the annulus to the sinotubular junction – when describing aortic valve functionality.

As blood decelerates in the aorta at the end of systole, vortexes in the sinuses of Valsalva behind the AV cusps facilitate valve closure. These vortexes help funnel oxygenated blood into the coronary arteries and create a small pressure gradient across the leaflet, which helps bring the leaflets to a smooth and efficient closure.

The ability to prevent reverse flow of the aortic valve depends on the stretching and molding of the three cusps to fill the orifice during the closed phase of the cardiac cycle, during which back pressure from the blood is present in the aorta. Simultaneously, the valve annulus expands, pulling the cusps and thus preventing collapse (Thubrikar et al, 1980).

A further increase in the annular radius at end diastole and into the isovolumic contraction phase of the cardiac cycle pulls the cusps from their commissures such that a small stellate orifice results, even without the presence of transvalvular flow (Butcher et al, 2011). The valve orifice changes quickly from stellate, to triangular, and finally a to a circular pattern, as blood is ejected from the ventricle. The aortic root adjusts from a conical to a cylindrical shape during ejection, providing optimal hemodynamics at the larger flow volume

(Thubrikar et al, 1979). The aortic valve closes much more gradually than it opens. The total surface area of the three cusps is approximately 40% larger than the cross-sectional area of the aortic root at the annular level. This allows each cusp to bow slightly towards the left ventricular outflow tract, which prevents the cusp from inverting during diastole (Ho, 2009). The normal aortic valve orifice area (AVA) is 2.6-3.5 cm^2, however depends on the body mass area of the individual (Fowler, 1979).

2.3 Aortic valve structure

The structure of the aortic valve cusps is organized into three layers: (i) the *zona ventricularis*, closest to the left ventricle chamber and composed largely of elastin, which can extend in diastole and recoil in systole to minimize cusp area; (ii) the *zona fibrosa*, closest to the outflow surface, rich in densely packed collagen organized in radial and circumferential direction, which provides the strength and stiffness of the cusps and is mainly responsible for bearing diastolic stress; and (iii) the centrally located *zona spongiosa*, which consists mainly of glycosaminoglycans (GAGs) that accommodate shear forces of the cuspal layers, and absorbs shock during the valve cycle (Schoen, 2008). (Figure 1)

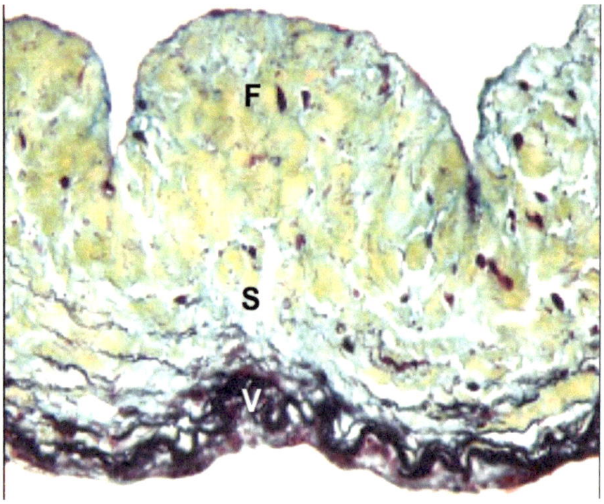

Fig. 1. Human normal aortic valve histopathology depicts a tri-layered structure (F) - fibrosa, (S) - spongiosa and (V) - ventricularis. Modified from Aikawa E. et al, Circulation, 2006

This organization of the aortic native heart valve allows for certain unique qualities. First, accordion-like folds called corrugations, present in the valve cusps, allow for the cuspal shape and dimensions to vary with the cardiac cycle. Second, microscopic collagen folding (also known as *crimp*) allows lengthening of the valve at minimal stress. Cusp tissue also displays anisotropy, the quality conferred by collagen architecture that permits differences in radial and circumferential extensibility. Finally, the macroscopic collagen alignment enables forces from the cusps to transfer to the aortic wall (De Hart et al, 2004). By employing these properties, the native heart valve avoids excess stress concentration on the cusps and supporting tissues and can withstand biomechanical loads caused by repetitive deformations. In addition, biomechanical stress may induce the remodelling and repair of connective tissue (Breuer et al, 2004). The aortic valve tissue possesses a cellular make-up that withstands a large amount of pressures and stresses.

2.4 Aortic valve biology

The native aortic heart valve consists of two types of cells: valvular interstitial cells (VICs) that permeate the entire valve tissue, and valvular endothelial cells (VECs) that cover the surface. The components of the extracellular matrix (ECM) are synthesized, degraded, and maintained by VICs, which seem to have adaptive characteristics. In the healthy aortic valve, they have primarily quiescent fibroblast-like properties, but they can change to an activated phenotype during valvular remodelling, response to injury, or pathology. VECs regulate immune and inflammation responses and provide the native heart valve with its nonthrombogenic properties (Butcher et al, 2004). Small populations of smooth muscle cells (Cimini et al, 2003) and nerve cells have also been described (Chester et al, 2008, Marron et al, 1996).

2.4.1 Valvular interstitial cells

VICs remodel ECM proteins in the aortic valve leaflet, and are of mesenchymal origin. Different phenotypes of VICs are present in the mature native valve. Five identifiable phenotypes of VICs have been described: embryonic mesenchymal cells, quiescent VICs (qVICs), activated VICs (aVICs), progenitor VICs (pVICs), and osteoblastic VICs (oVICs) (Yperman et al, 2004, Taylor et al, 2003, Liu et al, 2007, Rabkin-Aikawa et al, 2004, Rabkin et al, 2001). qVICs are at rest in the valvular interstitium and maintain normal valve physiology by becoming activated in response to injury or disease. This process leads to the differentiation of VICs into activated VICs, demonstrating a fibroblast-like phenotype. More specifically, aortic valve VICs secrete and turn over proteins at an increased rate compared to other cell types in vivo, which indicates that VICs continually repair mechanically induced tissue micro-damage to enable long-term durability. ECM remodelling results from the synthesis of ECM-degrading enzymes by VICs, such as matrix metalloproteinases (e.g., MMP-1, MMP-2, MMP-9, and MMP-13) and cathepsins (e.g., cathepsins S, K, and B), and tissue inhibitors (e.g., tissue inhibitors of metalloproteinases [TIMP] Rabkin et al, 2001, Schoen, 2008). The cellular and molecular mechanisms that control this phenotype differentiation also participate in aortic valve pathology. In particular, VICs become activated when stimulated by mechanical loading, and mediate connective tissue remodelling to restore a normal stress profile in the tissue (Aikawa et al, 2006).

The pressure load applied to the leaflet causes an increase in circumferential and radial leaflet length, which increases strain on the tissue (Butcher et al, 2008). Valve strain seems highest at areas where leaflets attach to the aortic wall; these locations are also where calcification begins in CAVD (Thubrikar et al, 1986b, Levitt et al, 1984). Mechanical forces acting on the valve translate into biological responses at the tissue level, which in turn lead to a VIC response at the cellular level – which causes constant synthesis and renewal of the ECM (Mulholland and Gotlieb, 1996). Intracellular signaling leads to changes that include increased VIC stiffness and increased ECM biosynthesis. Concurrently, the higher valvular pressure gradients on the left side of the heart lead to larger local tissue stress on VICs, which in turn lead to higher VIC stiffness and collagen biosynthesis in the left-sided valves (Merryman et al, 2006).

2.4.2 Endothelial cells

The surface of the aortic valve is lined with a single monolayer of VECs that maintain non-thrombogenicity. VECs are similar to arterial endothelial cells in the expression of von

Willebrand factor because they produce nitric oxide and have prostacyclin activity (Butcher et al, 2008). Cell junctions between VECs are also similar to those of arterial endothelial cells. VECs however seem to be phenotypically different from arterial endothelial cells (Jaffee, 1967), based on the observation that VECs originate developmentally from sources different from arterial endothelial cells. In addition, VECs are oriented circumferentially across leaflets, perpendicular to the direction of the blood flow, in contrast to vascular endothelium, which aligns parallel to flow (Deck, 1986; Schoen, 2008). Comparing valvular and vascular endothelium in a static culture has led to the identification of significantly different genes (Butcher et al, 2006). In addition, although VECs and arterial endothelial cells are both prone to calcification, different mechanisms lie at the heart of the process. VECs show an increased expression of genes involved in chondrogenic differentiation, while arterial endothelial cells more strongly express osteogenic genes (Butcher et al., 2011).

Due to their location at the surface of the aortic valve, VECs are important in relation to the hemodynamic forces exerted on the heart valve. The ventricularis part of the valve (inflow) is exposed to rapid, pulsatile, unidirectional shear stress. In contrast, the fibrosa part of the valve (outflow) experiences a lower, almost oscillatory shear stress (Kilner et al, 2000). Interestingly, recent evidence suggests that different transcriptional profiles are expressed by the endothelium on the opposite faces (ventricularis vs. fibrosa) of a normal adult pig aortic valve. (Simmons et al, 2005) Studies have demonstrated that high pulsatile shear stress on the fibrosa side of the aortic valve increases inflammatory receptors and the expression of bone morphogenic protein (BMP) (Sucosky et al, 2009), but also decreases the expression of inhibitors of fibrosis and calcification, including osteoprotegerin (OPG), C-type natriuretic peptide (CNP), and chordin (Yip et al, 2009). In addition, *in vivo* studies have demonstrated that CAVD initiates on the fibrosa side of the valve (Mohler et al, 2001, Mohler, 2004). Investigators have hypothesized that these differences in endothelium between opposite sides of the aortic valve may contribute to the typical predominant localization of pathologic aortic valve calcification near the outflow surface (*zona fibrosa*) (Simmons et al, 2005). In addition, a recent study has demonstrated that mechanical stress may induce the osteogenic potential of VECs, providing evidence that the valvular endothelium harbours a reserve of progenitor cells that can repopulate the leaflet with osteogenic-like interstitial cells (New & Aikawa, 2011, Wylie-Sears et al, 2011). Future studies are needed to show whether this mechanism, in combination with pro-inflammatory factors, contributes to valve calcification.

2.4.3 Cellular interaction

VICs and VECs exist in close communication, which indicates that cellular interaction is vital for leaflet biology. Studies have demonstrated that VECs interact with VICs in a complex hemodynamic and mechanical environment to maintain aortic valve cusp tissue integrity. Additionally, VECs regulate VIC function through paracrine signals, such as controlling VIC contractility and leaflet mechanics (El-Hamamsy et al, 2009). More specifically, valvular endothelial dysfunction has been implicated as the initiator of inflammatory reactions, blood clots, and even calcification (Butcher & Nerem, 2006). The interaction between vascular endothelial cells and vascular smooth muscle cells, and its importance to normal vessel function, has been well documented. Such interaction likely exists between valvular endothelium and VICs.

VIC–VEC co-culture studies have corroborated that VECs help maintain a qVIC phenotype (Butcher & Nerem, 2006). Moreover, when exposed to shear stress, the presence of endothelium stabilized VIC proliferation, increased the synthesis of ECM proteins by VICs, and decreased GAG loss (Butcher & Nerem, 2006). These results suggest that damage to or loss of valvular endothelium leads to VIC hyperplasia and myofibroblast activation. When the endothelial layer of aortic valve explants was removed, it promoted the formation of calcific nodules (Mohler et al, 1999). Studies also have demonstrated that neurogenic dilation of aortic valve cusps only occurred only when the endothelium was intact (Chester et al, 2008). The communication between VECs and VICs is fundamental in normal and pathological signalling, but more work is needed to further delineate these relationships.

3. Clinical aspects of calcific aortic valve disease

CAVD is a progressive disease that begins with initial changes in the cell biology of valve leaflets, develops into atherosclerotic lesions and aortic sclerosis, that eventually leads to calcification of the valve, which causes left ventricular outflow tract obstruction. This is known as calcific aortic stenosis, which is viewed as the critical end stage of this disease process, and is associated with poor outcomes.

3.1 Epidemiology

CAVD is the most common cause of aortic stenosis in the developed world. Increased aortic valve cusp thickness due to fibrosis and lipid accumulation, but without left ventricular outflow tract obstruction, is known as *aortic valve sclerosis*. Aortic valve sclerosis and aortic stenosis are generally viewed as the early stage and late stage, respectively, of the CAVD pathological process. Aortic sclerosis is common in the elderly population; the prevalence in the general population is 29% (Stewart et al, 1997). A landmark study (Stewart et al, 1997) identified 26% of study population older than 65 years having aortic sclerosis, indicating that aortic sclerosis associates with age. In the same population, 2% had aortic stenosis. These numbers increase with age – those over 74 years old, 37% had aortic sclerosis, and almost 3% had aortic stenosis. Importantly, approximately 16% of patients with aortic sclerosis will develop aortic stenosis within 6 to 8 years (Cosmi et al, 2002). Other studies have reported that up to 33% of patients with aortic sclerosis developed aortic stenosis within 4 years of follow-up (Faggiano et al, 2003). No known therapies slow aortic valve disease progression, and surgical valve replacement currently is the only effective treatment for aortic stenosis. In addition, aortic valve sclerosis increases the risk of myocardial infarction or cardiovascular death by 50% (Lloyd-Jones, 2009). As such, aortic valve disease has a serious impact on general health.

3.2 Risk factors

Calcific aortic stenosis shares nearly identical risk factors with atherosclerosis. Clinical risk factors for calcific aortic stenosis include age, male sex, hypertension, smoking, elevated serum levels of lipoprotein (A), and low-density lipoprotein (LDL) levels (Stewart et al, 1997). Other studies have demonstrated that traditional risk factors that are important in atherosclerosis, including the metabolic syndrome and renal failure, also associate with calcifc aortic stenosis (Aronow et al, 1987, Katz et al, 2009, Otto et al, 1997, Fox et al, 2006). This overlapping of risk factors has led to the hypothesis that calcific aortic valve disease and atherosclerosis have similar etiologies, but there are epidemiological discrepancies, as demonstrated by the inconsistency in coexisting prevalence between calcific aortic stenosis and coronary artery disease. Only 50% of patients with severe calcific aortic stenosis have significant coronary artery disease, and the majority of patients with coronary artery disease have no calcific aortic stenosis (Otto & O'Brien, 2001). Furthermore, metabolic diseases such as hyperparathyroidism (secondary to chronic renal failure, Paget's disease) have also associated with accelerated progression of aortic valve calcification and stenosis (Horl, 2004, Hultgren, 1998). Further studies are needed to understand the differences between the pathophysiologies of atherosclerosis and aortic valve disease.

3.3 Pathophysiology and diagnosis

A discrepancy exists between the onset of symptoms and the onset of disease. Symptoms usually do not occur until calcific aortic stenosis has developed. The symptoms and clinical signs of CAVD are better understood by discussing the physiological changes that occur. Calcific aortic stenosis leads to left ventricular outflow tract obstruction, which causes several physiological changes, best described in a left ventricular pressure-volume loop. Ventricular emptying is impaired by outflow tract resistance, which results from a reduced aortic valve orifice area during systole. This, in turn, causes a large pressure gradient over the aortic valve – which means that ventricular pressure needs to exceed the increased aortic pressure gradient, causing increased peak systolic pressure and subsequent aortic valve closure due to an increased end-systolic volume. Consequently, stroke volume decreases. Higher end-systolic volume raises the afterload, and thus the incoming venous return, leading to increased end-diastolic volume. This process activates the Frank-Starling mechanism, which increases contraction force and thus maintains a normal stroke volume when the aortic stenosis is mild. Stenosis severity correlates with the increase of left ventricular outflow tract obstruction and afterload. When the end-systolic volume increases more than the end-diastolic volume, stroke volume will decrease, leading to a reduction in arterial pressure. The cardiovascular system will strive to maintain arterial pressure, increasing peripheral vascular resistance. In addition, the left ventricular heart muscle will demonstrate hypertrophy to compensate for a chronic increase of afterload. Most cardiovascular systems can compensate for aortic stenosis until the orifice diameter is less than 0.6 cm^2/m^2 (~1.0 cm^2). The patient will remain relatively asymptomatic up to this point, due to adequate physiological compensatory mechanisms. Symptoms generally appear when the valve orifice is around 1.0 cm^2, and typically include shortness of breath, syncope, and chest pain. Left ventricular hypertrophy combined with a stenotic aortic valve may lead to impaired blood flow to the heart muscle, in turn causing increased oxygen demand by the heart muscle and leading to angina pectoris. Aortic stenosis can present itself clinically with a systolic ejection murmur at the right upper sternal border, often radiating to the neck. Peaking of the murmur late in systole, a palpable delay of the carotid upstroke, and a soft second heart sound can all point to aortic stenosis. Aortic stenosis is usually confirmed using ultrasound echocardiography (Nakamura et al, 1984, Braun & Comeau, 1951). The severity of aortic valve dysfunction is determined by the combination of the following hemodynamic indices: peak ejection velocity, effective orifice area, and mean transvalvular pressure gradient (Nakamura et al, 1984). As described earlier, CAVD progression involves the narrowing of the valve orifice and increased ventricular ejection velocities and pressure gradients. Mild aortic valve stenosis is generally defined by restricted opening of the valve cusps, with a mean transvalvular pressure gradient of less than 25 mm Hg; moderate aortic valve stenosis by a mean gradient between 25 and 40 mm Hg; and severe aortic valve stenosis by a mean gradient of 40 mm Hg or more (Cosmi et al, 2002). Because direct imaging of the aortic valve still involves technical challenges, echocardiography remains the gold standard for assessing aortic valve dysfunction (Aikawa & Otto, 2011).

3.4 Treatment

3.4.1 Surgical treatment

Unless discovered during monitoring for other conditions, patients rarely exhibit detectable symptoms of aortic valve disease until after it has already progressed to an advanced stage (Rosenhek et al, 2000). Patients with severe aortic stenosis have a life expectancy of less than 10 years if untreated. Of these patients with concomitant heart failure, 50% will die within a year (Carabello & Paulus, 2009). Aortic valve replacement is the only effective treatment, but optimal timing for surgery in asymptomatic patients remains unclear (Stout & Otto, 2007). Asymptomatic patients have good survival without surgery, and combined with the surgical risk for operative mortality and post-operative complications, surgeons are reluctant to perform valve replacement in these patients (Owen & Henein, 2011). Replacement valves, be they mechanical or bioprosthetic, have several shortcomings. The body recognizes a mechanical valve as foreign material, giving rise to thromboembolic compications that require lifelong anticoagulation therapy. (Hammermeister et al, 2000). Bioprosthetic valves are prone to reduced durability (~20 years) because of structural dysfunction resulting from progressive leaflet deterioration and calcification, eventually requiring reoperation (Hammermeister et al, 2000, Bloomfield et al, 1991). Bioprosthetic valves are the conduits of choice for patients over 60–65 years who are relatively physically inactive, and when there is a contraindication for anticoagulation therapy. Mechanical valves are chosen for active patients under 60 years, who can tolerate anticoagulation therapy.

3.4.2 Pharmacological treatment

The need for alternatives to surgery is emphasized by the increasing age of the general population and the rising prevalence of CAVD. Therapeutic strategies to restrict disease progression are needed to delay and possibly avoid surgical valve replacement. Because CAVD and atherosclerosis have similar disease progression and risk factors, pharmacological treatment of CAVD mostly has been focused on lipid-lowering agents (statins) and angiotensin-converting enzyme (ACE) inhibitors (Stewart et al, 1997, O'Brien et al, 2002). LDLs are present in human aortic valve lesions. In addition, studies have demonstrated the presence of oxidized lipids in calcifying areas of aortic valves. (Olsson et al, 1999) Statins inhibit the pathway for synthesizing cholesterol in the liver and lower plasma cholesterol levels. Animal studies and retrospective clinical studies have demonstrated that statins could potentially slow CAVD progression (Rosenhek et al, 2004, Novaro et al, 2001, Shavelle et al, 2002, Moura et al, 2007). However, large clinical trials have demonstrated that statins do not affect CAVD in general valve disease population (Rosenhek et al, 2004, Novaro et al, 2001, Shavelle et al, 2002, Moura et al, 2007; Holme et al, 2010; Chan et al, 2010; Cowell et al, 2005). ACE, angiotensin II, and angiotensin II type 1 receptors have also been identified in aortic sclerotic lesions (O'Brien et al, 2002, Helske et al, 2004). Retrospective studies associate ACE inhibitors with a lower rate of aortic valve calcification, but ACE inhibitors do not inhibit CAVD progression (Rosenhek et al, 2004). Interestingly, angiotensin II type 1 antagonists have prevented aortic valve lesion formation in hypercholesterolemic rabbits (Arishiro et al, 2007). Trials are ongoing to elucidate further the effect of ACE inhibitors on the progression of CAVD. As we gain more information about the specific mechanisms of CAVD, different potential pharmaceutical targets surface. The valve endothelium has received a great deal of attention and could potentially be a drug delivery platform. A recently developed method tests for the presence or absence of diseased aortic valves in atherosclerotic mice using an anti-VCAM-1 peptide to target early-stage aortic valve disease endothelium (Aikawa et al, 2007a). We still generally lack clinically significant pharmacological therapies for CAVD, which indicates the importance of additional research to elucidate mechanisms of CAVD progression.

4. Pathology of calcific aortic valve disease

4.1 Pathology

CAVD is a progressive disorder that ranges from mild valve thickening to severe calcification with impaired leaflet motion or aortic valve stenosis (Freeman & Otto, 2005). Though CAVD traditionally was viewed as a passive degenerative disease resulting from years of stress, we now recognize it as an actively regulated disease, with evidence suggesting that it follows a mechanism akin to bone formation (Mohler et al, 2001). Pathologically, stenotic valves are characterized by the presence of chronic inflammatory cellular infiltrates such as macrophages and T-lymphocytes, by the accumulation of lipids, and by thickening of the *fibrosa* and mineralization (Otto et al, 1994). Early CAVD lesions are similar to atherosclerosis lesions, consisting of prominent LDL, lipoprotein (a), and apolipoproteins (O'Brien et al, 1996). Inflammatory cells and lipids in stenotic valve leaflets co-localize near the surface of CAVD lesions, supporting the notion that CAVD is an active inflammatory disease process.

The extent to which the mechanism of CAVD is similar to that of atherosclerosis remains unclear (Mohler, 2004, Rajamannan et al, 2007). Both CAVD and atherosclerosis seem to be initiated by endothelial dysfunction involving differentiation of underlying interstitial cells. In both diseases, endothelial dysfunction relates to disturbed blood flow, to bifurcations and sinuses in larger arteries, and to the outflow (*fibrosa*) side of the aortic valve (Porat et al, 2004). Both CAVD lesions and atherosclerotic lesions contain inflammatory cells, with advanced lesions containing calcium deposits (Hjortnaes et al, 2010). In addition, pathological studies of human stenotic valves have identified lesions similar to those in atherosclerotic plaques (Otto et al, 1994, Olsson et al, 1999), and similar lesions have been described in aortic valve leaflets of atherosclerosis in rabbits and mice (Tanaka et al, 2005, Aikawa et al, 2007b).

But differences exist between the pathologies of CAVD and atherosclerosis. First, CAVD can be present in younger patients — such as patients with bicuspid aortic valves, which usually are heavily calcified shortly after birth (Sabet et al, 1999). Second, discrepancies may exist between the pathological compositions of CAVD lesions and atherosclerosis lesions. Aortic plaques at the late stage of atherosclerosis contain lipid accumulations and fibrous tissue, and large calcific nodules mainly formed through apoptosis or matrix vesicles formation. Aortic valve lesions, in contrast, are pathologically composed of large, bone-like matrix nodules formed by osteoblast-like cells. In addition, calcified lesions in end-stage aortic valve disease progressively stiffen the valve leaflets, causing motion impairment. End-stage atherosclerotic lesions, however, demonstrate plaque ruptures and thrombotic occlusions. These differences support the notion that CAVD has characteristics that are different from those of atherosclerosis, which indicates the presence of potentially different and complex mechanisms.

The current pathological concept of CAVD is that mechanical stress, together with atherosclerotic risk factors, leads to valvular endothelial dysfunction, followed by the deposition of LDL particles and other compounds that trigger inflammation. The inflammatory state can lead to the activation of inflammatory signalling pathways, macrophage infiltration, and T-lymphocyte activation. Activation of inflammatory pathways contributes to the disease process, which in turn activates VICs to express osteoblastic phenotypes and cause calcium deposition. Our current understanding of the role of VECs and VICs in the disease process will be discussed later in this chapter.

4.2 Endothelial dysfunction

As described earlier, the surface of the aortic valve is lined with an endothelial monolayer. Although the exact initiating factors for the inflammatory process in CAVD are unclear, studies have demonstrated that the endothelium plays an important role. Because VECs are located at the surface of the aortic valve, the endothelium is subjected to hemodynamic forces. Different shear stresses are exerted on each side of the aortic valve. In vivo studies have demonstrated that early CAVD lesions initiate on the fibrosa (outflow) side of the valve (Sucosky et al, 2009). Endothelium subjected to abnormal blood flow seems more susceptible to inflammatory cytokines (Aikawa et al, 2006, Sacks & Yoganathan, 2007). Research has shown that high pulsatile shear stress on the *fibrosa* side of the aortic valve induces upregulation of inflammatory receptors by VECs for circulating cytokines and inflammatory monocytes, leukocytes and T-lymphocytes (Muller et al, 2000, Shavelle et al, 2008). In addition, elevated stretch loading on the aortic valve induced pro-inflammatory cytokine (bone morphogenetic protein [BMP2/4]) expression on the fibrosa part of the aortic valve. These results indicate the potential role of BMPs in early CAVD lesions {Balachandran et al, 2010}. Another mechanism proposed as an initiating factor in CAVD, but also in atherosclerosis, is the expression of pro-oxidant phenotypes (ROS) in VECs (Butcher et al, 2006, Sucosky et al, 2009, Sorescu et al, 2004). ROS, including oxidized lipids, can cause endothelial cell injury, which can lead to a loss of endothelial alignment and an increase the upregulation of cell adhesion molecules — permitting increased inflammatory infiltration (Mirzaie et al, 2003). These events may together or individually initiate and/or sustain chronic inflammation, and lead to the development of CAVD (Mohler, 2004). The expression of endothelial nitric oxide synthase (eNOS) — a vasodilator that protects blood vessels against atherosclerosis — is reduced in conditions with oxidative stress, such as disturbed blood flow, but is elevated by antioxidant signalling. Although its role in CAVD is less clear, eNOS expression is reduced on the VECs of the fibrosa side compared to the ventricularis side of the aortic valve. This reduction indicates that eNOS might be involved in the *fibrosa* susceptibility in CAVD pathogenesis (Butcher et al, 2006). Moreover, inhibition of eNOS expression results in increased cusp stiffness of the aortic valve (El-Hamamsy et al, 2009). Statins decreased the amount of calcification and increased VEC eNOS in rabbits, which suggests that eNOS may protect against CAVD. Our own studies, however, demonstrated an induction of eNOS expression on the fibrosa vs ventricularis sides during fetal valve development (Figure 2). Therefore, further studies are warranted to investigate these mechanisms.

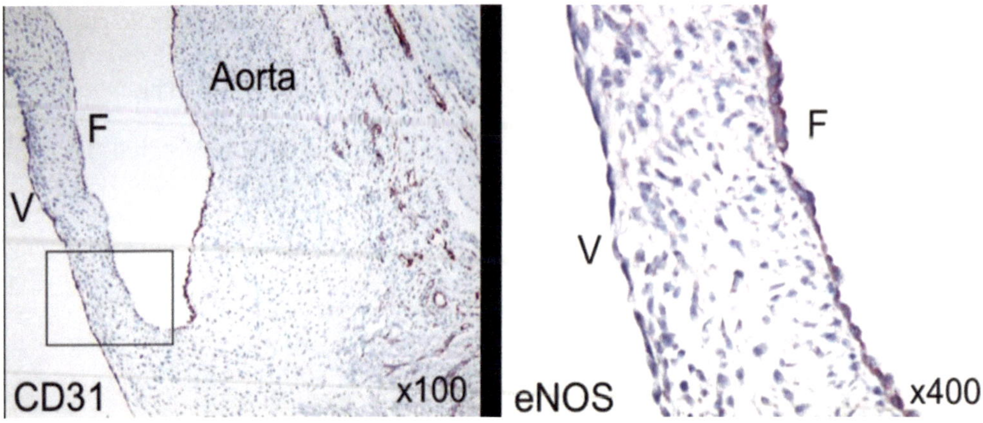

Fig. 2. Human fetal aortic valve section immunostained with anti-CD31 and anti-eNOS reveals side-specific expression of eNOS. (F) - fibrosa, (V) - ventricularis

4.3 Valvular interstitial cell remodelling and the role of the extracellular matrix

VICs are responsible for the physiological remodelling that maintains integrity and pliability in the aortic valve. In terms of CAVD, the general hypothesis is that VICs undergo myofibroblast differentiation to become osteoblast-like cells, which in turn deposit calcium in the aortic valve. This myofibroblast activation seems to be activated by invading inflammatory cells and activated endothelial cells that produce cytokines such as TGF-β1, BMP2/4, IL-1, IL- 6 and TNF-α. Increased α-smooth muscle actin (α-SMA) and smooth muscle myosin (SMM), decreased vimentin, increased migration, and increased proliferation characterize myofibroblast activation of VICs. (Taylor et al, 2003, Yip et al, 2009, Jian et al, 2003, Kaden et al, 2005b) Furthermore, studies have demonstrated that in CAVD, inflammatory cells and VICs secrete MMPs and cathepsins, which are involved in extracellular remodelling (Aikawa et al, 2009, Rabkin et al, 2001, Soini et al, 2001, Fondard et al, 2005). The exact role of the inhibitors of these proteins, such as TIMPs and cystatin C, which are also expressed by VICs in CAVD, remains to be established. In CAVD, the *zona fibrosa* is especially prone to this remodelling process, characterized by disruption and disorganization of collagen bundles, fragmentation of elastin, and an increase in proteoglycan deposition. The disruption of the ECM contributes to the release of growth factors such as TGF-β1, which consequently influences VIC differentiation (as described earlier). The osteoblast-like cell differentiation of VICs is subject to a number of mechanisms, which are described in the next section.

5. Cellular and molecular mechanisms of CAVD

CAVD is an active disease process characterized by progressive calcification of the valve leaflet by VICs and inflammatory cells. The cellular and molecular mechanisms are complex and involve growth factors, lipoproteins, and biomechanical factors. The molecular pathways that may participate in CAVD include Wnt, the angiotensin/kinin system, and the OPG/RANKL/RANK signalling pathways. Growth factors such as TGF–β (Jian et al, 2003) and cytokines (IL-6 and TNF-α) (O'Brien et al, 2002, Kaden et al, 2005b) also seem to affect the osteoblastic differentiation of VICs. Specific bone-cell phenotypes are present in calcifying human valves (Rajamannan et al, 2003). Increased levels of specific bone formation markers have been identified in CAVD. These include the non-collagenous bone matrix proteins such as osteopontin, osteocalcin, and bone sialoprotein (Kaden et al, 2004b, Mohler et al, 1997). The osteoblast transcription factor runx2 /cbfa1 has also been identified in calcified aortic valves (Caira et al, 2006). The LDL-receptor-related protein 5/wingless-type MMTC integration site family member 3 (Lrp5/Wnt3) signalling pathway regulates osteoblast differentiation in the aortic valve (Johnson & Rajamannan, 2006). Neoangiogenesis also has been implicated in the development of CAVD lesions (Chalajour et al, 2004). The exact cellular and molecular mechanisms of CAVD, however, remain scant.

5.1 Biomechanics

The roles of mechanical and hemodynamic factors have been well studied, considering the context of designing and analyzing prosthetic valves. CAVD associates with mechanical and hemodynamic factors, as demonstrated by the correlation of CAVD lesions with regions of disturbed blood flow. Mechanical forces are vital in valve homoeostasis, but deviations from normal mechanical stress patterns can exacerbate pathological differentiation, as seen in CAVD. Contrary to the traditional belief that mechanical forces contribute to valve disease in a wear-and-tear fashion, we now see a direct relationship between mechanics and the active regulation of the aortic valve cell phenotype. This relationship is corroborated by studies that describe a side-specific pathological susceptibility of CAVD, demonstrating that the *zona fibrosa* especially suffers from mechanically induced pathological development. This relationship also reflects the difference in cellular level strains in valve tissue layers when subjected to mechanical forces. Mechanical forces and hemodynamic changes associated with CAVD exert their influence on the cells with which they are in direct contact, namely endothelial cells. The exposure of shear stress to valve endothelial cells leads to the downregulation of genes associated with the activation and osteogenic differentiation of VICs (Butcher et al, 2006, Sucosky et al, 2009). VICs exposed to pathological cyclic strain demonstrated increased expression of (α-SMA, BMP2/4, MMP, and cathepsin activity (Balachandran et al, 2010). Similarly, hypertensive pressure showed increased VCAM-1 expression and decreased osteopontin (Warnock et al, 2006). Myofibroblast activation is also observed in autologous replacement valves implanted in an increased pressure environment, such as pulmonary autografts (Ross procedure) or tissue-engineered heart valves (Rabkin-Aikawa et al, 2004a, Rabkin et al, 2002). Moreover, increased mechanical stiffness of the ECM occurs due to changes resulting from CAVD, (Weinberg et al, 2009) and VICs cultured on stiff substrates demonstrate increased myofibroblast differentiation and calcification (Yip et al, 2009).

All in all, studies have demonstrated that changes in the mechanical environment and hemodynamic forces are important in the pathological process and changes occurring in CAVD. More specifically, biomechanics in the context of CAVD can catalyze the disease process, but are not an independent factor of osteoblastic differentiation.

5.2 Transcription growth factor–β

Transcription growth factor–β (TGF-β) regulates biological functions in various systems. In the aortic valve, TFG-β affects VIC differentiation, increasing the expression of α-SMA, smooth muscle myosin, and calponin (ten Dijke and Hill, 2004). TGF-β binds to its receptors (TGF-β receptors I and II), which initiates signalling through Smad proteins, which in turn interact with the transcription factors FoxH1, c-Jun, c-fos, and Gli-3. TGF-β can also initiate mitogen-activated protein kinase (MAPK) pathways. Both signalling pathways regulate cell cycle, proliferation, migration, cytokine secretion, and ECM synthesis and degradation – all of which are important in normal valvular biology (Walker et al, 2004). The ECM components heparin and fibronectin participate in the effect of TGF-β on VICs (Taipale et al, 1996). By binding TGF-β to the pericellular environment, heparin induces α-SMA expression in VICs. Heparin also induces new TGF-β synthesis by VICs. VICs express fibronectin, a major component of the ECM that can sequester TGF-β to activate VICs (Cushing et al, 2005). In CAVD, elevated VIC activation by TGF-β causes pathological remodelling of the ECM. More specifically, increased TGF-β1 expression increases collagen, glycosaminoglycan, and hyaluronic acid syntheses. In addition, studies of calcified valves have indicated increased expression of TGF-β in ECM. *In vitro* studies demonstrate that TGF-β promotes migration, aggregation, and formation of apoptotic alkaline phosphatase nodules. Anti-apoptotic agents prevent apoptosis and calcification in TGF-β-treated VICs. This indicates that TGF-β also promotes CAVD through a process involving apoptosis similar to atherosclerotic plaques (Jian et al, 2003).

5.3 Lipoproteins and the Wnt signalling pathway

Landmark studies of patient aortic valve specimens with CAVD demonstrated the presence of LDLs in the valvular tissue. It became clear that lipids participate in the calcification of aortic valves relate to events leading to the eventual osteoblast-like differentiation of VICs. Lipids induce oxidative stress in the endothelium. Similar to vascular disease, endothelial dysfunction predisposes LDL migration through the endothelium. The accumulation of LDL can recruit inflammatory cells, subsequently leading to the release of inflammatory cytokines, which can activate VICs to differentiate into osteoblast-like cells.

The active role of lipids in the calcification process is confirmed in humans and in animals, which show a higher rate and severity of CAVD (Aikawa et al, 2007b). Interestingly, studies have demonstrated a relation between the bone formation signalling pathway and the LDL metabolism pathway. More specifically, the regulation of the LRP5/Wnt signalling has been implicated in cardiovascular calcification (Caira et al, 2006, Rajamannan et al, 2005, Shao et al, 2005). LDL receptor-related protein (LRP) signalling in bone is regulated through the canonical Wnt pathway. Wnt, a growth factor involved in bone and heart development (Clevers, 2006, Chakraborty et al, 2008), binds to receptors composed of frizzled protein and either of LRP5 or LRP6. This inhibits β-catenin degradation and leads to its accumulation and subsequent entry into the cellular nucleus. Calcified valves express elevated LRP5 and β-catenin, compared to healthy controls (Caira et al, 2006, Rajamannan et al, 2005). β-catenin modulates the expression of several target genes, including cyclin D, Runx2/Cbfa1, and Sox9 (Shao et al, 2005). These transcription factors are crucial for myofibroblast differentiation to osteoblasts. The exact role of lipids in CAVD has yet to be elucidated. The recent failure in lipid-lowering pharmaceutical trials indicates that treating hyperlipidemia alone may not affect CAVD.

5.4 The OPG/RANKL/RANK signalling pathway

Calcified valves demonstrate the expression of RANKL (ligand of receptor activator of nuclear factor κ B, RANK) and osteoprotegerin (OPG), which also are parts of a cytokine system that regulates bone turnover (Kaden et al, 2004a, Kaden et al, 2004b). RANKL, a member of the TNF-α superfamily, is a transmembrane protein located on the surface of osteoblasts, stromal cells, T cells, and endothelial cells (Hofbauer & Schoppet, 2004). RANKL interacts with RANK, a transmembrane protein located on osteoclast precursors or mature osteoclasts, and induces osteoclastogenesis via NFκB. The interaction of RANKL with RANK also increases the binding of osteoblast transcription factor runx2/cbfa-1, which is essential for osteoblast differentiation (Kaden et al, 2004b). This interaction can be blocked by OPG, subsequently limiting the activation of RANK and thus preventing osteoclast differentiation. This pathway is critical in cardiovascular calcification, and provides a possible link between cardiovascular calcification and bone metabolism (Hjortnaes et al, 2010), but determining the exact mechanism will require further investigations. Studies have shown that RANK/RANKL are highly increased in stenotic valves (Steinmetz et al, 2008). In VICs, RANKL treatment induces an osteoblast-like phenotype, that favours bone formation, increased nodule formation, and increased alkaline phosphatase activity, along with elevated synthesis of matrix elements and enhanced DNA binding of Runx2/Cbfa-1 (Kaden et al, 2005a). Treatment of VICs with TNF-α causes similar effects (Kaden et al, 2005b).

Furthermore, mice deficient in OPG show calcification of large-sized and medium-sized vessels (Nanes, 2003), which supports the protective role of OPG against calcification. Interestingly, OPG has the opposite effect on skeletal bone, and inhibits bone resorption. Our recent study demonstrated that cardiovascular calcification inversely correlates with low bone mineral density of long bones in an animal model of CAVD (Hjortnaes et al, 2010). These results led to the hypothesis that calcium metabolites in the valve may originate from bone, and are mediated through inflammatory signalling. Further studies are needed to evaluate this hypothesis.

5.5 The renin-angiotensin system

Emerging evidence suggests that the renin-angiotensin system (RAAS) and the kallikrein-kinin system (KKS) are important in the regulation of heart valve homeostasis. In terms of CAVD, the RAAS/KKS balance seems to shift toward pro-fibrotic. ACE is a potent pro-fibrotic protein, capable of forming the equally pro-fibrotic angiotensin II (ATII) (Mehta & Griendling, 2007). ACE is produced by monocytes/macrophages and binds to circulating LDL particles. ACE can inactivate the anti-fibrotic enzyme bradykinin (BK), which is generated by the KKS (Helske et al, 2004). Studies have demonstrated the presence of ATII receptors on VICs in CAVD; the density of these receptors is significantly higher in CAVD than in healthy aortic valves. The importance of the RAAS is demonstrated in studies where the ATII type 1 antagonist olmesartan had similar protective effects as atorvastatin in CAVD in rabbits (Arishiro et al, 2007). Retrospective studies with ACE inhibitors also seem to slow calcification (Rosenhek et al, 2004), but randomized clinical trials are warranted.

5.6 Neoangiogenesis

Healthy human aortic valves are avascular and receive their nutrients through diffusion. In CAVD, however, neo-vessel formation or angiogenesis occurs, especially around calcified nodules. Histopathological studies have demonstrated the expression of vascular endothelial growth factor in calcified valves (Soini et al, 2003). Furthermore, endothelial progenitor cells localize in the *zona fibrosa* of calcified native and bioprosthetic valves, indicating that cells of extra-valvular origin contribute to CAVD (Skowasch et al, 2005). Whether VIC differentiation or inflammatory cells are involved in the neovascularization is unclear. Interestingly, the aortic valve also expresses anti-angiogenic factors, such as chondromodulin-1 and endostatin (Chalajour et al, 2004). This observation has led to the hypothesis that the aortic valve possesses mechanisms to inhibit neovascularization in the healthy native valve, but in CAVD these mechanisms are disrupted, adding to its pathological process. Further studies are needed to investigate the precise role of angiogenesis in CAVD.

5.7 Genetics

The potential involvement of genes in CAVD has received much attention. Lessons learned from studies of bicuspid aortic valves, which associate with relatively quick calcific deterioration, demonstrate the potential role of a genetic component – namely, NOTCH1 and eNOS. For instance, 40% of adult mice that lack eNOS develop bicuspid aortic valves (Lee et al, 2000). NOTCH1 is a receptor-based transcriptional activator and has been shown to promote endothelial-to-mesenchymal transformation (EMT) and valve formation during valvular development. NOTCH1 normally inhibits calcification by inducing the expression of its target genes Hey1 and Hey2, which in turn interact with and repress the activity of Runx2/Cbfa1. Inactivation or mutations of NOTCH1 catalyze the progression of Runx2/Cbfa1-mediated calcification (Rusanescu et al, 2008). Much research is still needed to elucidate the role of a genetic component in CAVD, but evidence indicates that its development could be multifactorial.

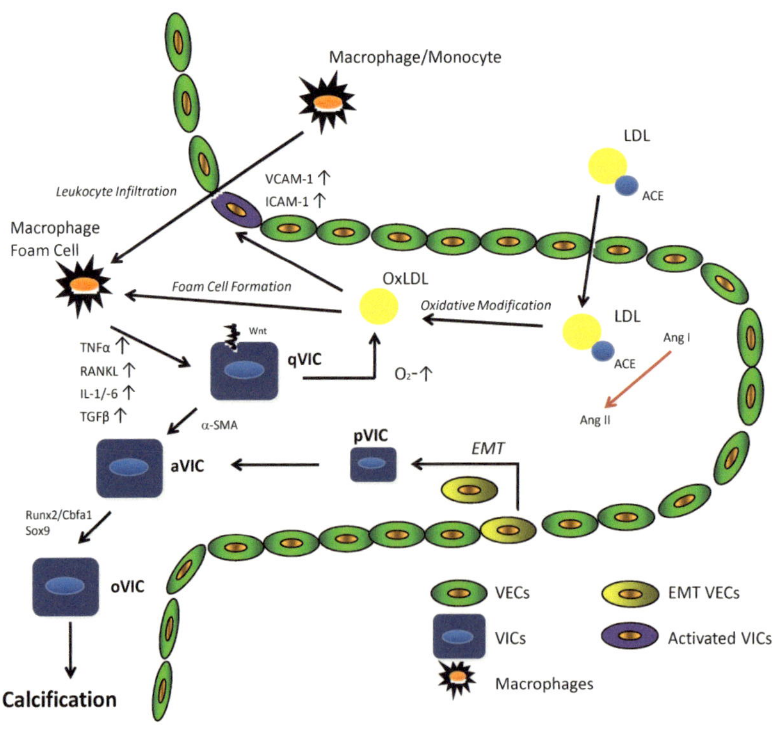

Fig. 3. Schematic depiction of cellular and molecular mechanisms in CAVD. qVIC - quiescent VICs, aVIC - activated VICs, pVIC - progenitor VICs, oVIC - osteoblastic VICs

5.8 Final common pathway

In summary, the previously discussed mechanisms lead to a final common pathway of CAVD – the active mineralization of valvular matrix by activated VICs that have differentiated into osteoblast-like cells (Figure 3). The calcification process initiates mainly in the *zona fibrosa*. The osteogenic differentiation of VICs is characterized by the presence of osteoblast-related genes such as osteocalcin, osteonectin, and the transcription factors runx2/cbfa1. The RANKL/RANK/OPG and Lpr5/Wnt signalling pathways can lead to the stimulation of runx2/cbfa1-mediated calcification of the aortic valve. Excess of circulatory LDL, accompanied by ACE, acts through the Lrp5/Wnt signalling pathway and induces mineralization of the valve stroma. Inflammation also stimulates VIC differentiation into osteoblast-like cells (Aikawa et al, 2007). Inflammatory cells produce cytokines that stimulate the RANKL/RANK/OPG pathway; ACE that acts through Wnt; and enzymes that degrade the ECM (e.g., MMPs, cathepsins). The inflammatory state and the degradation of ECM upregulates TGFβ, which stimulates the myofibroblast differentiation of VICs and further degrades ECM. Biomechanical forces, in which increased mechanical pressure environments can stimulate myofibroblast differentiation of VICs, also influence ECM homeostasis. CAVD should be considered a multifactorial disease for which the onset and progression to aortic valve stenosis mandate further investigations.

6. Animal models

Animal models are important in studying CAVD *in vivo* and in evaluating the effects of new therapies. The perfect animal model should be able to simulate the human disease. Murine, rabbit and porcine models are most commonly used in CAVD research. The main difference between these models is that mice require genetic manipulation to create disease, while rabbits and pigs, naturally susceptible to cardiovascular calcification, often suffice with diet-induced hyperlipidemia.

6.1 Murine models

Transgenic mouse models have proved very effective in recreating human disease. Apolipoprotein E (ApoE) knockout and low-density lipoprotein receptor (LDLr) knockout mice are the most commonly used animal models. ApoE is a protein that allows for receptor-mediated removal of very low-density lipoprotein (VLDL) from the circulation. Spontaneous hypercholesterolemia occurs in ApoE-/- mice, and as they age, they demonstrate increased transvalvular velocity, aortic regurgitation, and nodular calcification (Tanaka et al, 2005). When subjected to a hypercholesterolemic diet, accelerated early disease is observed, characterized by thickened leaflets, activated endothelial cells, and subendothelial lesions rich in macrophages, which co-localize with MMPs, cathepsins, α-SMA, ALP, Runx2/Cbfa1, and osteocalcin expression (Aikawa et al, 2007a, Aikawa et al, 2007b). Moreover, studies have shown that ApoE-/- mice display aortic valve sclerosis similar to that in humans. By knocking out the LDL receptor, the removal of circulatory LDL is inhibited, also leading to a hypercholesterolemic state. Fed a high-cholesterol diet, these mice develop extreme hyperlipidemia, hyperglycemia, and mineral deposition at 16 weeks of age. They also show increases in valve thickness, macrophage accumulation, activated myofibroblasts and osteoblasts, and ectopic mineralization (Matsumoto et al, 2010). An expansion of this model, the Reversa mouse, is achieved by inhibiting apolipoprotein B (ApoB) 100 and incorporating a conditional knockout of the microsomal triglyceride transfer protein (Mttp) under the control of an inducible Mx1-Cre+/+ gene (LDLr-/-, ApoB100/100, Mttp fl/fl, Mx1-Cre+/+) (Miller et al, 2009). Fed a high-cholesterol diet, these mice develop calcific aortic stenosis in 6 months; profibrotic signalling, myofibroblast activation, and procalcific signalling are also observed (Miller et al, 2009, Miller et al, 2010). Our recent studies have induced chronic renal disease (CRD) in ApoE-/- mice, to cause accelerated ectopic calcification (Aikawa et al, 2009, Hjortnaes et al, 2010).

6.2 Rabbit models

Rabbits are used in CAVD research because they have tri-layer aortic valve morphology, respond to a high-cholesterol diet, and show similarities to human lipoprotein metabolism. They also are susceptible to accelerated calcification with vitamin D2 and are available as transgenic strains (Otto et al, 1999, Fan & Watanabe, 2000). Their disadvantages, however, include the requirement of very high cholesterol levels to form atherosclerotic lesions, and vitamin D2 admission to cause accelerated calcification. Rabbits also seem to demonstrate atherosclerotic lesions different from those in humans. The standard rabbit model is the New Zealand white rabbit (NZWR), subjected to a high-cholesterol diet, a vitamin D2-supplemented diet or both. After 1 week, the subendothelial region of the fibrosa shows the accumulation of macrophages, collagen fibers, elastin fragmentation, and proteoglycan accumulation (Filip et al, 1987). After 8 weeks, myofibroblast proliferation, ACE, osteopontin, and osteoblast gene expression are increased (Rajamannan et al, 2002b). Calcification is present after 12 weeks (Rajamannan et al, 2005). Similar to murine models, the LDLr and apolipoproteins can be altered in rabbits, resulting in hypercholesterolemia. One such rabbit model used in CAVD research is the Watanabe heritable hyperlipidemic (WHHL) rabbit, characterized by a spontaneous LDLr mutation (Fan & Watanabe, 2000).

6.3 Porcine models

Pigs demonstrate many similarities to humans, such as hemodynamic environment, heart anatomy, tri-layered aortic valve leaflets, similar lipid profiles, and lipoprotein metabolism (Dixon et al, 1999, Gerrity et al, 2001). They are popular mostly in atherosclerosis research. Yorkshire swine and miniature pig breeds fed with high-cholesterol diets have been used in CAVD research. After 6 months, these pigs demonstrate small calcific nodules histologically, and subendothelial lipid infiltration in the *zona fibrosa* (Simmons et al, 2005). Atherosclerotic pigs demonstrate a similar inflammatory state, but this is observed only in vascular walls, not in valves (Gerrity et al, 2001). Mutations in LDLr and apolipoprotein genes have also yielded porcine models suitable for atherosclerosis and CAVD research, achieving complex lesions at 2 years old without a high-cholesterol diet (Prescott et al, 1991). Size is the main limitation of porcine models, requiring relatively high expenditures in animal care and maintenance.

7. "The point of no return"

An important discussion in the field of CAVD research involves whether the disease is reversible, whether there is a point of no return in the disease process, and where such a point may lie. Answers to these questions would have vital implications for therapeutic intervention, including determining the optimal timing of surgery. We would need to develop imaging tools that can evaluate the disease process in patients with risk factors. Traditional imaging modalities such as echocardiography and computerized tomography, albeit very suitable in identifying and quantifying calcification, are limited because they are unable to detect early CAVD lesions. Molecular imaging has emerged in the search for new technologies to allow early detection and offer insight into the mechanism of CAVD, as a successful tool that can detect pathobiological processes associated with inflammation and early stages of calcification *in vivo* at the cellular level (Nahrendorf et al, 2008, Aikawa et al, 2007b, Jaffer et al, 2007, Hjortnaes et al, 2010). Research into the mechanisms of CAVD has enabled the development of molecular imaging agents that can visualize key cellular and molecular processes. Studies have successfully detected pro-inflammatory, pro-osteogenic, and proteolytic activity in cardiovascular calcification *in vivo* (Aikawa et al, 2009, Aikawa et al, 2007b, Aikawa et al, 2006, Deguchi et al, 2006). Imaging agents use molecular processes to generate image contrast using high-resolution imaging technology. This approach has led to the discovery of imaging agents that chemically attach to an affinity ligand, such as a fluorochrome or magnetic compound (e.g., biphosphonate-conjugated fluorescent agents, cross-linked iron oxide fluorescent nanoparticles to detect macrophages). We can visualize enzyme activity in CAVD by employing molecular imaging agents to interact with enzymes that, when active, undergo a chemical change leading to signal amplification (Deguchi et al, 2006, Aikawa et al, 2007b). Currently, only optical imaging modalities can be used to detect calcification and early stages of the disease, due to limited signal detection by conventional imaging techniques such as CT and MRI. Visualizing pathways involved in early stages of CAVD is warranted in the pursuit of new therapeutic targets. Studies have successfully utilized multimodal molecular imaging to detect and monitor over time the dynamic changes in inflammation and ectopic calcification in mouse models of cardiovascular calcification (Aikawa et al, 2009, Aikawa et al, 2007b, Hjortnaes et al, 2010) (Figure 4). These changes are undetectable by conventional imaging techniques. In addition, molecular imaging provides the opportunity to effectively visualize biological processes simultaneously using different imaging agents. This research demonstrates the importance of developing imaging techniques able to detect early calcification before a "point of no return," and to establish the reversibility potential of CAVD.

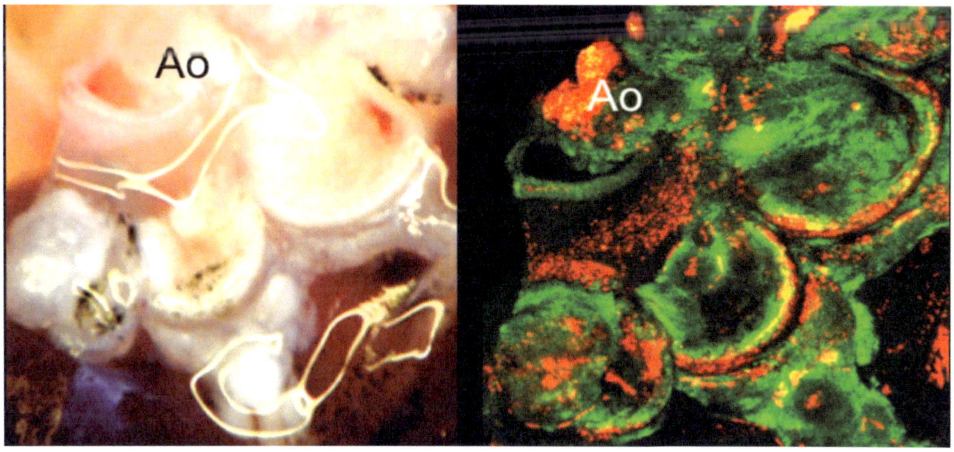

Fig. 4. Aortic valves of apoE−/− mice had characteristics of CAVD. Gross morphology of calcified aortic valve (left). Fluorescence microscopy (image stacks; right) visualized osteogenic activity (OsteoSense-680, red) in the areas of leaflet attachment to the aortic wall in inflamed valve (CLIO-750, green). Modified from Aikawa et al, Circulation, 2009

8. Conclusion

CAVD is a growing burden in the Western world. It is a progressive disease ranging from mild valve thickening to severe calcification with aortic valve stenosis. Despite its increasing prevalence and clinical significance, the mechanisms of CAVD are unclear. Fuelled by the absence of effective therapies other than aortic valve replacement, studies are needed to achieve a better understanding of CAVD – a complex disease in which multiple cellular and molecular mechanisms have been identified. The presence of additional comorbidities and clinical risk factors indicates a multifactorial pathogenesis.

The National Heart, Lung and Blood Institute Aortic Stenosis Working Group recently set out recommendations for CAVD research: 1) identification of genetic, anatomic, and clinical risk factors for the distinct phases of initiation and progression of CAVD; 2) development of high-resolution and high-sensitivity imaging modalities that can identify early and subclinical CAVD, including molecular imaging and other innovative imaging approaches; 3) understanding the basic science of CAVD, including signalling pathways and the roles of valve interstitial cells and endothelial cells, autocrine and paracrine signaling, the extracellular matrix and its stiffness, interacting mechanisms of calcification, biomechanics, and hemodynamics; 4) development of suitable multi-scale *in vitro*, *ex vivo*, and animal models; 5) identification of the relationship between CAVD and bone metabolism; 6) creation of tissue banks from valve tissue acquired from surgery, pathology, and autopsy, with and without CAVD; and 7) establishing clinical studies of CAVD to determine the feasibility of pharmacological intervention and optimal timing of surgical valve replacement.

9. References

Aikawa, E. and Otto CM. (2011) Look more closely at the valve. *Circulation,* PMID: 22090164.

Aikawa, E., Aikawa, M., Libby, P., Figueiredo, J. L., Rusanescu, G., Iwamoto, Y., Fukuda, D., Kohler, R. H., Shi, G. P., Jaffer, F. A. & Weissleder, R. (2009) Arterial and aortic valve calcification abolished by elastolytic cathepsin S deficiency in chronic renal disease. *Circulation,* 119, 1785-94.

Aikawa, E., Nahrendorf, M., Figueiredo, J. L., Swirski, F. K., Shtatland, T., Kohler, R. H., Jaffer, F. A., Aikawa, M. & Weissleder, R. (2007a) Osteogenesis associates with inflammation in early-stage atherosclerosis evaluated by molecular imaging in vivo. *Circulation,* 116, 2841-50.

Aikawa, E., Nahrendorf, M., Sosnovik, D., Lok, V. M., Jaffer, F. A., Aikawa, M. & Weissleder, R. (2007b) Multimodality molecular imaging identifies proteolytic and osteogenic activities in early aortic valve disease. *Circulation,* 115, 377-86.

Aikawa, E., Whittaker, P., Farber, M., Mendelson, K., Padera, R. F., Aikawa, M. & Schoen, F. J. (2006) Human semilunar cardiac valve remodeling by activated cells from fetus to adult: implications for postnatal adaptation, pathology, and tissue engineering. *Circulation,* 113, 1344-52.

Arishiro, K., Hoshiga, M., Negoro, N., Jin, D., Takai, S., Miyazaki, M., Ishihara, T. & HanaFUSA, T. (2007) Angiotensin receptor-1 blocker inhibits atherosclerotic changes and endothelial disruption of the aortic valve in hypercholesterolemic rabbits. *J Am Coll Cardiol,* 49, 1482-9.

Aronow, W. S., Ahn, C., Kronzon, I. & Goldman, M. E. (2001) Association of coronary risk factors and use of statins with progression of mild valvular aortic stenosis in older persons. *Am J Cardiol,* 88, 693-5.

Aronow, W. S., Schwartz, K. S. & Koenigsberg, M. (1987) Correlation of serum lipids, calcium, and phosphorus, diabetes mellitus and history of systemic hypertension with presence or absence of calcified or thickened aortic cusps or root in elderly patients. *Am J Cardiol,* 59, 998-9.

Balachandran, K., Sucosky, P., Jo, H. & Yoganathan, A. P. (2010) Elevated cyclic stretch induces aortic valve calcification in a bone morphogenic protein-dependent manner. *Am J Pathol,* 177, 49-57.

Bellamy, M. F., Pellikka, P. A., Klarich, K. W., Tajik, A. J. & Enriquez-Sarano, M. (2002) Association of cholesterol levels, hydroxymethylglutaryl coenzyme-A reductase inhibitor treatment, and progression of aortic stenosis in the community. *J Am Coll Cardiol,* 40, 1723-30.

Bloomfield, P., Wheatley, D. J., Prescott, R. J. & Miller, H. C. (1991) Twelve-year comparison of a Bjork-Shiley mechanical heart valve with porcine bioprostheses. *N Engl J Med,* 324, 573-9.

Braun, H. A. & Comeau, W. J. (1951) The importance of high-pitched squeaking systolic murmur in the diagnosis of aortic stenosis and calcification of the aortic valve. *N Engl J Med,* 244, 507-9.

Breuer, C. K., Mettler, B. A., Anthony, T., Sales, V. L., Schoen, F. J. & Mayer, J. E. (2004) Application of tissue-engineering principles toward the development of a semilunar heart valve substitute. *Tissue Eng,* 10, 1725-36.

Butcher, J. T., Mahler, G. J. & Hockaday, L. A. Aortic valve disease and treatment: The need for naturally engineered solutions. *Adv Drug Deliv Rev.*

Butcher, J. T., Mahler, G. J. & Hockaday, L. A. (2011) Aortic valve disease and treatment: The need for naturally engineered solutions. *Adv Drug Deliv Rev.*

Butcher, J. T. & Nerem, R. M. (2006) Valvular endothelial cells regulate the phenotype of interstitial cells in co-culture: effects of steady shear stress. *Tissue Eng,* 12, 905-15.

Butcher, J. T., Penrod, A. M., Garcia, A. J. & Nerem, R. M. (2004) Unique morphology and focal adhesion development of valvular endothelial cells in static and fluid flow environments. *Arterioscler Thromb Vasc Biol,* 24, 1429-34.

Butcher, J. T., Simmons, C. A. & Warnock, J. N. (2008) Mechanobiology of the aortic heart valve. *J Heart Valve Dis,* 17, 62-73.

Butcher, J. T., Tressel, S., Johnson, T., Turner, D., Sorescu, G., Jo, H. & Nerem, R. M. (2006) Transcriptional profiles of valvular and vascular endothelial cells reveal phenotypic differences: influence of shear stress. *Arterioscler Thromb Vasc Biol,* 26, 69-77.

Caira, F. C., Stock, S. R., Gleason, T. G., Mcgee, E. C., Huang, J., Bonow, R. O., Spelsberg, T. C., Mccarthy, P. M., Rahimtoola, S. H. & Rajamannan, N. M. (2006) Human degenerative valve disease is associated with up-regulation of low-density lipoprotein receptor-related protein 5 receptor-mediated bone formation. *J Am Coll Cardiol,* 47, 1707-12.

Carabello, B. A. & Paulus, W. J. (2009) Aortic stenosis. *Lancet,* 373, 956-66.

Chakraborty, S., Cheek, J., Sakthivel, B., Aronow, B. J. & Yutzey, K. E. (2008) Shared gene expression profiles in developing heart valves and osteoblast progenitor cells. *Physiol Genomics,* 35, 75-85.

Chalajour, F., Treede, H., Ebrahimnejad, A., Lauke, H., Reichenspurner, H. & ERGUN, S. (2004) Angiogenic activation of valvular endothelial cells in aortic valve stenosis. *Exp Cell Res,* 298, 455-64.

Chan, K. L., Teo, K., Dumesnil, J. G., Ni, A. & Tam, J. (2010) Effect of Lipid lowering with rosuvastatin on progression of aortic stenosis: results of the aortic stenosis progression observation: measuring effects of rosuvastatin (ASTRONOMER) trial. *Circulation,* 121, 306-14.

Chester, A. H., Kershaw, J. D., Sarathchandra, P. & Yacoub, M. H. (2008) Localisation and function of nerves in the aortic root. *J Mol Cell Cardiol,* 44, 1045-52.

Cimini, M., Rogers, K. A. & Boughner, D. R. (2003) Smoothelin-positive cells in human and porcine semilunar valves. *Histochem Cell Biol,* 120, 307-17.

Clevers, H. (2006) Wnt/beta-catenin signaling in development and disease. *Cell,* 127, 469-80.

Cosmi, J. E., Kort, S., Tunick, P. A., Rosenzweig, B. P., Freedberg, R. S., Katz, E. S., Applebaum, R. M. & Kronzon, I. (2002) The risk of the development of aortic stenosis in patients with "benign" aortic valve thickening. *Arch Intern Med,* 162, 2345-7.

Cowell, S. J., Newby, D. E., Prescott, R. J., Bloomfield, P., Reid, J., Northridge, D. B. & Boon, N. A. (2005) A randomized trial of intensive lipid-lowering therapy in calcific aortic stenosis. *N Engl J Med,* 352, 2389-97.

Cushing, M. C., Liao, J. T. & Anseth, K. S. (2005) Activation of valvular interstitial cells is mediated by transforming growth factor-beta1 interactions with matrix molecules. *Matrix Biol,* 24, 428-37.

De Hart, J., Peters, G. W., Schreurs, P. J. & Baaijens, F. P. (2004) Collagen fibers reduce stresses and stabilize motion of aortic valve leaflets during systole. *J Biomech,* 37, 303-11.

Deck, J. D. (1986) Endothelial cell orientation on aortic valve leaflets. *Cardiovasc Res,* 20, 760-7.

Deguchi, J. O., Aikawa, M., Tung, C. H., Aikawa, E., Kim, D. E., Ntziachristos, V., Weissleder, R. & Libby, P. (2006) Inflammation in atherosclerosis: visualizing matrix metalloproteinase action in macrophages in vivo. *Circulation,* 114, 55-62.

Dixon, J. L., Stoops, J. D., Parker, J. L., Laughlin, M. H., Weisman, G. A. & Sturek, M. (1999) Dyslipidemia and vascular dysfunction in diabetic pigs fed an atherogenic diet. *Arterioscler Thromb Vasc Biol,* 19, 2981-92.

El-Hamamsy, I., Balachandran, K., Yacoub, M. H., Stevens, L. M., Sarathchandra, P., Taylor, P. M., Yoganathan, A. P. & Chester, A. H. (2009) Endothelium-dependent regulation of the mechanical properties of aortic valve cusps. *J Am Coll Cardiol,* 53, 1448-55.

Faggiano, P., Antonini-Canterin, F., Erlicher, A., Romeo, C., Cervesato, E., Pavan, D., Piazza, R., Huang, G. & Nicolosi, G. L. (2003) Progression of aortic valve sclerosis to aortic stenosis. *Am J Cardiol,* 91, 99-101.

Fan, J. & Watanabe, T. (2000) Cholesterol-fed and transgenic rabbit models for the study of atherosclerosis. *J Atheroscler Thromb,* 7, 26-32.

Filip, D. A., Nistor, A., Bulla, A., Radu, A., Lupu, F. & Simionescu, M. (1987) Cellular events in the development of valvular atherosclerotic lesions induced by experimental hypercholesterolemia. *Atherosclerosis,* 67, 199-214.

Fondard, O., Detaint, D., Iung, B., Choqueux, C., Adle-Biassette, H., Jarraya, M., Hvass, U., Couetil, J. P., Henin, D., Michel, J. B., Vahanian, A. & Jacob, M. P. (2005) Extracellular matrix remodelling in human aortic valve disease: the role of matrix metalloproteinases and their tissue inhibitors. *Eur Heart J,* 26, 1333-41.

Fowler, N. O. (1979) Clinical aspects of acquired valvular heart disease. *Semin Roentgenol,* 14, 83-95.

Fox, C. S., Larson, M. G., Vasan, R. S., Guo, C. Y., Parise, H., Levy, D., Leip, E. P., O'donnell C, J., D'agostino, R. B., Sr. & Benjamin, E. J. (2006) Cross-sectional association of kidney function with valvular and annular calcification: the Framingham heart study. *J Am Soc Nephrol,* 17, 521-7.

Freeman, R. V. & Otto, C. M. (2005) Spectrum of calcific aortic valve disease: pathogenesis, disease progression, and treatment strategies. *Circulation,* 111, 3316-26.

Gerrity, R. G., Natarajan, R., Nadler, J. L. & Kimsey, T. (2001) Diabetes-induced accelerated atherosclerosis in swine. *Diabetes,* 50, 1654-65.

Hammermeister, K., Sethi, G. K., Henderson, W. G., Grover, F. L., Oprian, C. & Rahimtoola, S. H. (2000) Outcomes 15 years after valve replacement with a mechanical versus a bioprosthetic valve: final report of the Veterans Affairs randomized trial. *J Am Coll Cardiol,* 36, 1152-8.

Helske, S., Lindstedt, K. A., Laine, M., Mayranpaa, M., Werkkala, K., Lommi, J., Turto, H., Kupari, M. & Kovanen, P. T. (2004) Induction of local angiotensin II-producing systems in stenotic aortic valves. *J Am Coll Cardiol,* 44, 1859-66.

Higashidate, M., Tamiya, K., Beppu, T. & Imai, Y. (1995) Regulation of the aortic valve opening. In vivo dynamic measurement of aortic valve orifice area. *J Thorac Cardiovasc Surg,* 110, 496-503.

Hjortnaes, J., Butcher, J., Figueiredo, J. L., Riccio, M., Kohler, R. H., Kozloff, K. M., Weissleder, R. & Aikawa, E. (2010) Arterial and aortic valve calcification inversely correlates with osteoporotic bone remodelling: a role for inflammation. *Eur Heart J,* 31, 1975-84.

Hjortnaes, J., Gottlieb, D., Figueiredo, J. L., Melero-Martin, J., Kohler, R. H., Bischoff, J., Weissleder, R., Mayer, J. E. & Aikawa, E. (2010) Intravital molecular imaging of small-diameter tissue-engineered vascular grafts in mice: a feasibility study. *Tissue Eng Part C Methods,* 16, 597-607.

Ho, S. Y. (2009) Structure and anatomy of the aortic root. *Eur J Echocardiogr,* 10, i3-10.

Hofbauer, L. C. & Schoppet, M. (2004) Clinical implications of the osteoprotegerin/RANKL/RANK system for bone and vascular diseases. *Jama,* 292, 490-5.

Horl, W. H. (2004) The clinical consequences of secondary hyperparathyroidism: focus on clinical outcomes. *Nephrol Dial Transplant,* 19 Suppl 5, V2-8.

Hultgren, H. N. (1998) Osteitis deformans (Paget's disease) and calcific disease of the heart valves. *Am J Cardiol,* 81, 1461-4.

Iung, B., Baron, G., Butchart, E. G., Delahaye, F., Gohlke-Barwolf, C., Levang, O. W., Tornos, P., Vanoverschelde, J. L., Vermeer, F., Boersma, E., Ravaud, P. & Vahanian, A.

(2003) A prospective survey of patients with valvular heart disease in Europe: The Euro Heart Survey on Valvular Heart Disease. *Eur Heart J*, 24, 1231-43.

Jaffee, O. C. (1967) The development of the arterial outflow tract in the chick embryo heart. *Anat Rec*, 158, 35-42.

Jaffer, F. A., Kim, D. E., Quinti, L., Tung, C. H., Aikawa, E., Pande, A. N., Kohler, R. H., Shi, G. P., Libby, P. & Weissleder, R. (2007) Optical visualization of cathepsin K activity in atherosclerosis with a novel, protease-activatable fluorescence sensor. *Circulation*, 115, 2292-8.

Jian, B., Narula, N., Li, Q. Y., Mohler, E. R., 3rd & Levy, R. J. (2003) Progression of aortic valve stenosis: TGF-beta1 is present in calcified aortic valve cusps and promotes aortic valve interstitial cell calcification via apoptosis. *Ann Thorac Surg*, 75, 457-65; discussion 465-6.

Johnson, M. L. & Rajamannan, N. (2006) Diseases of Wnt signaling. *Rev Endocr Metab Disord*, 7, 41-9.

Kaden, J. J., Bickelhaupt, S., Grobholz, R., Haase, K. K., Sarikoc, A., Kilic, R., Brueckmann, M., Lang, S., Zahn, I., Vahl, C., Hagl, S., Dempfle, C. E. & Borggrefe, M. (2004a) Receptor activator of nuclear factor kappaB ligand and osteoprotegerin regulate aortic valve calcification. *J Mol Cell Cardiol*, 36, 57-66.

Kaden, J. J., Bickelhaupt, S., Grobholz, R., Vahl, C. F., Hagl, S., Brueckmann, M., Haase, K. K., Dempfle, C. E. & Borggrefe, M. (2004b) Expression of bone sialoprotein and bone morphogenetic protein-2 in calcific aortic stenosis. *J Heart Valve Dis*, 13, 560-6.

Kaden, J. J., Dempfle, C. E., Grobholz, R., Fischer, C. S., Vocke, D. C., Kilic, R., Sarikoc, A., Pinol, R., Hagl, S., Lang, S., Brueckmann, M. & Borggrefe, M. (2005a) Inflammatory regulation of extracellular matrix remodeling in calcific aortic valve stenosis. *Cardiovasc Pathol*, 14, 80-7.

Kaden, J. J., Kilic, R., Sarikoc, A., Hagl, S., Lang, S., Hoffmann, U., Brueckmann, M. & Borggrefe, M. (2005b) Tumor necrosis factor alpha promotes an osteoblast-like phenotype in human aortic valve myofibroblasts: a potential regulatory mechanism of valvular calcification. *Int J Mol Med*, 16, 869-72.

Katayama, S., Umetani, N., Sugiura, S. & Hisada, T. (2008) The sinus of Valsalva relieves abnormal stress on aortic valve leaflets by facilitating smooth closure. *J Thorac Cardiovasc Surg*, 136, 1528-35, 1535 e1.

Katz, R., Budoff, M. J., Takasu, J., Shavelle, D. M., Bertoni, A., Blumenthal, R. S., Ouyang, P., Wong, N. D. & O'brien, K. D. (2009) Relationship of metabolic syndrome with incident aortic valve calcium and aortic valve calcium progression: the Multi-Ethnic Study of Atherosclerosis (MESA). *Diabetes*, 58, 813-9.

Kilner, P. J., Yang, G. Z., Wilkes, A. J., Mohiaddin, R. H., Firmin, D. N. & Yacoub, M. H. (2000) Asymmetric redirection of flow through the heart. *Nature*, 404, 759-61.

Lee, T. C., Zhao, Y. D., Courtman, D. W. & Stewart, D. J. (2000) Abnormal aortic valve development in mice lacking endothelial nitric oxide synthase. *Circulation*, 101, 2345-8.

Levitt, L. C., Thubrikar, M. J. & Nolan, S. P. (1984) Patterns and pathogenesis of calcification in pathologic human aortic valves. *Curr Surg*, 41, 17-9.

Liu, A. C., Joag, V. R. & Gotlieb, A. I. (2007) The emerging role of valve interstitial cell phenotypes in regulating heart valve pathobiology. *Am J Pathol,* 171, 1407-18.

Lloyd-Jones, D., Adams, R., Carnethon, M., De Simone, G., Ferguson, T. B., Flegal, K., Ford, E., Furie, K., Go, A., Greenlund, K., Haase, N., Hailpern, S., Ho, M., Howard, V., Kissela, B., Kittner, S., Lackland, D., Lisabeth, L., Marelli, A., Mcdermott, M., Meigs, J., Mozaffarian, D., Nichol, G., O'donnell, C., Roger, V., Rosamond, W., Sacco, R., Sorlie, P., Stafford, R., Steinberger, J., Thom, T., Wasserthiel-Smoller, S., Wong, N., Wylie-Rosett, J. & Hong, Y. (2009) Heart disease and stroke statistics--2009 update: a report from the American Heart Association Statistics Committee and Stroke Statistics Subcommittee. *Circulation,* 119, 480-6.

Marron, K., Yacoub, M. H., Polak, J. M., Sheppard, M. N., Fagan, D., Whitehead, B. F., De Leval, M. R., Anderson, R. H. & Wharton, J. (1996) Innervation of human atrioventricular and arterial valves. *Circulation,* 94, 368-75.

Matsumoto, Y., Adams, V., Jacob, S., Mangner, N., Schuler, G. & Linke, A. (2010) Regular exercise training prevents aortic valve disease in low-density lipoprotein-receptor-deficient mice. *Circulation,* 121, 759-67.

Mehta, P. K. & Griendling, K. K. (2007) Angiotensin II cell signaling: physiological and pathological effects in the cardiovascular system. *Am J Physiol Cell Physiol,* 292, C82-97.

Merryman, W. D., Youn, I., Lukoff, H. D., Krueger, P. M., Guilak, F., Hopkins, R. A. & Sacks, M. S. (2006) Correlation between heart valve interstitial cell stiffness and transvalvular pressure: implications for collagen biosynthesis. *Am J Physiol Heart Circ Physiol,* 290, H224-31.

Miller, J. D., Weiss, R. M., Serrano, K. M., Brooks, R. M., 2nd, Berry, C. J., Zimmerman, K., Young, S. G. & Heistad, D. D. (2009) Lowering plasma cholesterol levels halts progression of aortic valve disease in mice. *Circulation,* 119, 2693-701.

Miller, J. D., Weiss, R. M., Serrano, K. M., Castaneda, L. E., Brooks, R. M., Zimmerman, K. & Heistad, D. D. (2010) Evidence for active regulation of pro-osteogenic signaling in advanced aortic valve disease. *Arterioscler Thromb Vasc Biol,* 30, 2482-6.

Mirzaie, M., Schultz, M., Schwartz, P., Coulibaly, M. & Schondube, F. (2003) Evidence of woven bone formation in heart valve disease. *Ann Thorac Cardiovasc Surg,* 9, 163-9.

Mohler, E. R., 3RD (2004) Mechanisms of aortic valve calcification. *Am J Cardiol,* 94, 1396-402, A6.

Mohler, E. R., 3rd, Adam, L. P., Mcclelland, P., Graham, L. & Hathaway, D. R. (1997) Detection of osteopontin in calcified human aortic valves. *Arterioscler Thromb Vasc Biol,* 17, 547-52.

Mohler, E. R., 3rd, Chawla, M. K., Chang, A. W., Vyavahare, N., Levy, R. J., Graham, L. & Gannon, F. H. (1999) Identification and characterization of calcifying valve cells from human and canine aortic valves. *J Heart Valve Dis,* 8, 254-60.

Mohler, E. R., 3rd, Gannon, F., Reynolds, C., Zimmerman, R., Keane, M. G. & Kaplan, F. S. (2001) Bone formation and inflammation in cardiac valves. *Circulation,* 103, 1522-8.

Moura, L. M., Ramos, S. F., Zamorano, J. L., Barros, I. M., Azevedo, L. F., Rocha-Goncalves, F. & Rajamannan, N. M. (2007) Rosuvastatin affecting aortic valve endothelium to slow the progression of aortic stenosis. *J Am Coll Cardiol,* 49, 554-61.

Mulholland, D. L. & Gotlieb, A. I. (1996) Cell biology of valvular interstitial cells. *Can J Cardiol,* 12, 231-6.

Muller, A. M., Cronen, C., Kupferwasser, L. I., Oelert, H., Muller, K. M. & Kirkpatrick, C. J. (2000) Expression of endothelial cell adhesion molecules on heart valves: up-regulation in degeneration as well as acute endocarditis. *J Pathol,* 191, 54-60.

Nahrendorf, M., Sosnovik, D., Chen, J. W., Panizzi, P., Figueiredo, J. L., Aikawa, E., Libby, P., Swirski, F. K. & Weissleder, R. (2008) Activatable magnetic resonance imaging agent reports myeloperoxidase activity in healing infarcts and noninvasively detects the antiinflammatory effects of atorvastatin on ischemia-reperfusion injury. *Circulation,* 117, 1153-60.

Nakamura, T., Hultgren, H. N., Shettigar, U. R. & Fowles, R. E. (1984) Noninvasive evaluation of the severity of aortic stenosis in adult patients. *Am Heart J,* 107, 959-66.

Nanes, M. S. (2003) Tumor necrosis factor-alpha: molecular and cellular mechanisms in skeletal pathology. *Gene,* 321, 1-15.

New, S. E. & Aikawa, E. (2011) Molecular imaging insights into early inflammatory stages of arterial and aortic valve calcification. *Circ Res,* 108, 1381-91.

Novaro, G. M., Tiong, I. Y., Pearce, G. L., Lauer, M. S., Sprecher, D. L. & Griffin, B. P. (2001) Effect of hydroxymethylglutaryl coenzyme a reductase inhibitors on the progression of calcific aortic stenosis. *Circulation,* 104, 2205-9.

O'brien, K. D., Reichenbach, D. D., Marcovina, S. M., Kuusisto, J., Alpers, C. E. & Otto, C. M. (1996) Apolipoproteins B, (a), and E accumulate in the morphologically early lesion of 'degenerative' valvular aortic stenosis. *Arterioscler Thromb Vasc Biol,* 16, 523-32.

O'brien, K. D., Shavelle, D. M., Caulfield, M. T., Mcdonald, T. O., Olin-Lewis, K., Otto, C. M. & Probstfield, J. L. (2002) Association of angiotensin-converting enzyme with low-density lipoprotein in aortic valvular lesions and in human plasma. *Circulation,* 106, 2224-30.

Olsson, M., Thyberg, J. & Nilsson, J. (1999) Presence of oxidized low density lipoprotein in nonrheumatic stenotic aortic valves. *Arterioscler Thromb Vasc Biol,* 19, 1218-22.

Otto, C. M. (2008) Calcific aortic stenosis--time to look more closely at the valve. *N Engl J Med,* 359, 1395-8.

Otto, C. M., Burwash, I. G., Legget, M. E., Munt, B. I., Fujioka, M., Healy, N. L., Kraft, C. D., Miyake-Hull, C. Y. & Schwaegler, R. G. (1997) Prospective study of asymptomatic valvular aortic stenosis. Clinical, echocardiographic, and exercise predictors of outcome. *Circulation,* 95, 2262-70.

Otto, C. M., Kuusisto, J., Reichenbach, D. D., Gown, A. M. & O'brien, K. D. (1994) Characterization of the early lesion of 'degenerative' valvular aortic stenosis. Histological and immunohistochemical studies. *Circulation,* 90, 844-53.

Otto, C. M., Lind, B. K., Kitzman, D. W., Gersh, B. J. & Siscovick, D. S. (1999) Association of aortic-valve sclerosis with cardiovascular mortality and morbidity in the elderly. *N Engl J Med,* 341, 142-7.

Otto, C. M. & O'brien, K. D. (2001) Why is there discordance between calcific aortic stenosis and coronary artery disease? *Heart,* 85, 601-2.

Owen, A. & Henein, M. Y. (2011) Challenges in the management of severe asymptomatic aortic stenosis. *Eur J Cardiothorac Surg.*

Porat, R. M., Grunewald, M., Globerman, A., Itin, A., Barshtein, G., Alhonen, L., Alitalo, K. & Keshet, E. (2004) Specific induction of tie1 promoter by disturbed flow in atherosclerosis-prone vascular niches and flow-obstructing pathologies. *Circ Res,* 94, 394-401.

Prescott, M. F., Mcbride, C. H., Hasler-Rapacz, J., Von Linden, J. & Rapacz, J. (1991) Development of complex atherosclerotic lesions in pigs with inherited hyper-LDL cholesterolemia bearing mutant alleles for apolipoprotein B. *Am J Pathol,* 139, 139-47.

Rabkin-Aikawa, E., Aikawa, M., Farber, M., Kratz, J. R., Garcia-Cardena, G., Kouchoukos, N. T., Mitchell, M. B., Jonas, R. A. & Schoen, F. J. (2004a) Clinical pulmonary autograft valves: pathologic evidence of adaptive remodeling in the aortic site. *J Thorac Cardiovasc Surg,* 128, 552-61.

Rabkin-Aikawa, E., Farber, M., Aikawa, M. & Schoen, F. J. (2004b) Dynamic and reversible changes of interstitial cell phenotype during remodeling of cardiac valves. *J Heart Valve Dis,* 13, 841-7.

Rabkin, E., Aikawa, M., Stone, J. R., Fukumoto, Y., Libby, P. & Schoen, F. J. (2001) Activated interstitial myofibroblasts express catabolic enzymes and mediate matrix remodeling in myxomatous heart valves. *Circulation,* 104, 2525-32.

Rabkin, E., Hoerstrup, S. P., Aikawa, M., Mayer, J. E., Jr. & Schoen, F. J. (2002) Evolution of cell phenotype and extracellular matrix in tissue-engineered heart valves during in-vitro maturation and in-vivo remodeling. *J Heart Valve Dis,* 11, 308-14; discussion 314.

Rajamannan, N. M., Bonow, R. O. & Rahimtoola, S. H. (2007) Calcific aortic stenosis: an update. *Nat Clin Pract Cardiovasc Med,* 4, 254-62.

Rajamannan, N. M., Sangiorgi, G., Springett, M., Arnold, K., Mohacsi, T., Spagnoli, L. G., Edwards, W. D., Tajik, A. J. & Schwartz, R. S. (2001) Experimental hypercholesterolemia induces apoptosis in the aortic valve. *J Heart Valve Dis,* 10, 371-4.

Rajamannan, N. M., Springett, M. J., Pederson, L. G. & Carmichael, S. W. (2002a) Localization of caveolin 1 in aortic valve endothelial cells using antigen retrieval. *J Histochem Cytochem,* 50, 617-28.

Rajamannan, N. M., Subramaniam, M., Caira, F., Stock, S. R. & Spelsberg, T. C. (2005) Atorvastatin inhibits hypercholesterolemia-induced calcification in the aortic valves via the Lrp5 receptor pathway. *Circulation,* 112, I229-34.

Rajamannan, N. M., Subramaniam, M., Rickard, D., Stock, S. R., Donovan, J., Springett, M., Orszulak, T., Fullerton, D. A., Tajik, A. J., Bonow, R. O. & Spelsberg, T. (2003) Human aortic valve calcification is associated with an osteoblast phenotype. *Circulation,* 107, 2181-4.

Rajamannan, N. M., Subramaniam, M., Springett, M., Sebo, T. C., Niekrasz, M., Mcconnell, J. P., Singh, R. J., Stone, N. J., Bonow, R. O. & Spelsberg, T. C. (2002b) Atorvastatin inhibits hypercholesterolemia-induced cellular proliferation and bone matrix production in the rabbit aortic valve. *Circulation,* 105, 2660-5.

Roberts, W. C. (1970) The structure of the aortic valve in clinically isolated aortic stenosis: an autopsy study of 162 patients over 15 years of age. *Circulation,* 42, 91-7.

Rosenhek, R., Binder, T., Porenta, G., Lang, I., Christ, G., Schemper, M., Maurer, G. & Baumgartner, H. (2000) Predictors of outcome in severe, asymptomatic aortic stenosis. *N Engl J Med,* 343, 611-7.

Rosenhek, R., Rader, F., Loho, N., Gabriel, H., Heger, M., Klaar, U., Schemper, M., Binder, T., Maurer, G. & Baumgartner, H. (2004) Statins but not angiotensin-converting enzyme inhibitors delay progression of aortic stenosis. *Circulation,* 110, 1291-5.

Rossebo, A. B., Pedersen, T. R., Boman, K., Brudi, P., Chambers, J. B., Egstrup, K., Gerdts, E., Gohlke-Barwolf, C., Holme, I., Kesaniemi, Y. A., Malbecq, W., Nienaber, C. A., Ray, S., Skjaerpe, T., Wachtell, K. & Willenheimer, R. (2008) Intensive lipid lowering with simvastatin and ezetimibe in aortic stenosis. *N Engl J Med,* 359, 1343-56.

Rusanescu, G., Weissleder, R. & Aikawa, E. (2008) Notch signaling in cardiovascular disease and calcification. *Curr Cardiol Rev,* 4, 148-56.

Sabet, H. Y., Edwards, W. D., Tazelaar, H. D. & Daly, R. C. (1999) Congenitally bicuspid aortic valves: a surgical pathology study of 542 cases (1991 through 1996) and a literature review of 2,715 additional cases. *Mayo Clin Proc,* 74, 14-26.

Sacks, M. S. & Yoganathan, A. P. (2007) Heart valve function: a biomechanical perspective. *Philos Trans R Soc Lond B Biol Sci,* 362, 1369-91.

Schoen, F. J. (2005) Cardiac valves and valvular pathology: update on function, disease, repair, and replacement. *Cardiovasc Pathol,* 14, 189-94.

Schoen, F. J. (2008) Evolving concepts of cardiac valve dynamics: the continuum of development, functional structure, pathobiology, and tissue engineering. *Circulation,* 118, 1864-80.

Shao, J. S., Cheng, S. L., Pingsterhaus, J. M., Charlton-Kachigian, N., Loewy, A. P. & Towler, D. A. (2005) Msx2 promotes cardiovascular calcification by activating paracrine Wnt signals. *J Clin Invest,* 115, 1210-20.

Shavelle, D. M., Katz, R., Takasu, J., Lima, J. A., Jenny, N. S., Budoff, M. J. & O'brien, K. D. (2008) Soluble intercellular adhesion molecule-1 (sICAM-1) and aortic valve calcification in the multi-ethnic study of atherosclerosis (MESA). *J Heart Valve Dis,* 17, 388-95.

Shavelle, D. M., Takasu, J., Budoff, M. J., Mao, S., Zhao, X. Q. & O'brien, K. D. (2002) HMG CoA reductase inhibitor (statin) and aortic valve calcium. *Lancet,* 359, 1125-6.

Simmons, C. A., Grant, G. R., Manduchi, E. & Davies, P. F. (2005) Spatial heterogeneity of endothelial phenotypes correlates with side-specific vulnerability to calcification in normal porcine aortic valves. *Circ Res,* 96, 792-9.

Skowasch, D., Schrempf, S., Wernert, N., Steinmetz, M., Jabs, A., Tuleta, I., Welsch, U., Preusse, C. J., Likungu, J. A., Welz, A., Luderitz, B. & Bauriedel, G. (2005) Cells of primarily extra-valvular origin in degenerative aortic valves and bioprostheses. *Eur Heart J,* 26, 2576-80.

Soini, Y., Salo, T. & Satta, J. (2003) Angiogenesis is involved in the pathogenesis of nonrheumatic aortic valve stenosis. *Hum Pathol,* 34, 756-63.

Soini, Y., Satta, J., Maatta, M. & Autio-Harmainen, H. (2001) Expression of MMP2, MMP9, MT1-MMP, TIMP1, and TIMP2 mRNA in valvular lesions of the heart. *J Pathol,* 194, 225-31.

Sorescu, G. P., Song, H., Tressel, S. L., Hwang, J., Dikalov, S., Smith, D. A., Boyd, N. L., Platt, M. O., Lassegue, B., Griendling, K. K. & Jo, H. (2004) Bone morphogenic protein 4 produced in endothelial cells by oscillatory shear stress induces monocyte adhesion by stimulating reactive oxygen species production from a nox1-based NADPH oxidase. *Circ Res,* 95, 773-9.

Steinmetz, M., Skowasch, D., Wernert, N., Welsch, U., Preusse, C. J., Welz, A., Nickenig, G. & Bauriedel, G. (2008) Differential profile of the OPG/RANKL/RANK-system in degenerative aortic native and bioprosthetic valves. *J Heart Valve Dis,* 17, 187-93.

Stewart, B. F., Siscovick, D., Lind, B. K., Gardin, J. M., Gottdiener, J. S., Smith, V. E., Kitzman, D. W. & Otto, C. M. (1997) Clinical factors associated with calcific aortic valve disease. Cardiovascular Health Study. *J Am Coll Cardiol,* 29, 630-4.

Stout, K. K. & Otto, C. M. (2007) Indications for aortic valve replacement in aortic stenosis. *J Intensive Care Med,* 22, 14-25.

Sucosky, P., Balachandran, K., Elhammali, A., Jo, H. & Yoganathan, A. P. (2009) Altered shear stress stimulates upregulation of endothelial VCAM-1 and ICAM-1 in a BMP-4- and TGF-beta1-dependent pathway. *Arterioscler Thromb Vasc Biol,* 29, 254-60.

Taipale, J., Saharinen, J., Hedman, K. & Keski-Oja, J. (1996) Latent transforming growth factor-beta 1 and its binding protein are components of extracellular matrix microfibrils. *J Histochem Cytochem,* 44, 875-89.

Takkenberg, J. J., Rajamannan, N. M., Rosenhek, R., Kumar, A. S., Carapetis, J. R. & Yacoub, M. H. (2008) The need for a global perspective on heart valve disease epidemiology. The SHVD working group on epidemiology of heart valve disease founding statement. *J Heart Valve Dis,* 17, 135-9.

Tanaka, K., Sata, M., Fukuda, D., Suematsu, Y., Motomura, N., Takamoto, S., Hirata, Y. & Nagai, R. (2005) Age-associated aortic stenosis in apolipoprotein E-deficient mice. *J Am Coll Cardiol,* 46, 134-41.

Taylor, P. M., Batten, P., Brand, N. J., Thomas, P. S. & Yacoub, M. H. (2003) The cardiac valve interstitial cell. *Int J Biochem Cell Biol,* 35, 113-8.

Ten Dijke, P. & Hill, C. S. (2004) New insights into TGF-beta-Smad signalling. *Trends Biochem Sci,* 29, 265-73.

Thubrikar, M., Bosher, L. P. & Nolan, S. P. (1979) The mechanism of opening of the aortic valve. *J Thorac Cardiovasc Surg,* 77, 863-70.

Thubrikar, M., Nolan, S. P., Bosher, L. P. & Deck, J. D. (1980) The cyclic changes and structure of the base of the aortic valve. *Am Heart J,* 99, 217-24.

Thubrikar, M. J., Aouad, J. & Nolan, S. P. (1986a) Comparison of the in vivo and in vitro mechanical properties of aortic valve leaflets. *J Thorac Cardiovasc Surg,* 92, 29-36.

Thubrikar, M. J., Aouad, J. & Nolan, S. P. (1986b) Patterns of calcific deposits in operatively excised stenotic or purely regurgitant aortic valves and their relation to mechanical stress. *Am J Cardiol,* 58, 304-8.

Walker, G. A., Masters, K. S., Shah, D. N., Anseth, K. S. & Leinwand, L. A. (2004) Valvular myofibroblast activation by transforming growth factor-beta: implications for pathological extracellular matrix remodeling in heart valve disease. *Circ Res,* 95, 253-60.

Warnock, J. N., Burgess, S. C., Shack, A. & Yoganathan, A. P. (2006) Differential immediate-early gene responses to elevated pressure in porcine aortic valve interstitial cells. *J Heart Valve Dis,* 15, 34-41; discussion 42.

Weinberg, E. J., Schoen, F. J. & Mofrad, M. R. (2009) A computational model of aging and calcification in the aortic heart valve. *PLoS One,* 4, e5960.

Wylie-Sears, J., Aikawa, E., Levine, R. A., Yang, J. H. & Bischoff, J. (2011) Mitral valve endothelial cells with osteogenic differentiation potential. *Arterioscler Thromb Vasc Biol,* 31, 598-607.

Yip, C. Y., Chen, J. H., Zhao, R. & Simmons, C. A. (2009) Calcification by valve interstitial cells is regulated by the stiffness of the extracellular matrix. *Arterioscler Thromb Vasc Biol,* 29, 936-42.

Yperman, J., De Visscher, G., Holvoet, P. & Flameng, W. (2004) Molecular and functional characterization of ovine cardiac valve-derived interstitial cells in primary isolates and cultures. *Tissue Eng,* 10, 1368-75.

Part 5

Bioprosthetic Valve

8

Clinical and Hemodynamic Performance of the Sorin Mitroflow Pericardial Bioprosthesis

W. R. E. Jamieson[1], C. A. Yankah[2], R. Lorusso[3], O. Benhameid[1], R. I. Hayden[1], R. Forgie[4] and H. Ling[1]
[1]*University of British Columbia, Vancouver,*
[2]*Berlin,*
[3]*Brescia,*
[4]*Saint John,*
[1,4]*Canada*
[2]*Germany*
[3]*Italy*

1. Introduction

The Mitroflow aortic pericardial bioprosthesis has been available worldwide since 1982, except in the United States, Japan, and China. The original prosthesis was designated model 11, and the model 12, introduced in 1991, was approved in the United States in November 2007. The current model Mitroflow LX is available on the worldwide market, except for Japan and China.

The objective of this review is to document the clinical and hemodynamic performance of the Mitroflow pericardial bioprosthesis and to document the modifications of the Mitroflow LX model and the recently introduced calcium mitigation treatment of pericardial tissue.

2. Device specifications

The Mitroflow pericardial bioprosthesis has had three design changes since its introduction in 1982 (Figure 1A-J).

There are the general specifications of all three models of the prosthesis. The prosthesis is formulated with a single unit acetal homopolymer stent that provides flexibility and strength at implantation without the risk of residual distortion. The stent is low-profile to afford clearance of the coronary ostia, and to avoid interfering with the sinotubular junction in narrow aortic roots. The stent is also creep resistant. The stent is covered with surgical-grade polyester cloth and incorporates a tungsten impregnated radiopaque, medical-grade silicone sewing ring that is tiny and soft so it can be easily attached to the patient's tissue annulus. The silicone sewing ring also provides a secure hemostatic seal. The pericardium is mounted externally to maximize the flow area with wide, synchronous opening of the leaflets. The pericardium is used as a single component without critical stent-post sutures. The pericardial thickness is related to the size of the prosthesis. The pericardial tissue is selected for uniformity, and this tissue is sewn onto the external surface of the covered stent.

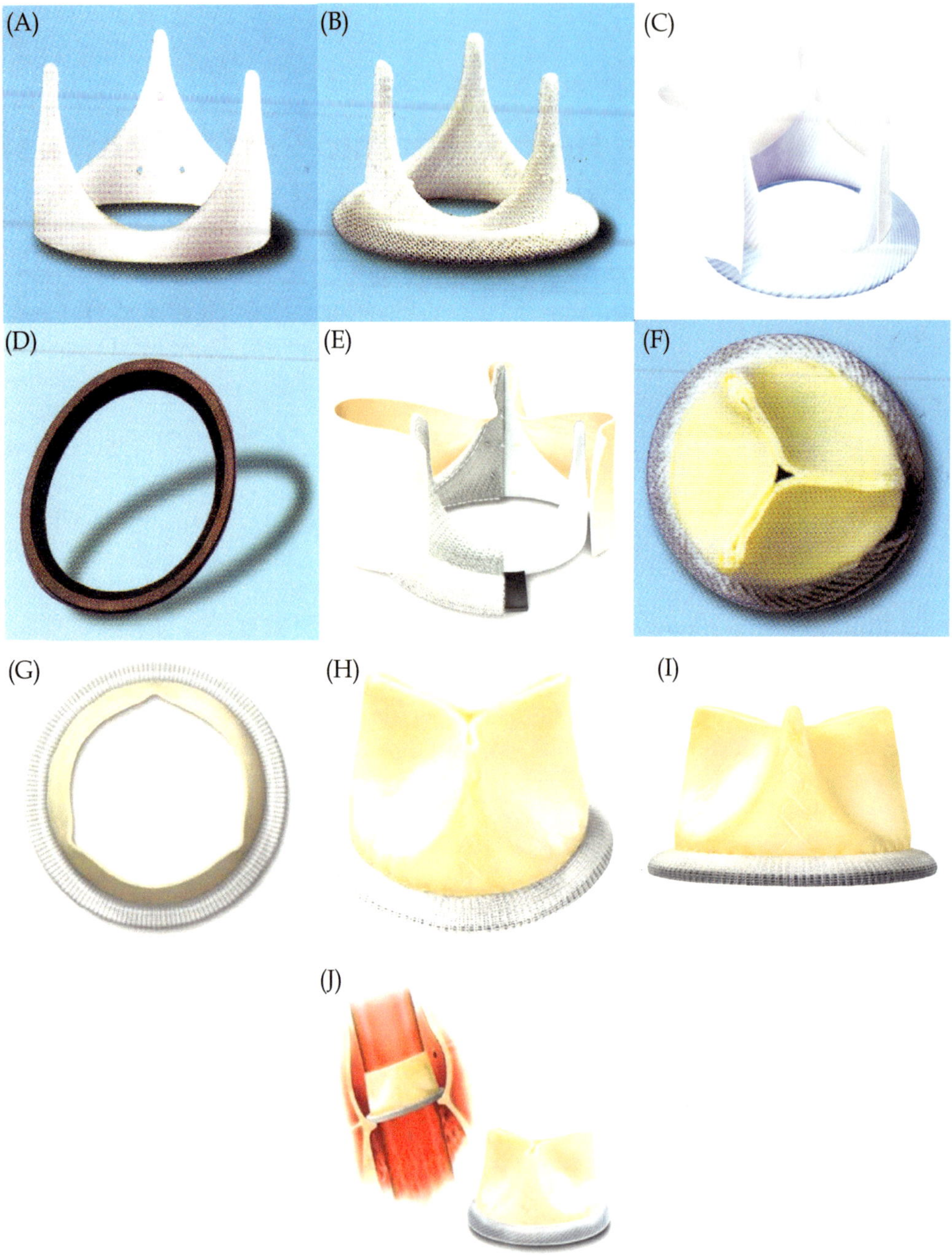

Fig. 1. (A) Acetyl homopolymer stent. (B) Stent covered polyester cloth. (C) Pericardium mounted externally. (D) Silicone sewing ring. (E) Cutaway of Prosthesis. (F) Aortic aspect of prosthesis. (G) Aortic aspect leaflets open. (H) Complete prosthesis - titled profile. (I) Complete prosthesis - lateral profile. (J) Supra-annular implantation of the prosthesis. Model 12 - B,C,F and Model LX - G,H,I

The pericardial tissue undergoes leaflet formation in the model 11 and 12 prostheses, and then fixation in 0.5% glutaraldehyde. The difference between model 11 and model 12 was that the polyester cloth was reversed so that the ribbed side was external rather than internal where there was a risk of abrasion.

The distinctive features of the initial models of the Mitroflow prostheses are inclusive in the current LX model. The design features of the various models are important when evaluating the current LX model. Model LX is a variation of model 12 with manufacturing modifications. The differences between the two models are related to manufacturing processes and minor design variations, but the material components remain the same as in model 12. The changes are these: because model LX uses automatic machine sewing instead of manual sewing for the fabric tube seam in the covered stent, there is a change in the fabric orientation of the covered stent. The number of sewing cuff base seams has been reduced to one seam. Model LX has changed tissue fixation with 0.2% glutaraldehyde of the bovine pericardium from postfixation (after stent application) to prefixation (before stent application) to facilitate tissue application on the stent. This change is from a manual leaflet formation method to an automated leaflet formation method. These manufacturing process improvements for model LX were implemented to increase manufacturing efficiencies, not to affect the design or performance of the prosthesis.

The next major change of the Mitroflow pericardial bioprosthesis is the addition of calcium mitigation therapy. Mitroflow models 11 and 12 did not have calcium mitigation therapy incorporated in the manufacturing process. The manufacturing processes are to control or reduce degeneration of biological tissue, induced by calcification, tissue stress, or both. The major contributing factors in the degeneration of biological tissue (porcine or pericardium) are considered to be residual aldehydes and the presence of phospholipids. The major manufacturers of bioprostheses have used chemical formulations to control one or both of these etiologies since the early 1980s.

The Sorin Group (Milan, Italy and Vancouver, Canada), manufacturer of the Mitroflow pericardial bioprosthesis, has recently completed an evaluation of incorporating calcium mitigation in the manufacturing process of the prosthesis and received market approval in Europe in July 2011 and subsequently in Canada. The Sorin Group has used methodology to control residual aldehydes in their other bioprostheses. This methodology is a detoxification process post-glutaraldehyde with homocysteic acid to neutralize unbound residual aldehydes. The methodology for the Mitroflow bioprosthesis is a chemical solution effective in reducing the phospholipid content of bovine pericardium (Figure 2).

The process has been named phospholipid reduction therapy (PRT), a patented chemical process that uses long-chain alcohol aqueous solutions to remove phospholipids from tissue materials. The process exposes the bovine pericardium to a buffered ethanolic solution containing long-chain aliphatic alcohol for specific times and temperatures. The PRT treatment is a sterile-filtered solution of 5% 1,2-Octanediol in ethanol and HEPES solutions. An evaluation of 5% 1,2-Octanediol in the rat subcutaneous model has revealed a very significant reduction of tissue calcium and phosphorus (Figure 2) (Pettenazzo et al., 2008). Incorporating PRT with homocysteic acid aldehyde control therapy is under consideration to control both known etiologies of tissue mineralization.

The Sorin Group (2011) has documented in their product literature the specifications and *in vitro* effective orifice areas (EOA) by valve size. The reported internal diameter/EOA for size 19 was 15.4 mm/1.7 cm^2; size 21, 17.3 mm/2.1 cm^2; size 23, 19.0 mm/2.8 cm^2; and size 25, 21.0 mm/3.2 cm^2.

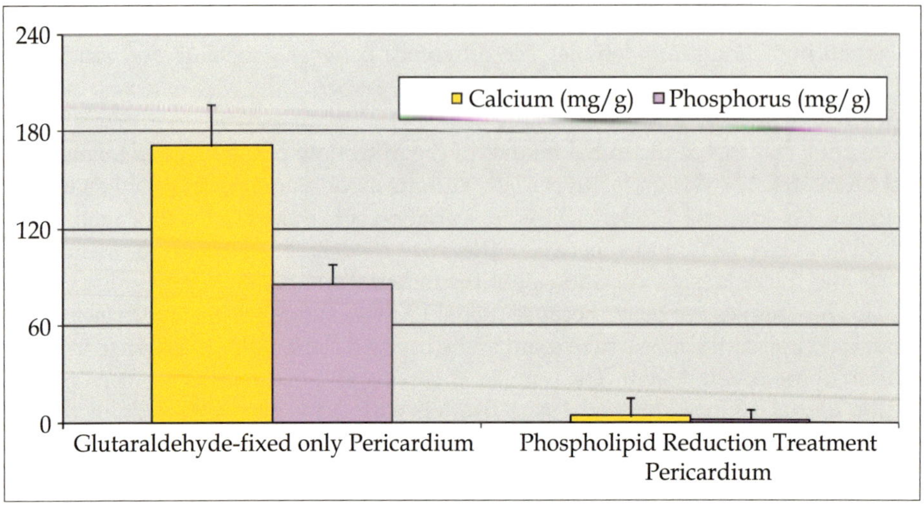

Fig. 2. Results of Phospholipid Reduction Therapy (PRT) in subcutaneous rat model Pettenazzo et al Eur J Cardiothorac Surg 2008

3. Implantation technique

The Mitroflow bioprosthesis can be implanted using either supra-annular or infra-annular techniques. The supra-annular technique is preferable to get the largest valve implanted and to optimize hemodynamic performance (Figure 1J). The supra-annular positioning facilitates a one-to-one annular match and optimal blood flow. The native annulus should be adequately debrided for placement of supra-annular suturing. Since the sewing cuff of the prosthesis is flat and non-scalloped, it may be optimal on some occasions, especially with bicuspid anatomy, to place non-pledgeted everting mattress sutures at the commissures and standard non-everting mattress sutures in the remainder of the annulus for supra-annular implantation.

4. Clinical performance

The clinical performance of the Mitroflow aortic bioprosthesis is comparable to that of other marketed porcine and pericardial bioprostheses (Jamieson, 2011).

The clinical performance of the Mitroflow pericardial bioprosthesis has been reported by several investigative groups (Table 1) (Benhameid et al., 2008; Minami et al., 2005; Yankah et al., 2008; Yankah et al., 2010; Jamieson et al., 2009; Alvarez et al., 2009; ISTHMUS investigators, 2011; Conte et al., 2010; Jamieson et al., 2009). Actuarial freedom from structural valve deterioration provides an assessment of durability while actual cumulative incidence analysis documents structural valve deterioration in patient groups, such as elderly patients, who are subject to competing risks of death. Actuarial freedom from structural valve deterioration (SVD) overestimates the incidence of SVD, while actual analysis provides the actual risk of failure in specific population groups.

Advancing life expectancy with the increased prevalence of aortic valve degenerative disease brings the need for an aortic bioprosthesis with excellent hemodynamic performance and comparable durability. The University of British Columbia and collaborating centers have published extensively on the Mitroflow pericardial bioprosthesis model 11 (Benhameid et al., 2008) and model 12 (Yankah, 2010; ISTHMUS Investigators, 2011, Lorusso, 2011 - Personal Communication - ISTHMUS Investigators).

Author	Prosthesis	Mean Age	Age Group	Freedom from SVD (%) Actuarial	Freedom from SVD (%) Actual	Time Interval (Years)
Jamieson et al. (2009)	Mitroflow		≥60	85.2 ± 3.9*	93.3 ± 1.8*	12
			≥65	85.0 ± 4.0*	94.2 ± 1.8*	12
			61-70	95.7 ± 4.3*	97.4 ± 2.6*	10
			>70	83.2 ± 4.6*	94.0 ± 1.9*	12
Yankah et al. (2008)	Mitroflow	73.2 ± 0.22				
			≥65	71.8 ± 6.0*	92.6 ± 4.6*	20
			≥70	84.8 ± 0.7*	96.6 ± 0.8*	20
ISTHMUS (2010)	Mitroflow	75.3 ± 6.8	<60	54.4 ± 3.4	60.9 ± 4.3	18
			61-70	62.0 ± 2.6	68.3 ± 3.3	18
			>70	78.2 ± 2.6	89.3 ± 2.5	18
			<60	75.4 ± 2.9**	87.4 ± 2.3**	18
			61-70	87.0 ± 1.6**	92.9 ± 0.4**	18
			>70	94.6 ± 0.6**	97.1 ± 0.5**	18

* *Reoperation,*
** *Reoperation, Autopsy & Echocardiography (non-prospective) Lorusso – Personal Communication 2011.*

Table 1. Freedom from Structural Valve Deterioration (SVD)

Benhameid et al. (2008) reported a satisfactory freedom from SVD after 15 years with model 11 for patients ≥70 years old. The majority of other publications provide information on the freedom from SVD in patient populations with model 11 (predominately) and 12 prostheses (Minami et al., 2006; Yankah et al., 2008). These reports provide support for use of the prosthesis in elderly patient populations. Yankah et al. (2008), documented in patients with predominately model 11 prostheses for 20 years, that freedom from SVD was 71.8 ± 6.0% for those ≥65 years old and 84.8 ± 0.7% for those ≥70 years old. Yankah et al. (2010) has since reported on 104 patients <60 years old (age range: 22-60 years) with a linearized rate of 1.9%/patient-year of SVD managed by reoperation with an actual risk of 12% at 10 years. Klieverik et al. (2007) concluded that the Mitroflow valve demonstrated an important complementary role to allograft and pulmonary autografts if implanted in appropriately selected patients.

The predominant publication on Mitroflow model 12 is Jamieson et al. (2009) (Figure 3A-D). This report provides preliminary support for using the prosthesis in patients 61-70 years old, as well as in patients >70 years old. The 12-year freedom from SVD (actual/actuarial) at explant was 94.4%/85.2% for those ≥60 years old, 94.2%/85.0% for those ≥65 years old, and 94.0%/83.2% for those >70 years old. For patients 61-70 years old, at 10 years, the freedom from SVD at explant was 97.4%/95.7%.

SVD at Explant

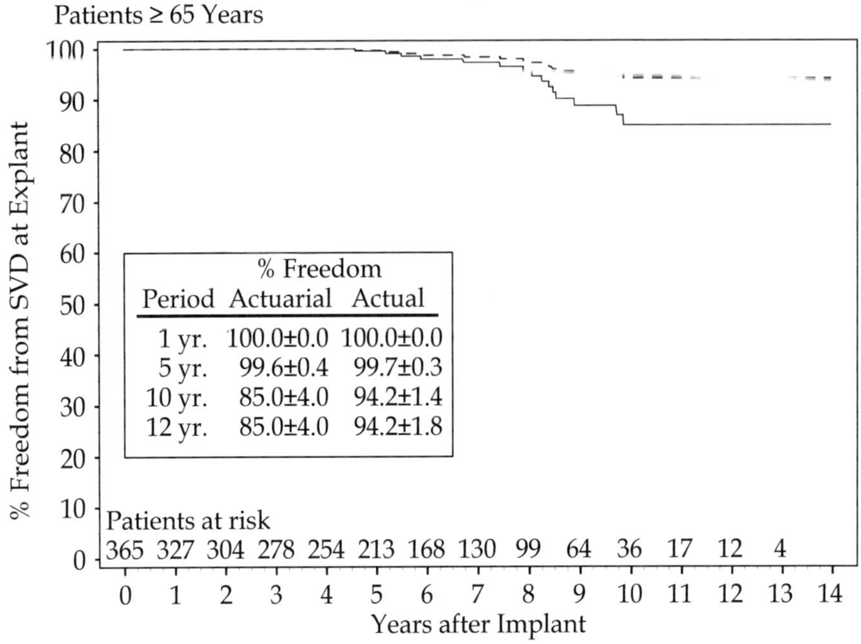

(A)

SVD at Explant

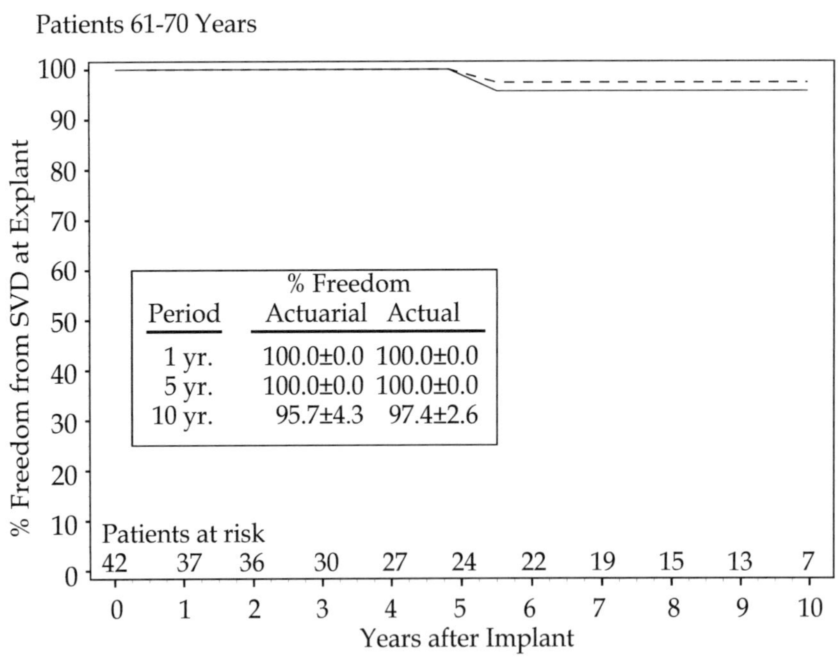

(B)

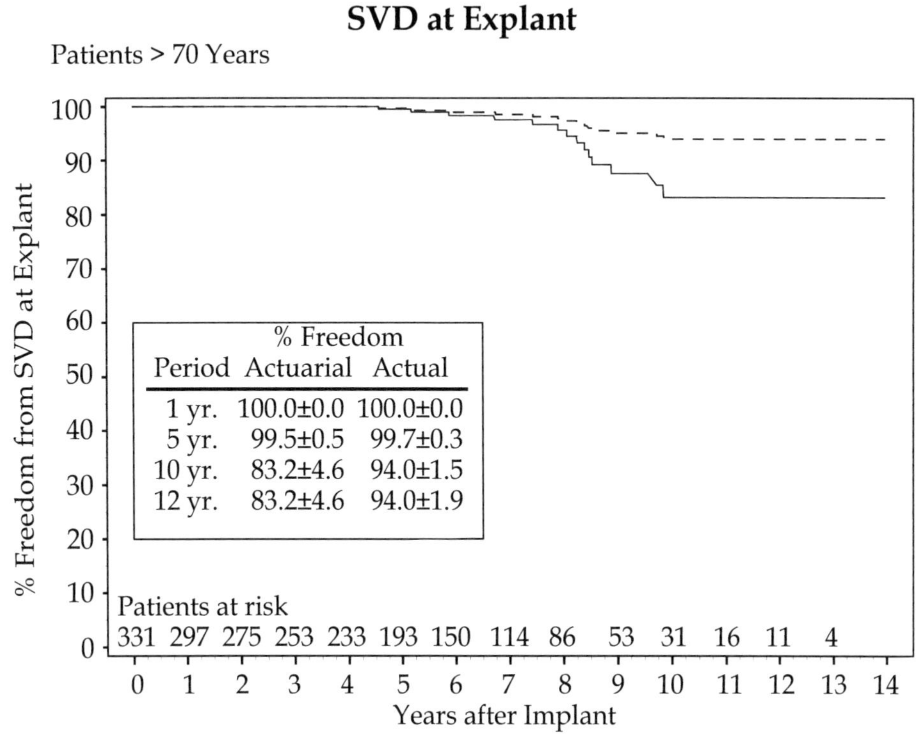

(C)

Fig. 3. Freedom from Structural Valve Deterioration (SVD) at Explant (A) ≥65 years, (B) 65-70 years, (C) >70 years

There always remains a concern about the true incidence of SVD unless there is a prospective echocardiographic program, because elderly patients may not be evaluated for prosthesis failure or presented for reoperation. The results in the 61-70 years old age group is encouraging, even though small in number, because patients with a failed prosthesis because of SVD in that age group would more likely to be referred for reoperative surgery.

In another recent report on the Mitroflow model 12, Alvarez et al. (2009) reported the freedom from SVD by reoperation, as well as the freedom from bioprosthesis degeneration determined from prospective echocardiographic assessment. These authors report their freedom from SVD at an advanced interval with a minimal number of patients at risk. The freedom from SVD at a more appropriate interval seems to be very similar to that documented in Jamieson et al. (2009). We believe that because Alvarez et al. (2009) did a prospective echocardiographic study, some patients had prophylactic reoperative surgery.

The most extensive published report is the multicenter ISTHMUS study (2011) on 1591 patients, of which 91% had model 12 prostheses. The study reported on SVD by actuarial analysis of echocardiographic diagnoses that used the American Association for Thoracic Surgery (AATS), Society of Thoracic Surgeons (STS), and European Association for Cardio-Thoracic Surgeons (EACTS) guidelines. Personal communication from the ISTHMUS

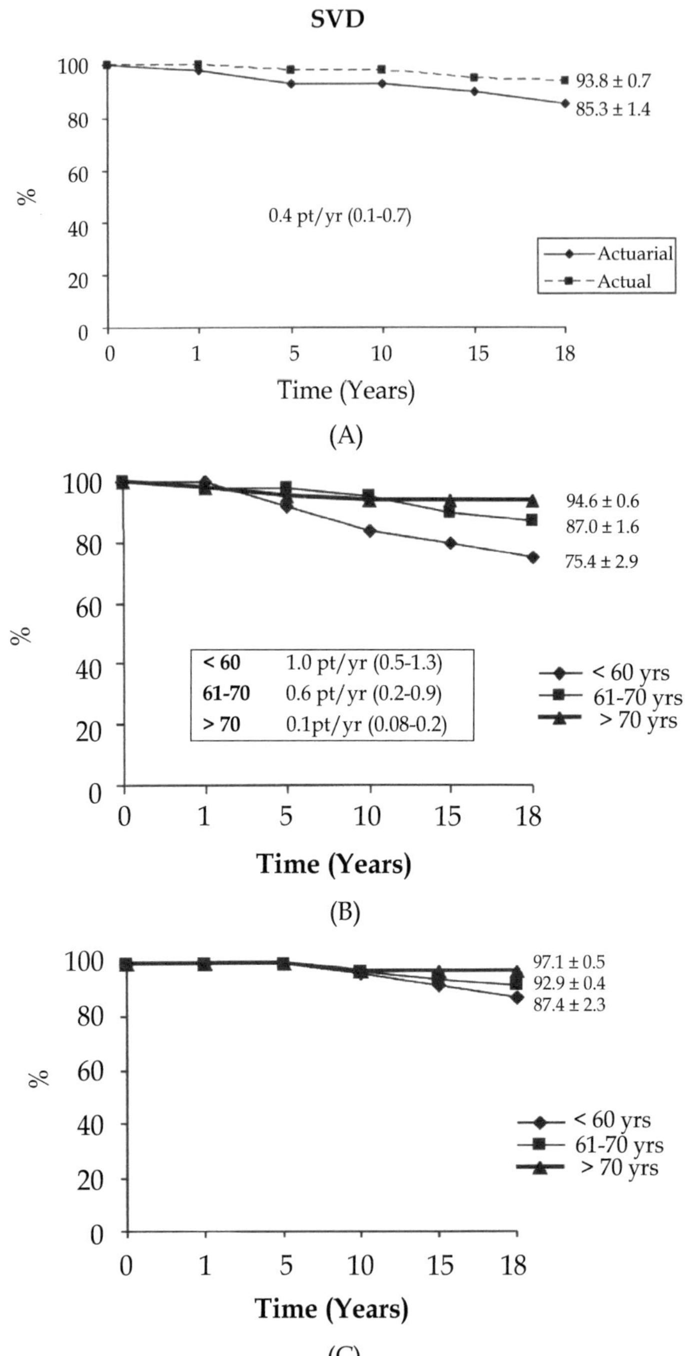

Fig. 4. Freedom from Structural Valve Deterioration (SVD) by clinical relevant symptoms, explantation or autopsy. (A) Overall freedom from SVD Actuarial and Actual. (B) Actuarial freedom from SVD. (C) Actual freedom (cumulative incidence) from SVD. ISTHMUS Investigators - Lorusso (Personal Communication - 2011)

authors (R Lorusso) has provided actual documentation incorporating clinical symptoms, explantation, echocardiographic examination, and autopsy assessment. The 18-year actual/actuarial freedom from SVD incorporating clinical symptoms, explantation, echocardiographic examination and autopsy examination for patients <60 years old was 87.4%/75.4%, for patients 61-70 years old was 92.9%/87.0%, and for patients >70 years old was 97.1%/94.6%.

4. Hemodynamic performance

The hemodynamic performance of the Mitroflow aortic bioprosthesis is considered excellent and very important in optimizing management for the small aortic annulus (Table 2).

	Size				
Author	19 mm	21 mm	23 mm	25 mm	27 mm
Yankah et al. (2008)	1.4	1.5	1.85		
Jamieson et al. (2009)	1.4	1.4	1.8	1.8	
Conte et al. (2010)	1.05	1.22	1.37	1.60	1.82

Table 2. Hemodynamic Orifice Areas (cm^2) for Mitroflow Aortic Bioprostheses

These three studies show excellent hemodynamic performance of the prosthesis. Jamieson et al. (2009) reported that the *in vivo* effective orifice areas by valve size provide the opportunity of avoiding obstructive characteristics for all valve sizes, including optimizing the management of the small aortic annulus. The EOA for the 19-mm and 21-mm prostheses is 1.4 cm^2, and for the 23-mm and 25-mm prostheses is 1.8 cm^2. These EOAs in the population reported prevented prosthesis-patient mismatch in all valve sizes with indexed EOAs ranging from 0.8 to 1.0 cm^2/m^2.

In their study on the hemodynamic performance of 1513 isolated aortic valve replacements, primarily model 11, Yankah et al. (2008) reported that the EOA for size 19-mm prosthesis was 1.4 cm^2; the 21-mm, 1.5 cm^2; and the 23-mm, 1.85 cm^2.

The Conte et al. (2010) study of the Mitroflow model 12 prosthesis reported very satisfactory hemodynamic performance. The effective orifice areas for the 19-mm prosthesis was 1.05 cm2; the 21-mm, 1.22 cm^2; the 23-mm, 1.37 cm^2; the 25-mm, 1.60 cm^2; and the 27-mm, 1.82 cm^2. The mean gradient for the 19-mm prosthesis was 13.4mm Hg.; the 21-mm, 11.5mm Hg.; the 23-mm, 10.6mm Hg.; the 25-mm, 8.6mm Hg.; and 27-mm, 7.3mm Hg.

The Mitroflow LX external mounted pericardial bioprosthesis will continue to provide optimization of hemodynamics regardless of valve size, especially in the small aortic annulus. The addition of anticalcification therapy to the manufacturing process will provide the opportunity to retard or prevent structural valve deterioration of the bioprosthesis and may improve its long-term durability; this prosthesis has clinically been shown to be comparable in durability to other bovine pericardial aortic bioprostheses (Jamieson et al., 2009; Alvarez et al., 2009; ISTHMUS Investigators, 2011).

5. References

Pettenazzo E., Valente M., Thiene G. Octanediol treatment of glutaraldehyde fixed bovine pericardium: evidence of anticalcification efficacy in the subcutaneous rat model. *Eur J Cardothorac Surg* 2008;34;418-422.

Sorin Group. Sorin Mitroflow - Aortic pericardial heart valve. Hemodynamics, durability and ease of implant in one valve. Sorin Group (Marketing Pamphlet). Available at: <http://www.sorin.com/product/mitroflowreg>
and
<http://www.sorin.com/product/mitroflowreg-aortic-pericardial-heart-valve>
Accessed 15 August 2011.

Jamieson WRE. Biological prostheses: current options and clinical performance. In: *Cardiothoracic Surgery Review*, Franco KL & Thourani VH (Eds.). Philadelphia, PA: Lippincott Williams & Wilkins, 2011 (In Press).

Benhameid O, Pomar JL, Jamieson WRE, Germann E, Castella M, Pellerin M, Carrier M, Brownlee RT. CarboMedics Mitroflow pericardial aortic bioprosthesis: performance in patients with ≥ 60 years of age. *Thorac Cardiovasc Surg*. 2008:56;1-5.

Minami K, Zittermann A, Schulte-Eistrup S, Koertke H, Korfer R. Mitroflow Synergy prostheses for aortic valve replacement: 19 years experience in 1,516 patients. *Ann Thorac Surg* 2005;80:1699-1705.

Yankah CA, Pasic M, Musci M, Stein J, Detschades C, Siniawski H, Hetzer R. Aortic valve replacement with the Mitroflow pericardial bioprosthesis: durability results up to 21 years. *J Thorac Cardiovasc Surg* 2008;136:688-696.

Yankah CA. Mitroflow pericardial aortic bioprosthesis in patients younger than 60 years. *J Thorac Cardiovasc Surg* 2010;140;e83-e84.

Klieverik LM, Takkenberg JJ, Bekkers JA, Roos-Hesselink JW, Witsenburg M, Bogers AJ. The Ross operation; a Trojan horse? *Eur Heart J* 2007;28(16):1993-2000.

Jamieson WRE, Koerfer R, Yankah CA, Dolman W, Zitterman A, Minami K, Hayden RI Ling H, Hetzer R. Mitroflow Aortic Pericardial Bioprosthesis– Clinical Performance. *Eur J Cardiothorac Surg*. 2009;36:818-824.

Alvarez RJ, Sierra J, Vega M, Adrio B, Martinez-Comendador J, Gude F, Martinez-Cerijo J, Garcia J. Early calcification of the aortic Mitroflow pericardial bioprosthesis in the elderly. *Interact Cardiovas Thorac Surg.*, 2009;9:842-846.

ISTHMUS Investigators. The Italian study on the Mitroflow postoperative results (ISTHMUS): a 20-year, multicentre evaluation of Mitroflow pericardial bioprosthesis. *Eur J Cardiothorac Surg,* 2011 Jan;39(1):18-26; discussion 26. Epub 2010 Jul 10.

Conte J, Weissman N, Dearani JA, Bavaria J, Heimansohn D, Dembitsky W, Doyle D. A North American, prospective, multicenter assessment of the Mitroflow aortic pericardial prosthesis. *Ann Thorac Surg* 2010;90:144-152.

Jamieson WRE, Forgie WR, Hayden RI, Langlois Y, Ling H, Stanford EA, Roberts KA, Brownlee RT, Moon BC, Dolman WB. Hemodynamic evaluation of the Mitroflow aortic pericardial bioprosthesis. *Thorac Cardiovasc Surg* 2009;57:1-6.

9

Influence of Prosthesis-Patient Mismatch on Survival with Aortic Valve Replacement

W.R. Eric Jamieson, Charlie Zhang,
Jennifer Higgins, Michael H. Yamashita and Jian Ye
University of British Columbia, Vancouver
British Columbia,
Canada

1. Introduction

Prosthesis-patient mismatch (PPM) was first described over 30 years ago (Rahimtoola, 1978) for aortic valve replacement: when the *in vivo* effective orifice area (EOA) of the prosthetic valve is less than that of the native, non-diseased, human valve. Extensive documentation on the role of PPM after aortic valve replacement (AVR) particularly addresses left ventricular mass regression and patient survival. Controversy continues about the influence of PPM on patient survival, both early and late mortality. Many studies (Pibarot and Dumesnil, 2000; Muneretto et al., 2004; Mohty et al., 2006; Tasca et al., 2006; Moon et al., 2006; Florath et al., 2008; Mohty et al., 2009; Blais et al., 2003) report PPM to be an independent predictor of mortality while others (Jamieson et al., 2010; Kato et al., 2007; Vicchio et al., 2008; Mascherbauer et al., 2008; Monin et al., 2007) showed no significant effect of PPM on patient outcome. There is also debate about whether the control of PPM reduces congestive heart failure and regression of the left ventricular mass, thereby contributing to improved survival. Several Canadian centers have been actively involved in this area of research, namely the Laval University group led by P. Pibarot, J.G. Dumesnil and D. Mohty, the UBC group led by W.R.E. Jamieson, and the University of Ottawa group led by M. Ruel and A. Kulik.

PPM is categorized by Pibarot and Dumesnil (2000), Mohty et al. (2009), and Jamieson et al. (2010) as normal (EOA index (EOAI) of > 0.85 cm^2 / m^2), mild-to-moderate (> 0.65 cm^2 / m^2 to ≤ 0.85 cm^2 / m^2), and severe (≤ 0.65 cm^2 / m^2). Tasca et al. (2006) defined PPM as an EOAI of ≤ 0.80 cm^2 / m^2, Moon et al. (2006) as an EOAI of < 0.75 cm^2 / m^2, while Ruel et al. (2004), Kulik et al. (2006), Kato et al. (2007), and Monin et al. (2007) as EOAI of ≤ 0.85 cm^2 / m^2; Florath et al. (2008) and Vicchio et al. (2008) chose 0.60 cm^2 / m^2 as the cutoff between moderate and severe PPM. As can be seen, there is no clear consensus on the exact definition of PPM; this lack of consensus may contribute at least in part to the observed discrepancies in the conclusions of the studies. The studies also differ in the length of their patient follow-up. Jamieson et al. (2010) report survival to 15 years, Moon et al. (2006) and Mohty et al. (2009) to 12 years, and the majority of the other publications on the topic of PPM report survival from 4 to 8 years (Mothy et al. 2006; Tasca et al., 2006; Florath et al., 2008; Kato et al., 2007; Mascherbauer et al., 2008; Monin et al., 2007). These differences may also contribute to the different conclusions reached.

It should be noted that the indication for surgical management of aortic stenosis is symptomatic severe aortic stenosis (< 1.0 cm^2 valve area). In the majority of patients, this is equivalent to an EOAI at or below the level of severe mismatch by our definition.

2. The influence of PPM on postoperative patient outcomes

The objective of our study (Jamieson et al., 2010) on 3,343 patients having AVR for severe aortic stenosis or mixed aortic stenosis/insufficiency was to determine the predictors for all levels of PPM on mortality and to determine if there is a relationship between PPM and other predictors of survival. The prostheses used were contemporary stented bioprostheses (2493) and mechanical prostheses (850). More specifically, 667 patients had Carpentier-Edwards PERIMOUNT pericardial prostheses (Edwards Lifesciences, Irvine, CA), 1250 patients had Carpentier-Edwards supra-annular porcine prostheses, 576 patients had Medtronic Mosaic porcine prostheses (Medtronic, Minneapolis, MN), 462 patients had St. Jude Medical mechanical prostheses (St. Jude Medical, St. Paul, MN), and 388 patients had CarboMedics mechanical prostheses (Sorin-CarboMedics, Saluggia, Italy) (Figure 1). There is a misconception with the Carpentier-Edwards supra-annular aortic valve for the early version (prior to 1985) of the mitral valve failed because of stent-post dehiscence due to excessive trimming of the aortic wall; however, this failure mode was identified in only one aortic prosthesis before the manufacturing trimming was changed (Jamieson et al., 2005; Jamieson et al, 2009). The level of PPM was classified for each patient based on reference EOAs and size for each prosthesis in the published literature. The patients considered for the study had their first aortic valve replacement. Patients who had a subsequent valvular replacement were censored alive on the date of the reoperative procedures. This concept was to avoid a hemodynamically different prosthesis at the time of reoperative explantation.

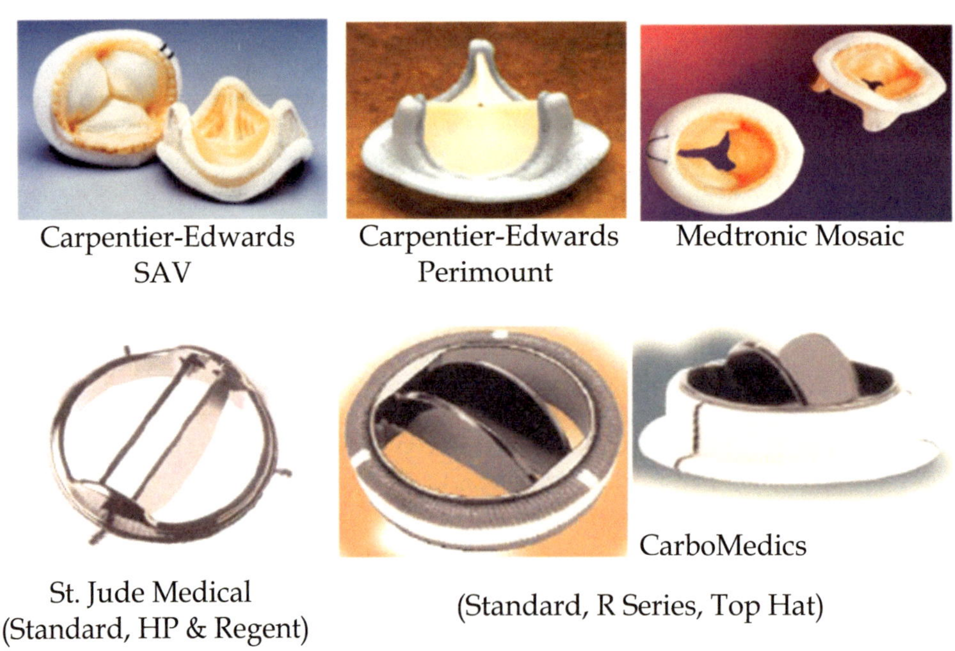

Fig. 1. Contemporary prostheses used in Jamieson et al. (2010)

The results of Jamieson et al. (2010) (N = 3343) are compared with those of Molty et al. (2009) (N = 2576); J.G. Dumesnil and P. Pibarot, two of the more prominent investigators in the area of PPM, were also authors of the 2009 study.

	Jamieson et al. 2010 (Overall) UBC Study			Mohty et al. 2009 (Late) Laval Study		
	NS PPM (N = 3343)	Moderate PPM (N = 1547)	Severe PPM (N = 212)	NS PPM (N = 1739)	Moderate PPM (N = 797)	Severe PPM (N = 40)
Pre-operative data						
Age, yrs	66 ± 11	69 ± 10	69 ± 12	68 ± 10	71 ± 9	69 ± 11
Female, %	29	36	57	33	50	67
BSA, m^2	1.8 ± 0.2	1.9 ± 0.2	2.0 ± 0.3	1.8 ± 0.2	1.8 ± 0.2	1.9 ± 0.3
BMI, kg/m^2	26 ± 4	28 ± 5	32 ± 8	26 ± 5	29 ± 5	32 ± 7
Hypertension	19	27	28	54	59	68
NYHA class III/IV	77	75	68	61	68	67
LVEF < 50%, %	19	19	18	19	17	18
Operative data						
Mechanical prosthesis, %	32	19	23	24	14	43
Prosthesis size ≤21mm, %	14	42	91	16	38	80
Concomitant CABG	40	47	44	43	46	58
EOAI, cm^2 / m^2	0.99 ± 0.15	0.76 ± 0.05	0.60 ± 0.04	1.10 ± 0.20	0.80 ± 0.05	± 0.04

NS = nonsignificant; PPM = prosthesis-patient mismatch (see text for description of the categories); BSA = body surface area; BMI = body mass index; NYHA = New York Heart Association; LVEF = left ventricular ejection fraction; CABG = coronary artery bypass grafting

Table 1. Descriptive preoperative and operative data of the two patient cohort studies: Overall (2010) and Late (2009)

As can be seen, the preoperative and operative characteristics of both cohorts are quite comparable, with the exception of hypertension and female gender, both of which higher in the Mohty et al. cohort. Also, 46.3% of patients were classified as having no PPM, 47.4% as mild-to-moderate PPM, and 6.3% as severe PPM in the Jamieson et al. cohort, whereas 67.5% of the patients had no PPM, 30.9% had moderate PPM, and 1.6% had severe PPM in the Mohty et al. cohort. The Jamieson et al. data analysis was based primarily on overall survival (early + late), whereas Mohty et al. took only late mortality into account because early mortality in the same cohort had already been analyzed by Blais et al. (2003).

Jamieson et al. found no significant difference in early mortality between the EOAI categories (no PPM: 3.4%, mild-to-moderate PPM: 3.5%, and severe PPM: 2.8%), or in late mortality (no PPM: 33.0%, moderate PPM: 30.2%, and severe PPM: 29.2%). The freedom from cardiac death by EOAI categories was also not significant (no PPM: 68.7 ± 2.4%, moderate PPM: 68.9 ± 2.6%, and severe PPM: 58.9 ± 9.7%, p = 0.699). In addition, the freedom from valve-related mortality was not significantly different by EOAI categories (no

PPM: 84.3 ± 2.0%, moderate PPM: 85.7% ± 1.9%, and severe PPM: 76.8 ± 9.6%, p = 0.998). The overall (early + late) survival, at 15 years, was 38.1 ± 2.1% for no PPM, 37.0 ± 2.2% for mild-moderate PPM, and 22.1 ± 6.5% for severe PPM (no PPM versus severe PPM: p=0.040) (Figure 2).

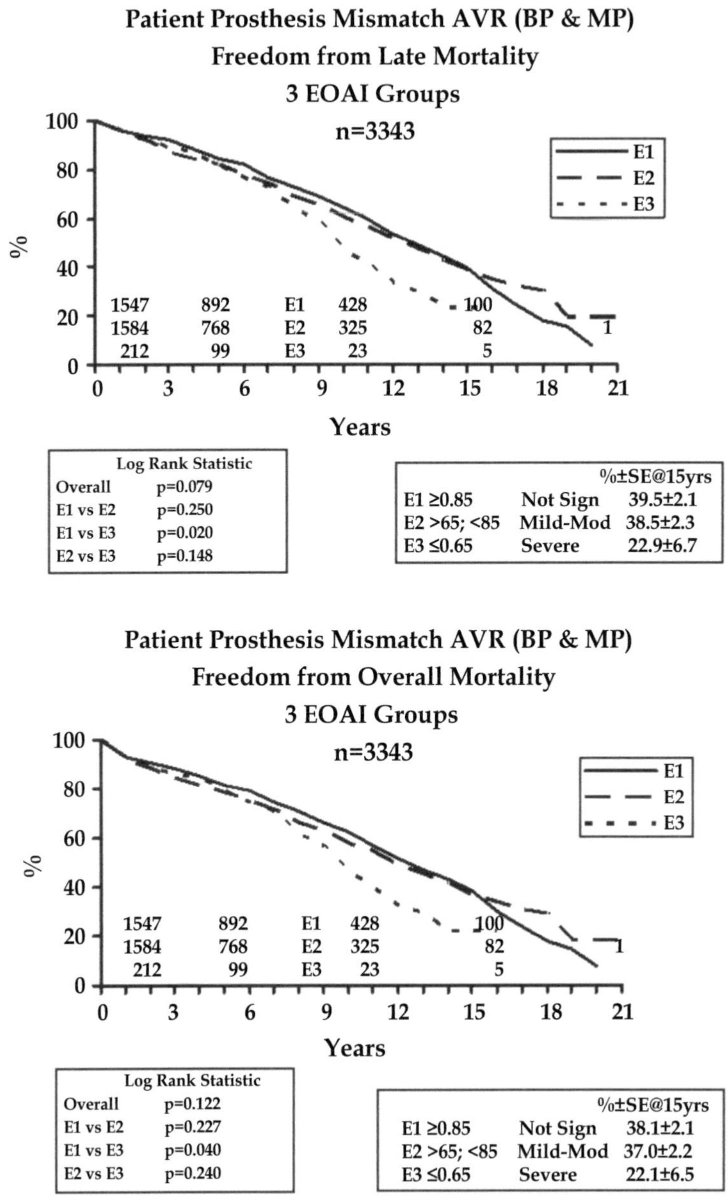

Fig. 2. Freedom from late and overall mortality by three effective orifice area index (EOAI) groups (N = 3343) (Jamieson et al., 2010). E1 (solid line), not significant; E2 (long-dash line), mild to moderate; and E3 (short-dash line), severe. (AVR = aortic valve replacement; BP = bioprosthesis; MP = mechanical prosthesis)

However, Mohty et al. found survival to be significantly lower for patients with severe PPM (5-year survival: no PPM: 84 ± 1%, moderate PPM: 81 ± 2%, severe PPM: 74 ± 8%; 10-year survival: no PPM: 61 ± 2%, moderate PPM: 57 ± 3%, severe PPM: 40 ± 10%). Freedom from cardiovascular-related death was also found to be significantly lower in patients with severe PPM (5-year survival: no PPM: 93 ± 1%, moderate PPM: 90 ± 1%, severe PPM: 78 ± 7%; 10-year survival: no PPM: 81 ± 2%, moderate PPM: 77 ± 3%, severe PPM: 50 ± 11%).

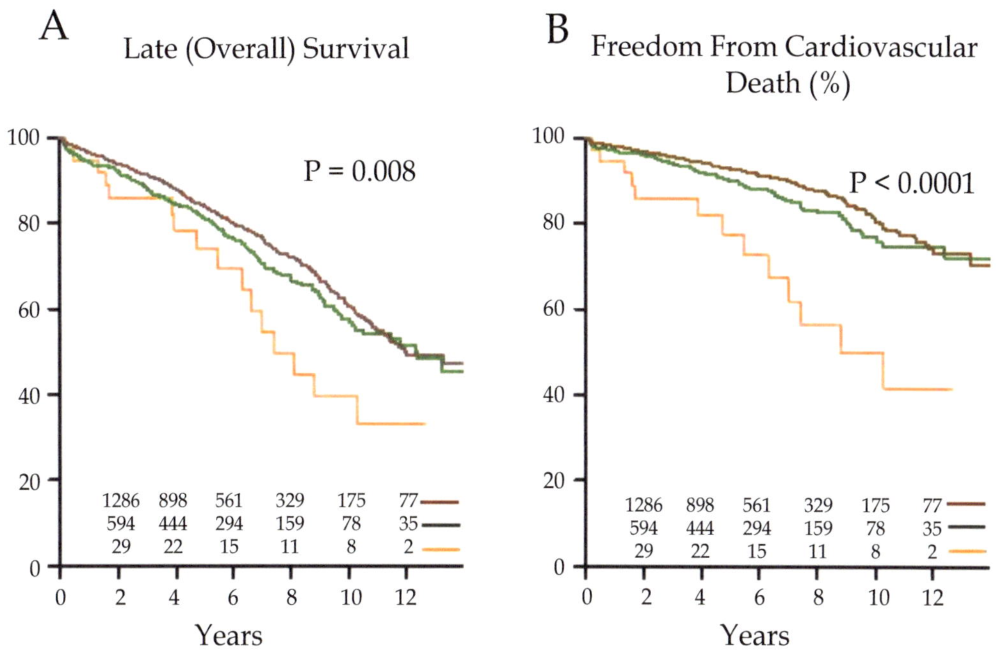

Fig. 3. Late overall survival and freedom from cardiovascular death (from Mohty et al., 2009). Brown line indicates nonsignificant prosthesis patient mismatch (PPM); green line indicates moderate PPM; orange line shows severe PPM

The conclusion by Mohty et al. that severe PPM is an independent predictor of late mortality in patients undergoing AVR differs from the conclusion by Jamieson et al. that PPM is not a predictor of survival. It should be noted that the severe PPM group consisted of 40 patients (1.6%) in the Mohty cohort whereas it consisted of 212 patients (6.3%) in the Jamieson cohort. The very small percentage of patients with severe PPM in the Mohty et al. study could be attributed to the fact that [1] only patients who survived through the short-term period following AVR were included (whereas all patients undergoing AVR was included in the Jamieson et al. study), and [2] the short-term mortality was much higher in the Mohty cohort (7 out of 27 patients with severe PPM, 25.9%), compared with the Jamieson cohort (6 out of 212, 2.8%), and therefore not as many patients in the severe PPM survived past the early period to be included in the Mohty et al. study. The finding of severe PPM as a significant predictor of survival may be purely related to the small group size. In other words, if the group had consisted of more patients, severe PPM may not have been found to be an independent predictor. The discrepancy between the findings of these two studies warrants further investigation.

In Jamieson et al., age, NYHA class III/IV, concomitant CABG, renal failure and dialysis, and emergent preoperative status were found to be predictors of early mortality (114/3343, 3.4%) on multivariate analysis. Because a univariate analysis of the various EOAI categories showed no significance in early mortality, there was no need for a multivariate analysis on PPM versus early mortality. A study by Blais et al. (2003) revealed LVEF < 40%, infectious endocarditis, emergent status, cardiopulmonary bypass time, chronic lung disease, and moderate-severe PPM to be independent predictors of early mortality (58/1266, 4.6%). Again, the short-term mortality in the severe PPM category was much higher in Blais et al. (7 out of 27 patients with severe PPM, 25.9%) than in Jamieson et al. (6 out of 212 patients, 2.8%), which may have contributed to the significant finding by Blais et al. that severe PPM was an independent predictor of survival (Figure 4). It is not clear why early mortality was so high in Blais et al.

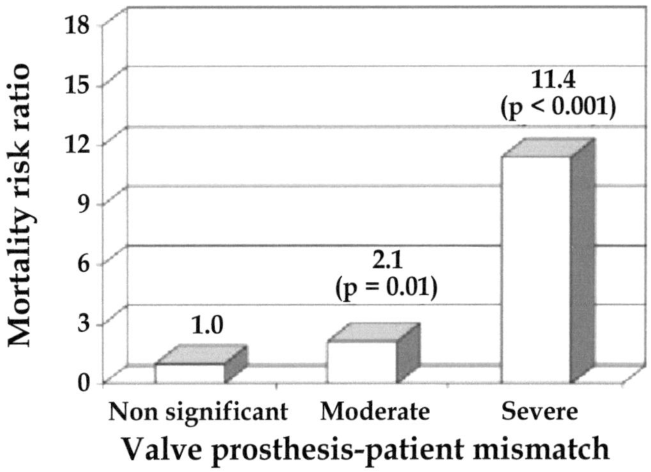

Fig. 4. Relative risk ratio for short-term mortality according to the presence and severity of valve prosthesis-patient mismatch (from Blais et al., 2003). Numbers above the bars indicate the relative risk ratio for mortality compared with the group with nonsignificant mismatch

The predictors for late mortality, identified in a multivariate analysis in Jamieson et al. were age, male gender, NYHA functional class III/IV, concomitant coronary artery bypass, LVEF < 35%, BMI < 18, BMI > 35, bioprosthesis, preoperative congestive heart failure, diabetes mellitus, renal failure, and chronic obstructive pulmonary disease. In comparison, Mohty et al. (2009) found age, coronary artery disease, diabetes, renal failure, chronic lung disease, mechanical prosthesis, and severe PPM to be multivariate predictors of late mortality.

Jamieson et al. found EOAI to have no predictive effect on survival, whether early, late, or overall, despite the survival curves differing by EOAI categories (38.1 ± 2.1% 15-year overall survival for no PPM, 37.0 ± 2.2% for mild-to-moderate PPM, and 22.1 ± 6.5% for severe PPM). The reasons for the differences in survival curves are related to the complexity of the patients in the three categories, especially the category of severe PPM for ≤ 60 years and ejection fraction ≤ 50%, rather than a direct contribution from PPM.

Survival was adjusted in Jamieson et al. to determine the effect of covariates (EOAI, age, BMI, and EF). Severe EOAI had no relationship on adjusted survival for the evaluated covariates, except for very low level of significance for EF > 50%.

The influence of BMI was further evaluated (Yamashita et al., personal communication). Overweight or mild-to-moderately obese patients had a lower risk of early mortality, while underweight and severely obese patients had a higher risk of late mortality. When patients were analyzed as normal/underweight or overweight/obese, those with a normal EOAI had better 15-year survival than those with severe PPM. After adjusting for EOAI, age > 60 years and EF ≤ 50% indicated a higher risk of overall (early + late) mortality within BMI categories. These results suggest that BMI is associated with survival after AVR and that PPM may modify the effect.

EOAI was also evaluated as a continuous variable (along with other variables except EF), as well as a categorical variable, which revealed that EOAI was not an independent risk factor for late (> 30 days) or overall mortality. The predictors, otherwise, were not different from the categorical modeling except for the elimination of valve size and the addition of BMI for early mortality. Valve type was eliminated for late mortality and overall mortality.

The survival curves in Jamieson et al. show that severe PPM (EOAI of ≤ 0.65 cm^2/m^2) reduces survival for patients > 60 years old but not for patients ≤ 60 years old, that severe PPM reduces survival for patients with a BMI ≥ 25kg/m^2 but not for those with a BMI < 25 kg/m^2, and that severe PPM reduces survival for patients with an ejection fraction > 50% but not for those with an EF ≤ 50% (Figure 5). In comparison, Mohty et al. found that severe PPM was associated with increased mortality in patients < 70 years old but not in older patients, and that it significantly affected survival in patients with a BMI < 30kg/m^2 but not in those with a BMI ≥ 30kg/m^2 (Figure 6A, 6B, 6C, 6D). They also found moderate-to-severe PPM to be an independent predictor of late mortality in patients with a pre-operative LVEF < 50% but not in those with preserved LV systolic function (Figure 6E, 6F). With regard to these discrepancies, it is worth noting that there were only 21 patients in the Jamieson et al. BMI < 25 kg/m^2 severe PPM group and 39 patients in the LVEF ≤ 50% severe PPM group, while for the severe PPM subset of the Mohty cohort, there were fewer than 20 patients in each of the < 70 years old, ≥ 70 years old, BMI < 30 kg/m^2, and BMI ≥ 30kg/m^2 subgroups. We therefore believe that the discrepancies in the above results may be purely due to random variations in the small data sets, and that if given an adequate number of cases in each of the categories, there may be no differences in the results between the Jamieson et al. and the Mohty et al. groups.

Ruel et al. (2006) found that PPM primarily affected patients with impaired left ventricular function at the time of AVR, and patients in whom PPM was associated with decreased overall long-term survival, lower freedom from heart failure, and diminished left ventricular mass regression. Also, an EOAI ≤ 0.85 cm^2 / m^2 did not have a significantly detrimental effect in patients with normal preoperative left ventricular function. However, the authors pointed out that PPM might have been found to have a significant effect in the normal LV function cohort had they evaluated cases with severe mismatch (≤ 0.65 cm^2 / m^2). An earlier study by Ruel et al. (2004) had shown that although PPM had significant effects on cardiac end points (occurrence of congestive heart failure, etc), it had no effect on overall survival after AVR. Kulik et al. (2006) found that patients with low-gradient aortic stenosis (LGAS, defined as an aortic valve area of < 1.2cm^2, a mean transvalvular pressure gradient of < 40 mmHg, and a LVEF of < 50%) have worse long-term outcomes after AVR, and that PPM further adversely affects the long-term outcomes of LGAS patients and should therefore be avoided in this population.

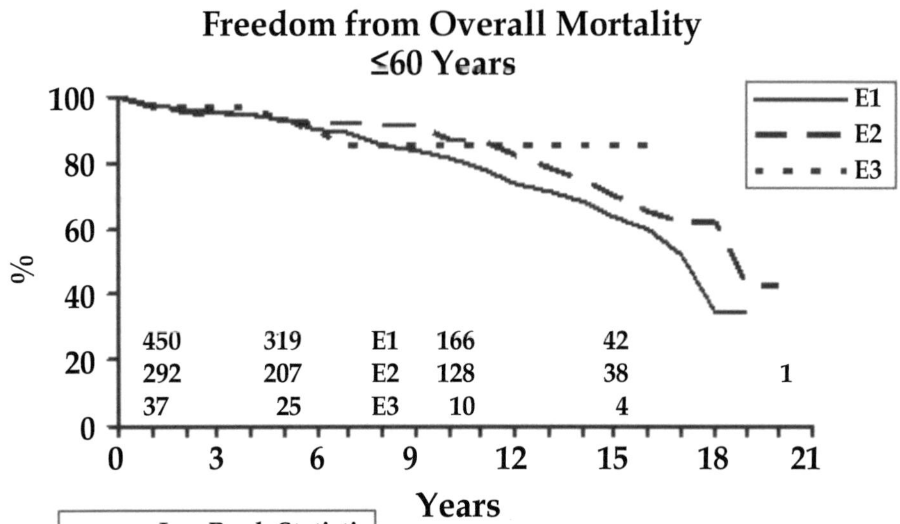

Log Rank Statistic	
Overall	p=0.171
E1 vs E2	p=0.090
E1 vs E3	p=0.301
E2 vs E3	p=0.662

		%±SE@15yrs
E1≥0.85	Not Sign	63.5±3.9
E2 >65; <85	Mild-Mod	69.8±4.5
E3 ≤0.65	Severe	85.0±7.0

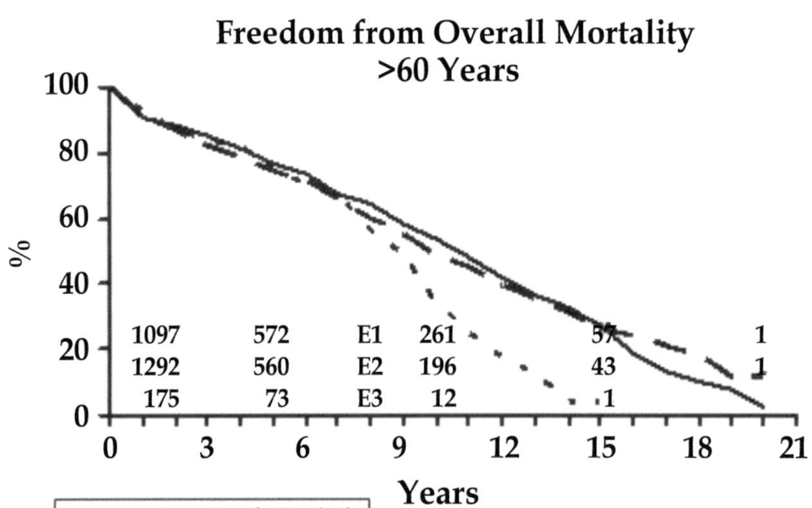

Log Rank Statistic	
Overall	p=0.128
E1 vs E2	p=0.432
E1 vs E3	p=0.025
E2 vs E3	p=0.139

		%±SE@15yrs
E1 ≥0.85	Not Sign	27.2±2.3
E2 >65; <85	Mild-Mod	26.6±2.4
E3 ≤0.65	Severe	4.2±3.9

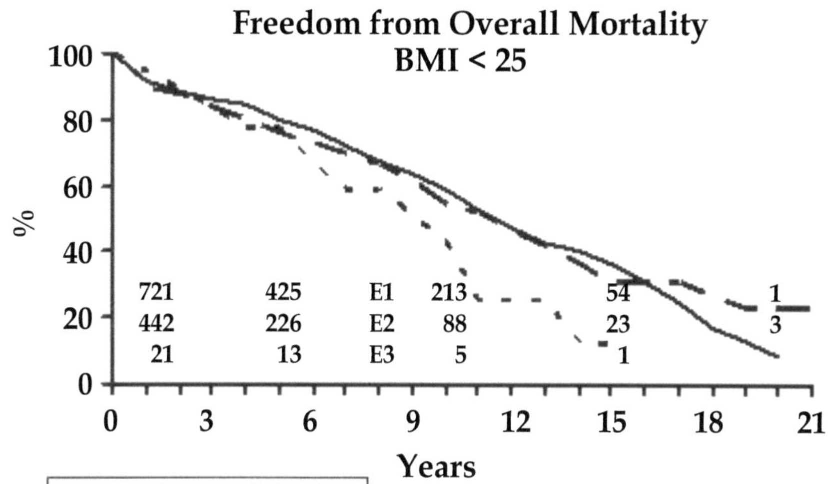

	Log Rank Statistic
Overall	p=0.357
E1 vs E2	p=0.523
E1 vs E3	p=0.169
E2 vs E3	p=0.282

		%±SE@15yrs
E1 ≥0.85	Not Sign	36.7±2.7
E2 >65; <85	Mild-Mod	31.0±3.9
E3 ≤0.65	Severe	12.7±10.9

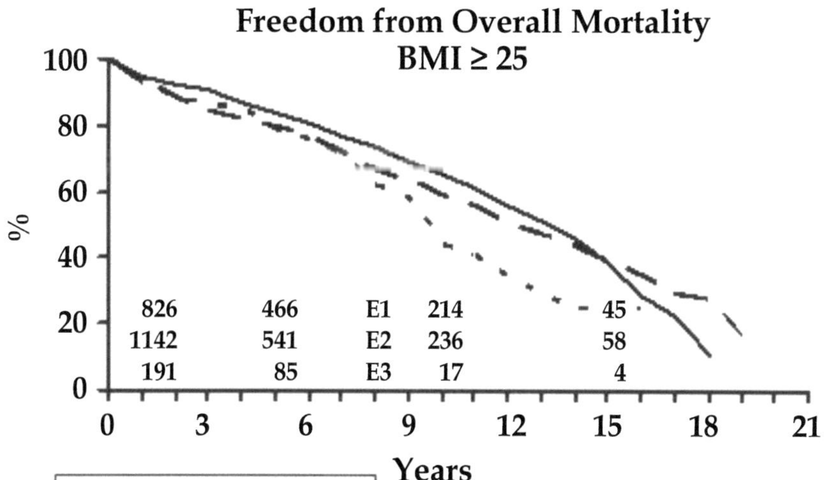

	Log Rank Statistic
Overall	p=0.089
E1 vs E2	p=0.114
E1 vs E3	p=0.031
E2 vs E3	p=0.339

		%±SE@15yrs
E1 ≥0.85	Not Sign	38.4±3.2
E2 >65; <85	Mild-Mod	39.7±2.6
E3 ≤0.65	Severe	24.5±7.7

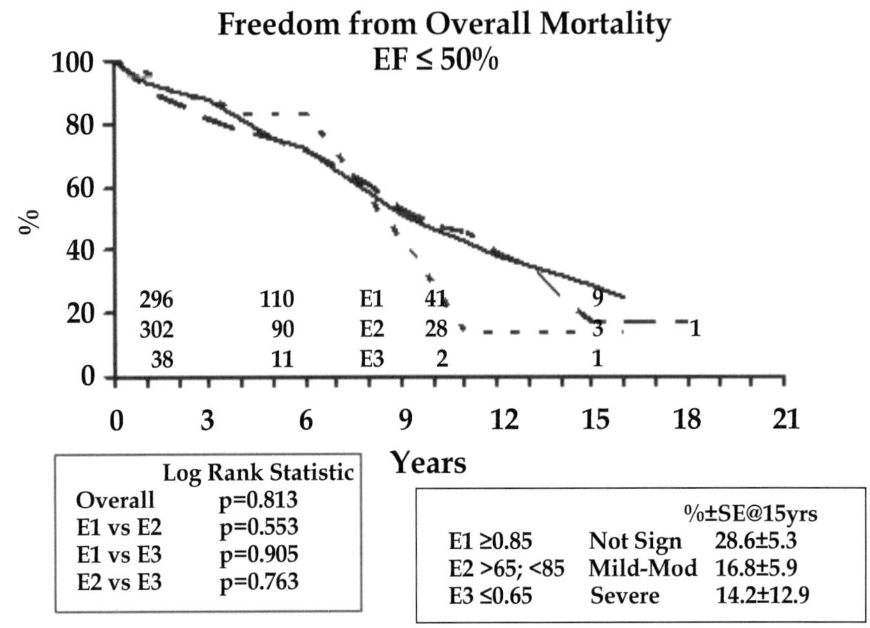

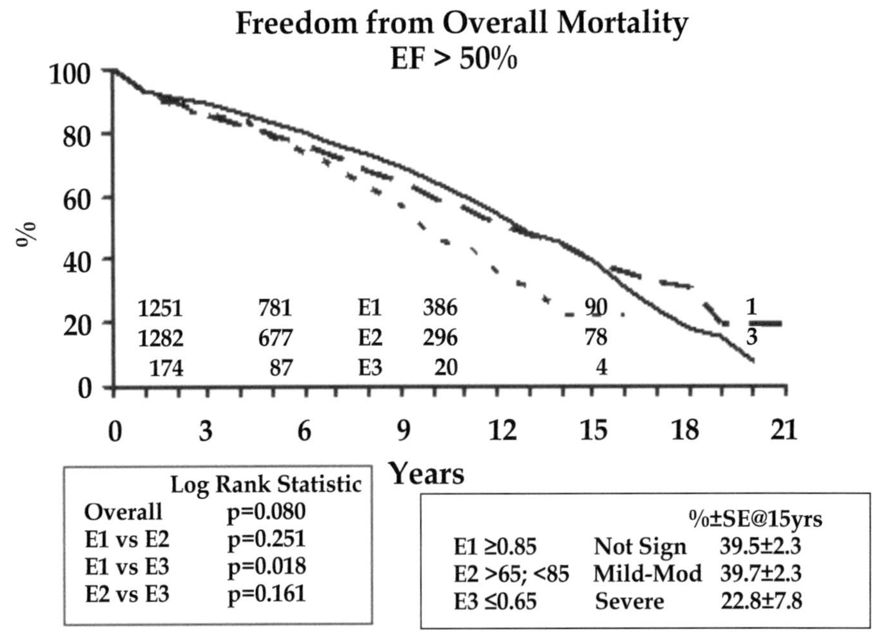

Fig. 5. Freedom from overall mortality in various subdivisions of the three effective orifice area index (EOAI) groups (Jamieson et al., 2010, and Jamieson, Personal Communication). E1 (solid line), not significant; E2 (long-dash line), mild to moderate; and E3 (short-dash line), severe. (EF = ejection fraction; BMI = body mass index)

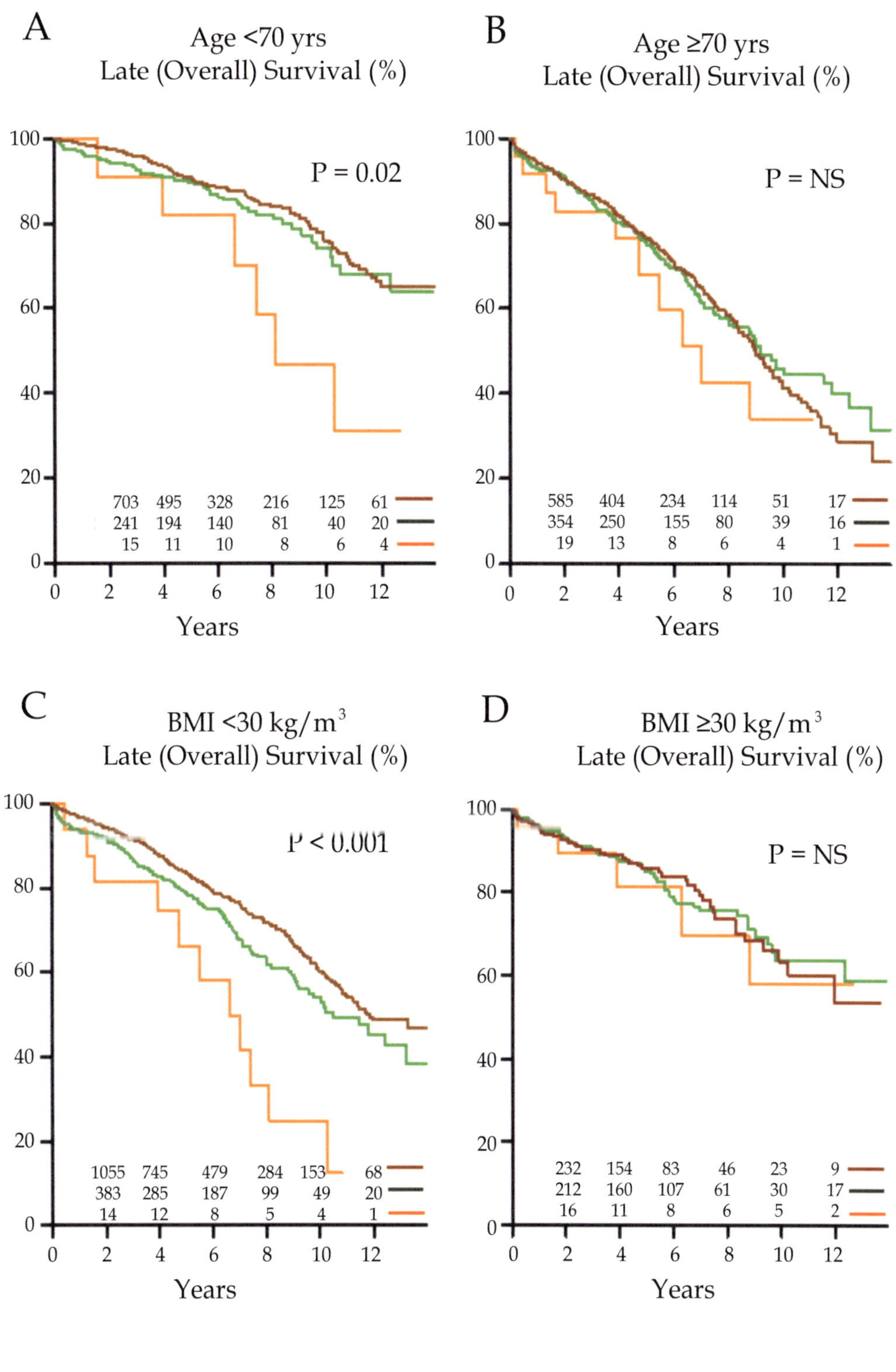
A
Age <70 yrs
Late (Overall) Survival (%)
P = 0.02
100
80
60
40
20
0
703 495 328 216 125 61
241 194 140 81 40 20
15 11 10 8 6 4
0 2 4 6 8 10 12
Years
B
Age ≥70 yrs
Late (Overall) Survival (%)
P = NS
585 404 234 114 51 17
354 250 155 80 39 16
19 13 8 6 4 1
Years
C
BMI <30 kg/m3
Late (Overall) Survival (%)
P < 0.001
1055 745 479 284 153 68
383 285 187 99 49 20
14 12 8 5 4 1
Years
D
BMI ≥30 kg/m3
Late (Overall) Survival (%)
P = NS
232 154 83 46 23 9
212 160 107 61 30 17
16 11 8 6 5 2
Years

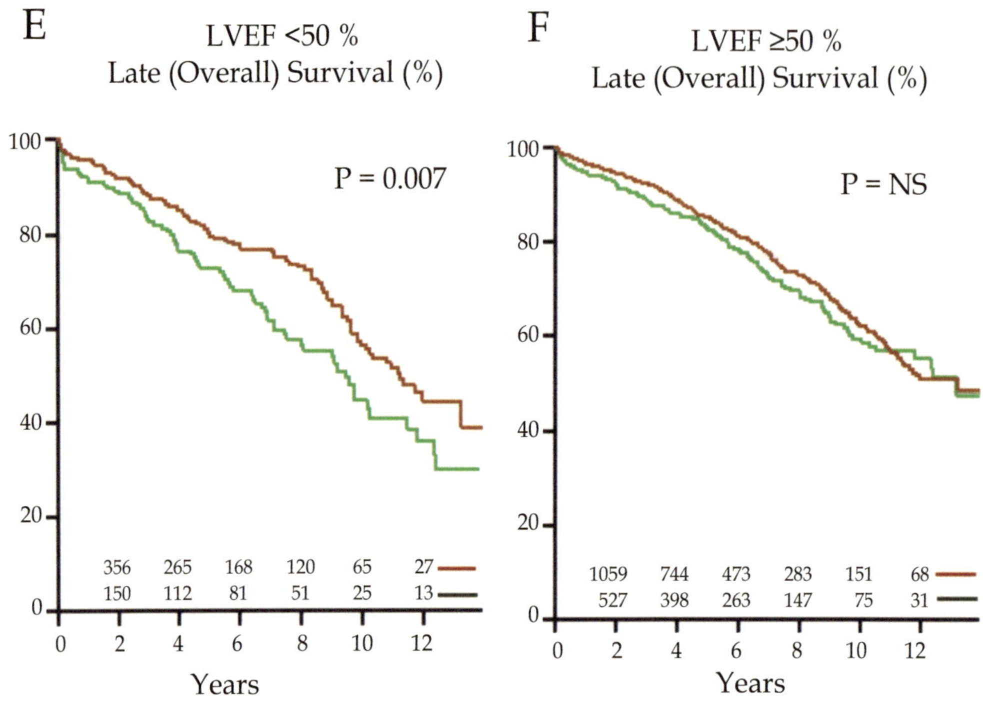

Fig. 6. Impact of prosthesis-patient mismatch on late overall survival (from Mohty et al. 2009, Figure 2). (A) Patients < 70 years old, (B) Patients ≥ 70 years old, (C) Body mass index (BMI) < 30 kg/m^2, (D) BMI ≥ 30 kg/m^2, (E) Pre-operative left ventricular ejection fraction (LVEF) < 50%, (F) LVEF ≥ 50%. Brown line indicates nonsignificant prosthesis-patient mismatch (PPM); green line indicates moderate PPM; orange line shows severe PPM

In the Jamieson et al. cohort of 3343 patients, an additional study (Higgins et al., 2011) that evaluated the influence of gender on early, late, and overall survival reported that the predictors of mortality after AVR for aortic stenosis differed between male and female patients. Female gender was a predictor of early mortality while male gender was a predictor of late (but not early or overall) mortality. Male gender increased the risk of late mortality, and a valve size ≤ 21 mm increased the risk of early and overall mortality among male patients only. These differences need to be taken into consideration preoperatively and require consideration during operative management.

The Jamieson et al. analysis indicated that severe PPM identified with an EOAI < 0.65 cm^2/m^2 is not an independent predictor of early mortality, late mortality, or overall mortality after AVR. These findings have been discussed in perspective with other studies that have and have not provided evidence of PPM as an independent predictor of survival. The independent influence of bioprostheses as a risk factor of late and overall mortality also needs extensive evaluation because currently bioprostheses are recommended for patients ≥ 60 years old to minimize serious valve-related morbidity and provide a relatively acceptable degree of valve-related reoperation for structural valve deterioration. Valve-related mortality is not influenced by valve type (bioprosthesis or mechanical prosthesis). The documented finding that AVR does not provide the same age/gender matched survival as in the general population allows this lower age threshold for bioprostheses in AVR (van Geldrop et al., 2009). This earlier failure threshold may be related to residual systolic dysfunction and more likely related to diastolic dysfunction concomitant with PPM (Nozohoor et al., 2008).

3. A suggested approach to PPM

Because the negative impact of severe PPM on postoperative survival, it is crucial to avoid leaving patients with severe PPM after valvular surgery. Pibarot and Dumesnil (2000) presented a 3-step approach for preventing PPM: [1] calculate the patient's body surface area from weight and height; [2] using a BSA versus EOAI table, find the minimal valve EOA (in cm^2) that will allow a given patient to have proper (ideally > 0.85 cm^2 / m^2) EOAI after surgery; and [3] select the type and size of prosthesis that has EOA reference values equal to or greater than the minimal valve EOA value obtained in step 2. The occurrence and severity of postoperative PPM can also be predicted before the operation from the patient's BSA and the reference EOA value of the selected prosthesis (Pibarot et al., 2001; Urso et al., 2010; Dumesnil and Pibarot, 2010).

In agreement with the above, despite failing to find severe PPM (< 0.65 cm^2 / m^2) as an independent predictor of early, late, or overall mortality after AVR, we recommend that surgeons do not leave patients with a severe mismatch (especially for bioprostheses, which may develop degenerative changes over time that would further reduce the EOAI). Surgeons should maintain a prospective strategy of implanting an adequately sized aortic prosthesis that will preclude patients from being in the category of severe mismatch (near equivalent to indications for intervention in severe aortic stenosis). However, a significant portion of patients undergoing AVR will have some level of mild-to-moderate PPM owing to the intrinsic obstructive nature of most prostheses, and Jamieson et al. (2010) should provide some confidence to surgeons and cardiologists that mild-to-moderate PPM is unlikely to be detrimental to survival.

Other than selecting a prosthesis with sufficient EOA, as described above, there are several more intraoperative options available to surgeons to prevent the occurrence of severe PPM. Aortic root enlargement may be considered in patients with an elevated risk of developing moderate-to-severe PPM at time of valvular replacement surgery (Mohty et al., 2006). Kulik et al. (2008) were able to insert larger prosthetic valves and achieve lower PPM by doing aortic root enlargement (ARE) at the time of AVR. They reported that the addition of an ARE to AVR increased the aortic cross-clamp time by 9.9 minutes, on average, and that there was no significant increase in perioperative morbidity or mortality associated with the added ARE. However, the lower incidence of PPM did not significantly affect long-term outcomes in their AVR + ARE cohort, once again coming back to the question of whether PPM significantly affects survival. The third option is a total aortic root replacement. Compared with a traditional stented bioprosthesis, total root replacement allows for optimal hemodynamics with no significant aortic regurgitation, improved regression of the LV mass, and less PPM in the small aortic root (Kon et al., 2002; Kincaid et al., 2007); however, total aortic root replacement comes at the cost of increased operative mortality, and a longer learning process. Several biological valves that allow for this procedure are the Medtronic

Freestyle (porcine, stentless), Edwards Prima Plus (porcine, stentless), and Sorin Pericarbon Freedom (pericardial, stentless) (Jamieson, 2010). Finally, a myectomy and a myotomy of the hypertrophied muscle are options for dealing with a small aortic root or a left ventricular outflow tract obstruction; they are safe and effective procedures without additional complications when done concomitantly with AVR (Kayalar et al., 2010). Myectomy-myotomy also has improved left ventricular mass regression after AVR for pure aortic stenosis (Tasca et al., 2003).

Among the three available intraoperative options available to surgeons to prevent the occurrence of severe PPM, the first option to consider for any patient should be to look for a valve with larger a EOAI and better hemodynamics. The On-X valve and the St. Jude Medical (SJM) Regent valve are mechanical valves with improved hemodynamics. The On-X valve by On-X Life Technologies Inc. also has improved hemodynamics (Palatianos et al., 2007; Chambers et al., 2005) and excellent postoperative EOA and transvalvular gradients (Moidl et al., 2002). The On-X valve was also designed to address the problems of occasional incidents of unexplained hemolytic anemia, tissue interference, excessive pannus overgrowth, and thrombotic complications (Moidl et al., 2002). The SJM Regent valve is an improvement on the SJM conventional valve, and has a wider valve area than the SJM HP valve (Sezai et al., 2010). With its supra-annular placement, several studies have suggested that using the Regent valve practically circumvents the need for root enlargement (Bach et al., 2002; Petracek, 2002). In a recent study (Okamura et al., 2010) in which 50 patients were given a small-sized (17-mm or 19-mm) St. Jude Regent mechanical valve, all patients improved to NYHA functional class II or better. Several biological valves with improved hemodynamics are the Carpentier-Edwards PERIMOUNT Magna Ease (pericardial), SJM Epic Supra (porcine), Sorin Soprano Armania (pericardial), and Medtronic Mosaic Ultra (porcine) valves (Jamieson, 2010). The Sorin Mitroflow (pericardial) and the St Jude Medical Trifecta (pericardial) (approved 2007 and 2010, respectively by the USFDA) are externally mounted pericardial bioprostheses and not amenable to increased diameter design.

For patients who have already developed moderate or severe postoperative PPM, reoperation may be an option to improve long-term survival (Girard et al., 2001). In Girard et al., there were no 30-day deaths for reoperations on 12 patients with isolated, severe PPM. However, 5 of the 9 patients who underwent concomitant major cardiac procedures at the time of valvular replacement died in-hospital, so there is a risk to reoperation. The benefit of relief from PPM must be weighed carefully against the risks of reoperation, and must be assessed on a patient-by-patient basis. When evaluating patients with mild-to-moderate PPM for the possibility of reoperation, we suggest that surgeons take into account the Jamieson et al. (2010) finding of the unlikelihood of mild-to-moderate PPM contributing to worse survival.

From the accumulated data from published literature, it is easy to see that the topic of prosthesis-patient mismatch remains controversial. The issue is further complicated by the fact that there are several levels of PPM (nonsignificant, mild, moderate, or severe), with different studies showing different outcomes for each level of PPM. There is also currently no clear consensus on the exact definitions of PPM and its categories.

A sensible approach to the issue of PPM is that we should avoid generalizations for any given level of PPM except for severe PPM, for which the data in the existing literature is more consistent; therefore, proactive measures should be taken to prevent its occurrence. For other levels of PPM, it is reasonable to evaluate each patient on an individual basis (i.e., moderate PPM being more acceptable for a sedentary elderly patient, but less so for someone who is younger and more active), and for surgical and postoperative management options to be dependent on the individualized assessment.

4. References

[1] Rahimtoola SH. The problem of valve prosthesis-patient mismatch. *Circulation.* 1978;58:20-4

[2] Pibarot P, Dumesnil JG. Hemodynamic and clinical impact of prosthesis-patient mismatch in the aortic valve position and its prevention. *J Am Coll Cardiol.* 2000;36:1131-41

[3] Muneretto C, Bisleri G, Negri A, Manfredi J. The concept of patient-prosthesis mismatch. *J Heart Valve Dis.* 2004;13:S59-S62

[4] Mohty D, Malouf JF, Girard SE, Schaff HV, Grill DE, Enriquez-Sarano ME, Miller FA Jr. Impact of prosthesis-patient mismatch on long-term survival in patients with small St Jude Medical mechanical prostheses in the aortic position. *Circulation.* 2006;113:420-6

[5] Tasca G, Mhagna Z, Perotti S, Centurini PB, Sabatini T, Amaducci A, Brunelli F, Cirillo M, Tomba MD, Quiani E, Troise G, Pibarot P. Impact of prosthesis-patient mismatch on cardiac events and midterm mortality after aortic valve replacement in patients with pure aortic stenosis. *Circulation.* 2006;113:570-6

[6] Moon MR, Pasque MK, Munfakh NA, Melby SJ, Lawton JS, Moazami N, Codd JE, Crabtree TD, Barner HB, Damiano RJ Jr. Prosthesis-patient mismatch after aortic valve replacement: impact of age and body size on late survival. *Ann Thorac Surg.* 2006;81:481-9

[7] Florath I, Albert A, Rosendahl U, Ennker IC, Ennker J. Impact of valve prosthesis-patient mismatch estimated by echocardiographic-determined effective orifice area on long-term outcome after aortic valve replacement. *Am Heart J.* 2008;155:1135-42

[8] Mohty D, Dumesnil JG, Echahidi N, Mathieu P, Dagenais F, Voisine P, Pibarot P. Impact of prosthesis-patient mismatch on long-term survival after aortic valve replacement. *J Am Coll Cardiol.* 2009;53:39-47

[9] Blais C, Dumesnil JG, Baillot R, Simard S, Doyle D, Pibarot P. Impact of valve prosthesis-patient mismatch on short-term mortality after aortic valve replacement. *Circulation.* 2003;108:983-8

[10] Jamieson WRE, Ye J, Higgins J, Cheung A, Fradet GJ, Skarsgard P, Germann E, Chan F, Lichtenstein SV. Effect of prosthesis-patient mismatch on long-term survival with aortic valve replacement: assessment to 15 years. *Ann Thorac Surg.* 2010;89:51-9

[11] Kato Y, Suehiro S, Shibata T, Sasaki Y, Hirai H. Impact of valve prosthesis-patient mismatch on long-term survival and left ventricular mass regression after aortic valve replacement for aortic stenosis. *J Cardiovasc Surg.* 2007; 22:314-9

[12] Vicchio M, Della Corte A, De Santo LS, De Feo M, Caianiello G, Scardone M, Cotrufo M. Prosthesis-patient mismatch in the elderly: survival, ventricular mass regression, and quality of life. *Ann Thorac Surg.* 2008;86:1791-7

[13] Mascherbauer J, Rosenhek R, Fuchs C, Pernica E, Klaar U, Scholten C, Heger M, Wollenek G, Maurer G, Baumgartner H. Moderate patient-prosthesis mismatch after valve replacement for severe aortic stenosis has no impact on short-term and long-term mortality. *Heart.* 2008;94:1639-45

[14] Monin JL, Monchi M, Kirsch ME, Petit-Eisenmann H, Baleynaud S, Chauvel C, Metz D, Adams C, Quere JP, Gueret P, Tribouilloy C. Low-gradient aortic stenosis: impact of prosthesis-patient mismatch on survival. *Eurn Heart J.* 2007;28(21):2620-6

[15] Ruel M, Rubens FD, Masters RG, Pipe AL, Bedard P, Hendry PJ, Lam BK, Burwash IG, Goldstein WG, Brais MP, Keon WJ, Mesana TG. Late incidence and predictors of persistent or recurrent heart failure in patients with aortic prosthetic valves. *J Thorac Cardiov Sur.* 2004;127:149-59

[16] Kulik A, Burwash IG, Kapila V, Mesana TG, Ruel M. Long-term outcomes after valve replacement for low-gradient aortic stenosis. *Circulation.* 2006;114:I553-8

[17] Jamieson WRE, Burr LH, Miyagishima RT, Germann E, Macnab JS, Stanford E, Chan F, Janusz MT, Ling H. Carpentier-Edwards supra-annular aortic porcine bioprosthesis: clinical performance over 20 years. *J Thorac Cardiov Sur.* 2005;130(4):994-1000

[18] Jamieson WRE, Gudas VM, Burr LH, Janusz MT, Fradet GJ, Ling H, Germann E, Lichtenstein SV. Mitral valve disease: if the mitral valve is not reparable/failed repair, is bioprosthesis suitable for replacement? *Eur J Cardio-thorac.* 2009;35(1):104-110

[19] Ruel M, Al-Faleh H, Kulik A, Chan K, Mesana TG, Burwash IG. Prosthesis-patient mismatch after aortic valve replacement primarily affects patients with pre-existing left ventricular dysfunction: impact on survival, freedom from heart failure, and left ventricular mass regression. *J Thorac Cardiov Sur.* 2006;131:1036-44

[20] Higgins J, Jamieson WRE, Benhameid O, Ye J, Cheung A, Skarsgard P, Germann E, Chan F, Lichtenstein SV. Influence of patient gender on mortality after aortic valve replacement for aortic stenosis. *J Thorac Cardiov Sur.* 2011;142:595-601

[21] van Geldorp MW, Jamieson WRE, Kappetein AP, Ye J, Fradet GJ, Eijkemans MJ, Grunkemeier GL, Bogers AJ, Takkenberg JJ. Patient outcome after aortic valve replacement with a mechanical or biological prosthesis: weighing lifetime anticoagulant-related event risk against reoperation risk. *J Thorac Cardiov Sur.* 2009;137(4):881-6,

[22] Nozohoor S, Nilsson J, Luhrs C, Roijer A, Sjogren J. Influence of prosthesis-patient mismatch on diastolic heart failure after aortic valve replacement. *Ann Thorac Surg.* 2008;85:1310-8.

[23] Pibarot P, Dumesnil JG, Cartier PC, Metras J, Lemieux MD. Patient-prosthesis mismatch can be predicted at the time of operation. *Ann Thorac Surg.* 2001;71:S265-8

[24] Urso S, Sadaba R, Monleón-Getino T, Aldamiz-Echevarría G. Moderate patient-prosthesis mismatch has no independent effect on 30-day mortality after isolated valve replacement [Spanish]. *Rev Esp Cardiol.* 2010;63:409-14

[25] Dumesnil JG, Pibarot P. Prevention of moderate prosthesis-patient mismatch: individualization versus generalization. *Rev Esp Cardiol.* 2010;63(4):387-9

[26] Kulik A, Al-Saigh M, Chan V, Masters RG, Bedard P, Lam BK, Rubens FD, Hendry PJ, Mesana TG, Ruel M. Enlargement of the small aortic root during aortic valve replacement: is there a benefit? *Ann Thorac Surg.* 2008;85(1)94-100

[27] Kon ND, Riley RD, Adair SM, Kitzman DW, Cordell AR. Eight-year results of aortic root replacement with the freestyle stentless porcine aortic root bioprosthesis. *Ann Thorac Surg.* 2002;73:1817-21

[28] Kincaid EH, Cordell AR, Hammon JW, Adair SM, Kon ND. Coronary insufficiency after stentless aortic root replacement: risk factors and solutions. *Ann Thorac Surg.* 2007;83:964-968

[29] Jamieson WRE. Update on technologies for cardiac valvular replacement, transcatheter innovations, and reconstructive surgery. In: Szabó, Z., Coburg, A.J., Reich, H., Yamamoto, M., Brem, H., Hartwin, S.F. (Eds.) *Surgical Technology International, XX.* 2010. San Francisco: Universal Medical Press; pp. 255-281

[30] Kayalar N, Schaff HV, Daly RC, Dearani JA, Park SJ. Concomitant septal myectomy at the time of aortic valve replacement for severe aortic stenosis. *Ann Thorac Surg.* 2010;89:459-64

[31] Tasca G, Amaducci A, Parrella PV, Troise G, Dalla Tomba M, Magna Z, Quaini E. Myectomy-myotomy associated with aortic valve replacement for aortic stenosis: effects on left ventricular mass regression. *Ital Heart J.* 2003;4:865-71

[32] Palatianos GM, Laczkovics AM, Simon P, Pomar JL, Birnbaum DE, Greve HH, Haverich A. Multicentered European study on safety and effectiveness of the On-X prosthetic heart valve: intermediate follow-up. *Ann Thorac Surg.* 2007;83(1):40-6

[33] Chambers J, Roxburgh J, Blauth C, O'Riordan J, Hodson F, Rimington H. A randomized comparison of the MCRI On-X and CarboMedics Top Hat bileaflet mechanical replacement aortic valves: early postoperative hemodynamic function and clinical events. *J Thorac Cardiov Sur.* 2005;130(3):759-64

[34] Moidl R, Simon P, Wolner E. The On-X prosthetic heart valve at five years. *Ann Thorac Surg.* 2002;74(4):S1312-7

[35] Sezai A, Kasamaki Y, Abe K, Hata M, Sekino H, Shimura K, Minami K. Assessment of the St Jude Medical Regent prosthetic valve by continuous-wave Doppler and dobutamine stress echocardiography. *Ann Thorac Sur.* 2010;89(1):87-92

[36] Bach DS, Sakwa MP, Goldbach M, Petracek MR, Emery RW, Mohr FW. Hemodynamics and early clinical performance of the St. Jude Medical Regent mechanical aortic valve. *Ann Thorac Surg.* 2002;74(6):2003-9

[37] Petracek MR. Assessing options for the small aortic root. *J of Heart Valve Dis.* 2002;S1:S50-5

[38] Okamura H, Yamaguchi A, Noguchi K, Naito K, Yuri K, Adachi H. Hemodynamics and outcomes of aortic valve replacement with a 17- or 19-mm valve. *Asian Cardiovas Thorac.* 2010;18(5):450-5

[39] Girard SE, Miller FA, Montgomery S, Edwards WD, Tazelaar HD, Malouf JF, Seward JB, Orszulak TA. Outcome of reoperation for aortic valve prosthesis-patient mismatch. *Am J Cardiol.* 2001;82:111-114

Part 6

Transcatheter Aortic Valve Implantation

10

Current Indications for Transcatheter Aortic Valve Implantation

Ibrahim Akin, Stephan Kische, Henrik Schneider, Tim C. Rehders, Christoph A. Nienaber and Hüseyin Ince
University of Rostock
Germany

1. Introduction

Rising life expectancy results in an increase of degenerative and neoplastic diseases. Population-based observational studies report that 1% to 2% of patients older than 65 years have moderate-to-severe aortic stenosis (AS) (Nkomo *et al.*, 2006). Surgical aortic valve replacement (AVR) dates back to 1960 and is currently the only treatment option for severe AS that has been shown to improve survival, regardless of age (Kvidal *et al.*, 2000). In the ideal candidate, surgical AVR has an estimated operative mortality of 4% (Kvidal *et al.*, 2000). Unfortunately, up to one-third of patients with severe AS are ineligible for corrective valve surgery, either because of advanced age or the presence of multiple comorbidities (Iung *et al.*, 2005). Current treatment options for those patients not offered surgery include medical treatment or percutaneous balloon aortic valvuloplasty, although neither has been

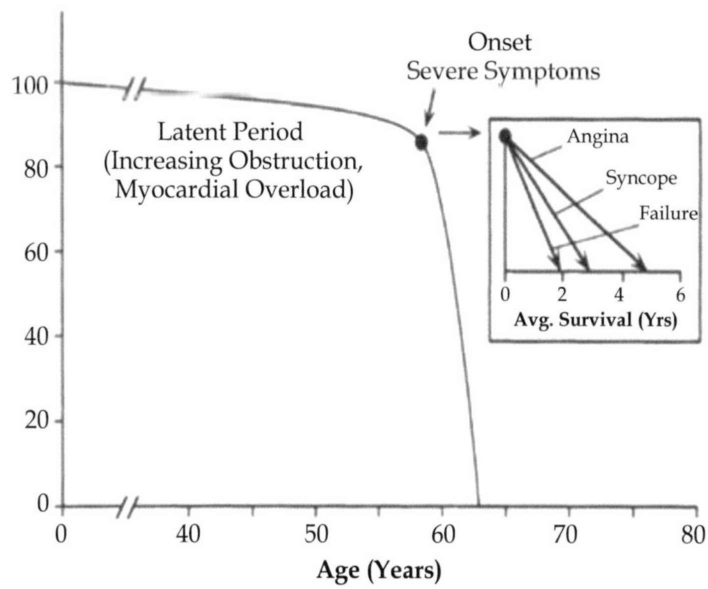

Fig. 1. Survival of medically treated symptomatic AS (Ross J Jr. & Braunwald E, 1965)

shown to reduce mortality. Medically treated patients with symptomatic AS have 1- and 5-year survival of 60% and 32%, respectively (Varadarajan *et al.*, 2006) (Figure 1). With the introduction of percutaneous aortic valve implantation in 2002, there seems to be an alternative for these patients.

2. Selection of patient

Due to the existence of tried and tested surgical AVR with good long-term results, the selection of patients for transcatheter aortic valve implantation (TAVI), which should done in a multidisciplinary consultation between cardiologists, surgeons, imaging specialists, and anesthesiologists, involves several critical steps (Vahanian *et al.*, 2008). Candidates considered for TAVI must have severe symptomatic AS in addition to a formal contraindication to surgery or other characteristics that would limit their surgical candidacy because of excessive mortality or morbidity (Figure 2). The procedure should be offered to patients who have a potential for functional improvement after valve replacement. It is not recommended for patients who simply refuse surgery on the basis of personal preference.

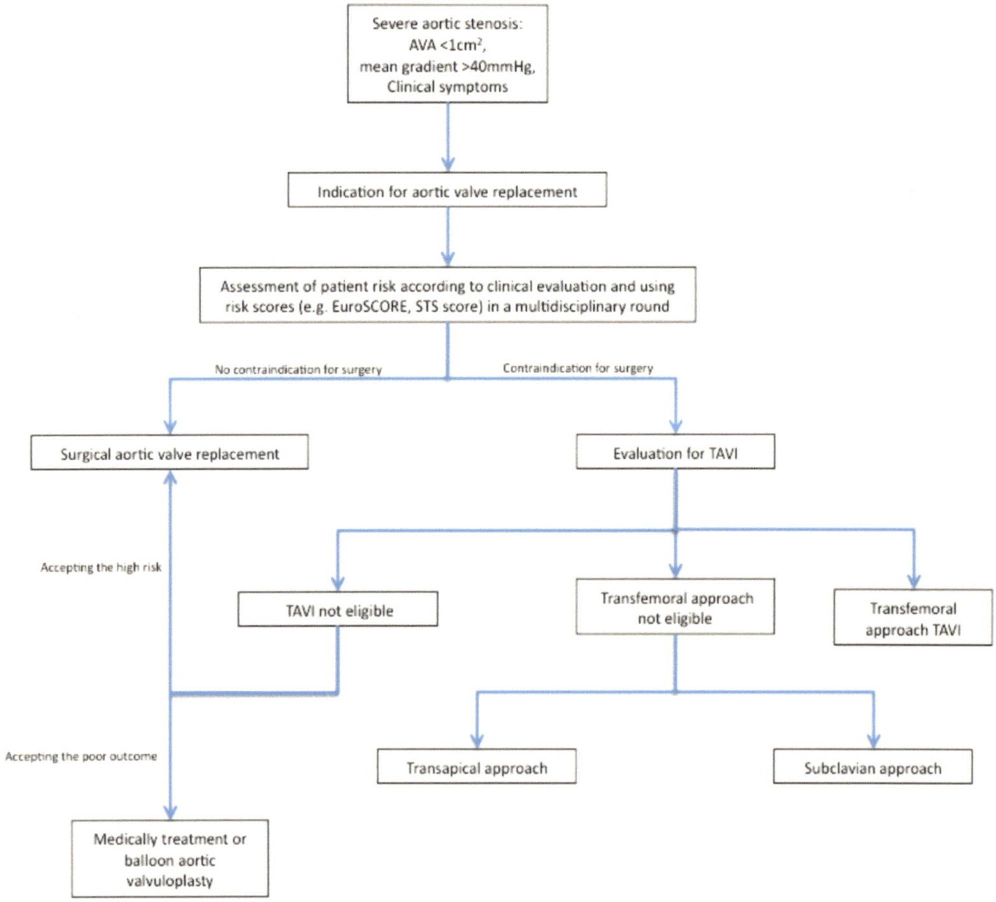

Fig. 2. Algorithm to determine the treatment options of patients with severe AS. (AVA: aortic valve area; TAVI: transcatheter aortic valve implantation)

3. Confirming the severity of aortic stenosis

Actually, TAVI is indicated only for patients with calcified pure or predominant symptomatic AS. The different imaging modalities can assist in the selection process by providing important information on the aortic valve, coronary arteries, and vascular structures. First, the severity of AS should be assessed. Both transthoracic (TTE) and transesophageal (TEE) Doppler echocardiography are the preferred tools (Figure 3).

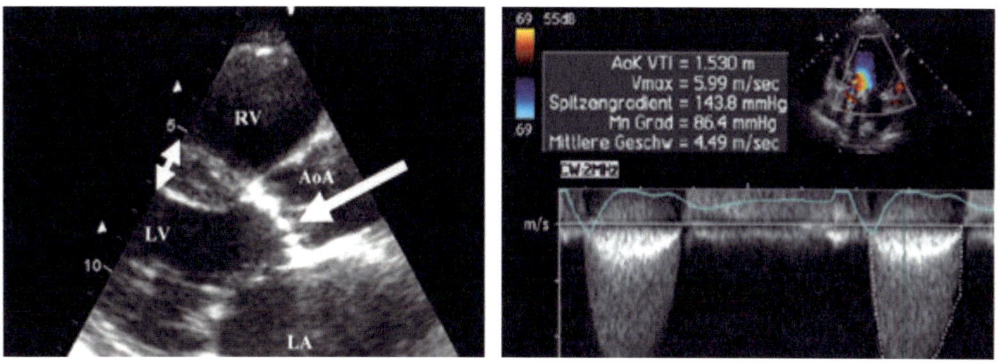

Fig. 3. TTE in the assessment of severe AS

In addition, the exact anatomy of the aortic valve should be assessed. Echocardiography, multislice CT (MSCT), and magnetic resonance imaging (MRI) can all help to distinguish between a bicuspid and a tricuspid aortic valve. It is important to point out that implantation of available percutaneous prostheses is contraindicated in the case of a bicuspid aortic valve, because of the risk of incomplete deployment, significant paravalvular regurgitation, and displacement of the prosthesis (Vahanian *et al.*, 2008; Zegdi *et al.*, 2008) (Figure 4).

A severely calcified aortic valve may result in the inability to cross the native valve with the catheter. Bulky leaflets and calcifications on the free edge of the leaflets may increase the risk of occlusion of the coronary ostia during aortic valve implantation. Therefore, the extent and exact location of calcifications should be carefully assessed before the implantation procedure. Assessing coronary anatomy is also important in the selection process. Conventional coronary angiography, which remains the "gold standard", should be done to exclude the presence of significant coronary artery disease (Figure 5).

4. Analysis of surgical risk and evaluation of life expectancy and quality of life

The precise evaluation of surgical risk in a specific patient is not easy and involves an attempt at individualization based on statistical data from databases containing a large number of procedures. The most accepted and validated algorithms that are widely available today are the EuroSCORE, the STS (Society of Thoracic Score) score,and the Parsonnet score. These algorithms predict the surgical risk by assigning weight to various factors that affect the clinical result, but it is clear that they can underestimate or overestimate the risk in certain groups of patients who are not represented satisfactorily in the population used to generate the algorithm (Roques *et al.*, 2001). There is some evidence in the literature of the incorrect prediction of aortic AVR outcome using the EuroSCORE model (Grossi *et al.*, 2008). The key element for establishing whether patients are at high risk for surgery is multidisciplinary clinical judgment, which should be used in association with a more quantitative assessment, based on the combination of several scores (for example, expected mortality >20% with the EuroSCORE and >10% with STS score). This approach allows the team to take into account risk factors that are not covered in scores but often seen in practice, such as chest radiation, previous aortocoronary bypass with patent grafts, porcelain aorta, liver cirrhosis.

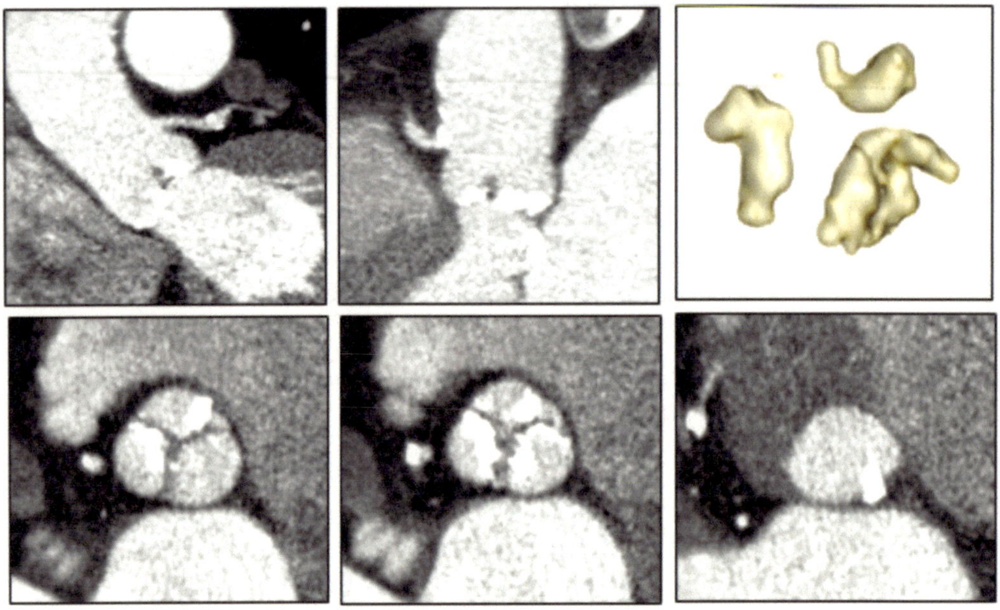

Fig. 4. ECG-gated CT-scan in a patient with severe aortic valve stenosis (the upper right panel shows the isolated calcification of the tricuspid aortic valve)

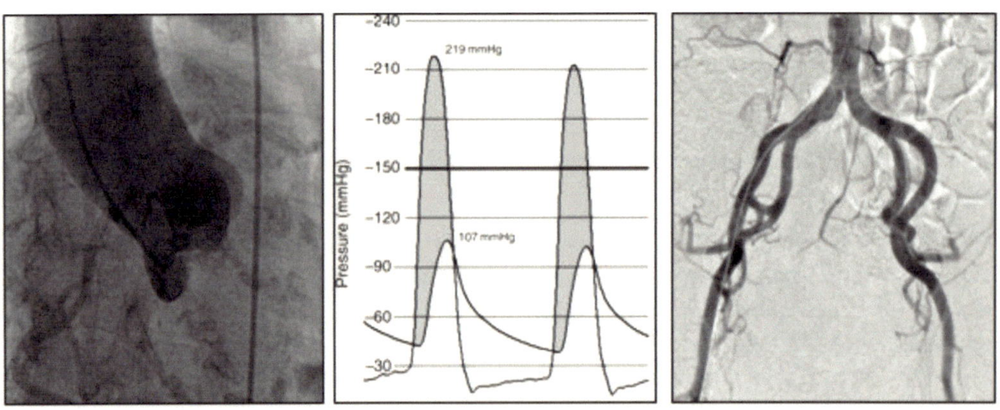

Fig. 5. Invasive diagnostic prior TAVI, including aortography and access vessels as well as transvalvular gradient

5. Assessment of feasibility and exclusion of contraindications for TAVI

After criteria of severe symptomatic aortic valve stenosis and high surgical risk are evaluated, the technical evaluation of the patient's suitability for the percutaneous implantation technique begins (Table 1).

Indication for Transcatheter aortic valve implantation
Severe aortic stenosis (AVA: $<1cm^2$,mean gradient >40mmHg, severe symptoms)
Contraindication for surgical valve replacement
Contraindication for Transcatheter aortic valve implantation
Mild to moderate aortic stenosis
Asymptomatic patients
Life expectancy <1 year
Surgical aortic valve replacement possible, but patient refused
Aortic anulus <18 or >25mm (balloon-expandable) and <20 or >27mm (self-expandable)
Bicuspid aortic valve
Asymetric heavy valvular calcification
Aortic root >45mm at the aortotubular junction
Presence of left ventricular apical thrombus
Contraindication for transfemoral approach
Severe calcification, tortuosity, small diameter of the iliac arteries
Previous aortofemoral bypass
Severe angulation, severe atheroma of the aorta
Coarctation of the aorta
Aneurysm of the aorta with protruding mural thrombus
Contraindication for transapical approach
Previous surgery of the left ventricle using a patch
Calcified pericardium
Severe respiratory insufficiency
Non-reachable left ventricular apex

Table 1. Actually proposed indications and contraindications for TAVI

The two most basic parameters are the suitability of the peripheral arteries and the size of the aortic valve annulus. Contrast angiography is needed to assess the former, while the latter requires an initial assessment of the diameter of the aortic annulus on a TTE. In general terms, a large artery with dominant elastic elements should have a diameter up to 1 mm smaller than the external diameter of the sheath that has to be introduced for the valve implantation. Thus, current systems with an external sheath diameter of 28 F (SAPIEN 26 mm, Edwards Lifescience LLC, Irvine, CA), 25 F (SAPIEN 23 mm, Edwards) and 22 F (CoreValve, Medtronic, Inc., Minneapolis, MN) require minimum diameters of 8, 7, and 6 mm, respectively. Apart from the minimum diameter, the existence of significant vessel tortuosity (>90°), especially when combined with wall calcifications, makes advancing the large sheath problematic, with a high risk of vascular complications that could potentially affect the final outcome. In addition, the existence of extensive circumferential calcifications limits the elastic dilation of the artery; thus, the minimum diameters referred to above are underestimated. Patients who do not meet the criteria of suitable peripheral arterial access may still be candidates for transapical implantation. For the assessment of aortic annulus diameter, we should keep in mind that TTE underestimates its size by a mean of 1.4 mm compared with TEE (Babaliaros *et al.*, 2008; Vahanian *et al.*, 2008), while the latter method also underestimates the size by 1.2 mm compared with intraoperative measurement (Babaliaros *et al.*, 2008). Therefore, in order to avoid undesirable and often catastrophic displacement of the prosthesis, there should be a margin of at least 1-2 mm between the diameter of the valve and the size of the aortic annulus estimated using TEE, so that the former may be successfully and safely anchored within the latter. Computed tomography scan aortography and angiography of the ascending aorta are the most appropriate examinations for investigating these aspects. Those examinations will also be used for the measurement of the dimensions of the ascending aorta and the aortic arch, which are essential for checking eligibility for the CoreValve (the most important being the diameter of the ascending aorta, which should be <4.3 cm) (Figure 6).

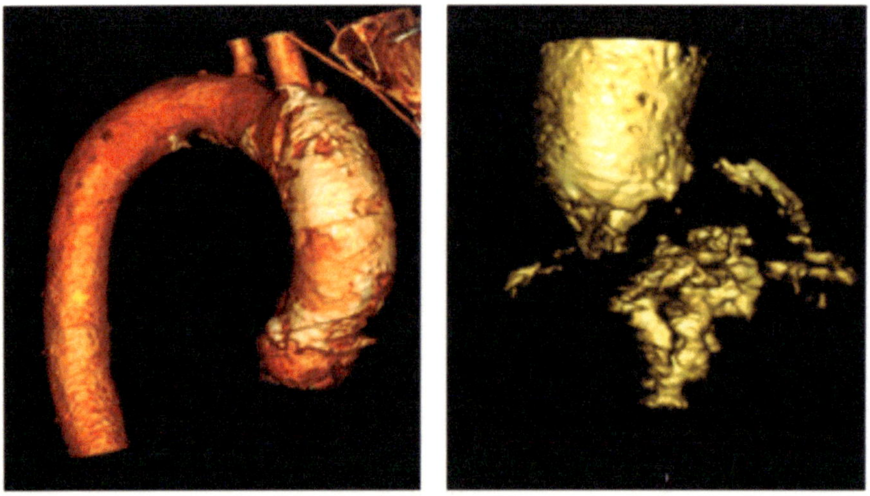

Fig. 6. ECG-gated CT-scan of a patient with severe aortic valve stenosis and porcelain aorta after radiation exposure

The anatomy of the thoracic aorta (any chance of porcelain aorta) and the abdominal aorta should be studied by some imaging method for the existence of extensive atheromatosis, mural thrombi and aneurysm.

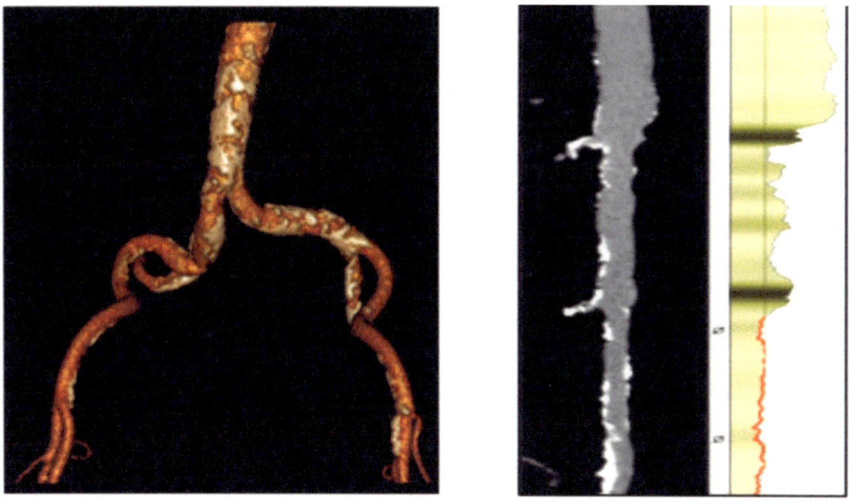

Fig. 7. Three-dimensional reconstruction of contrast-enhanced CT angiography to assess morphology of femoral arteries (left) and centerline stretched view (right)

6. Different transcatheter aortic valves

On the basis of first results from clinical trials, CoreValve Revalving System and Edwards Lifescience SAPIEN obtained CE mark approval in 2007 with the specification that these valves are intended for patients with a high or prohibitive risk for surgical valve replacement or who cannot undergo AVR. The first generation balloon-expandable valve was entitled Cribier-Edwards valve (Edwards Lifesciences), whereas at present the Edwards SAPIEN valve (Edwards) is commercially available (Figure 8). The Edwards Lifesciences SAPIEN THV device is a balloon-expandable valve. It consists of bovine pericardium that is firmly mounted within a tubular, slotted, stainless steel balloon-expandable stent. Two

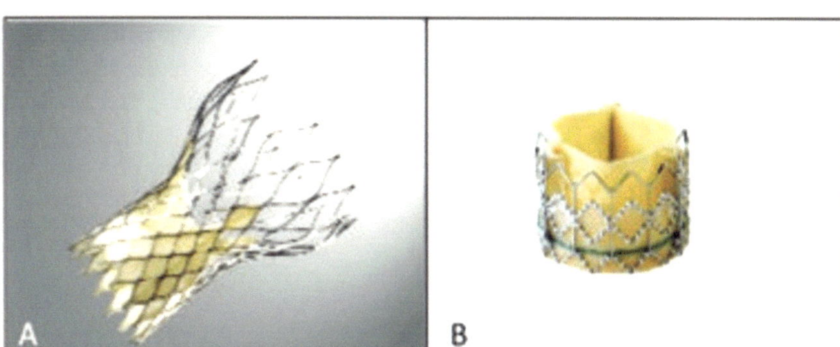

Fig. 8. Profile of the CoreValve Revaving System (A) and Edwards SAPIEN Transcatheter Heart Valve (B)

valve sizes have been developed (23mm and 26mm). At present, available prosthesis sizes are 23 and 26 mm for aortic annulus diameters between 18–22 mm and 21–25 mm, respectively. The CoreValve Revalving device is a self-expanding frame-valve prosthesis (Figure 2). It consists of a porcine pericardial tissue valve that is mounted and sutured in a multilevel self-expanding nitinol frame. It is available in 26 and 29 mm sizes. The device has a broader upper segment (outflow aspect), which yields proper orientation to the blood flow. The first-generation valve used bovine pericardial tissue and was constrained within a 25 French (F) delivery catheter. The second-generation valve was built with porcine pericardial tissue within a 21 F catheter to allow access through smaller-diameter vascular beds. The third-generation of the device features a catheter with a valve delivery sheath size of 18 F and a follow-on shaft of 12 F.

Newer devices that have first-in-man application include Paniagua (Endoluminal Technology Research, Miami, FL), Enable (ATS, Minneapolis, MN), AoTx (Hansen Medical, Mountain View, CA), Perceval (Sorin Group, Arvada, CO), Jena (JenaValve Technology, Wilmington, DE), Lotus Valve (Sadra Medical, Campbell, CA), and Direct Flow percutaneous aortic valve (Direct Flow Medical, Inc., Santa Rosa, CA). TAVI represents a unique challenge for anesthesiologists. As with other invasive procedures, a careful preoperative assessment, appropriate intraoperative monitoring and imaging, meticulous management of hemodynamics, and early treatment of expected side effects and complications is of utmost importance. An unexpected decrease or increase in systemic vascular resistance resulting in decreased coronary perfusion pressure or acute heart failure by elevated left ventricular end-diastolic pressure should be avoided by maintaining a normotensive blood pressure and heart rate between 60 bpm and 100 bpm. The choice of anesthetic technique, either local anesthesia with mild sedation promoting spontaneous respiration, deep intravenous sedation with insertion of a laryngeal mask, or general anesthesia, varies among centers and is probably not associated with a significant difference in outcome. Post valvuloplasty and implantation, which were done under rapid right ventricular pacing due to reduce left ventricular ejection and cardiac motion, may require some additional inotropic support. Tracheal extubation can usually be done at the end of the procedure. Close postoperative monitoring is necessary, and admission to an intensive care unit is required. However, at present a retrograde approach through the femoral artery is used. During the procedure, a balloon valvuloplasty is first done to facilitate passage of the native aortic valve. During rapid right ventricular pacing, the prosthesis is positioned and deployed under fluoroscopy and echocardiographic guidance. Alternatively, in patients with difficult vascular access because of extensive calcifications or tortuosity of the femoral artery or aorta, a transapical approach can be used. After a partial thoracotomy, direct puncture of the apical portion of the left ventricular free wall is done to gain catheter access to the left ventricle and aortic valve. The prosthesis is subsequently positioned and deployed, similar to the antegrade approach.

7. Implantation approaches

With regard to the delivery systems and their introduction into ascending aorta, two specific pathways have been explored so far: the antegrade pathway, which uses direct transapical access, and the retrograde pathway, which uses either transfemoral or trans-subclavian or trans-axillary access (De Robertis *et al*, 2009).

7.1 The transapical approach

The main advantages of using transapical procedures are: [1] the feasibility does not rely on the absence of a concomitant peripheral vascular disease or previous aortic surgery; [2] the delivery system seems to be more "steady" and the procedure itself more "straightforward"; and [3] this access potentially reduces the risk of calcium dislodgement due to the passage of a stiff transfemoral device into a diseased aortic arch. A transapical approach can be used in the operating room, in a hybrid room, or in a catheterization laboratory with a patient under general anesthesia. Regardless of where the transapical approach is done, it is a prerequisite that high-quality fluoroscopic imaging must be guaranteed. Apical bleeding is very rare, mostly related to patient tissue fragility or to the team learning curve, and represents the most dangerous complication related to transapical access itself. In transapical TAVI, the cardiac apex is prepared through a small left anterolateral mini-thoracotomy using a purse-string or a crossing suture reinforced by pledgets and, after the procedure, a chest tube is routinely inserted into the left pleura with pain releasers injected in the intercostal tissue (Figure 9).

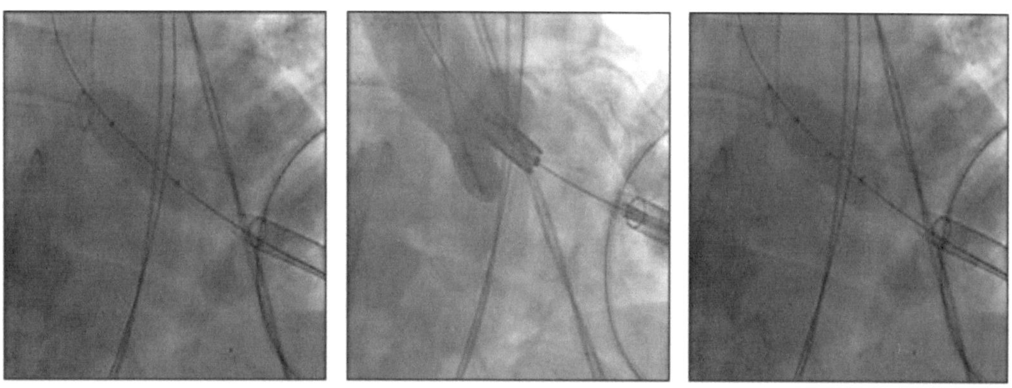

Fig. 9. TAVI using the transapical approach

7.2 The transfemoral approach

The transfemoral approach is used mostly in cardiac catheterization laboratory or a hybrid room. One of the main advantages of this technique is that it allows fully percutaneous implantation in conscious patients, as long as the peripheral vessels are of an adequate caliber (more than 6mm diameter), there are no very tortuous vessels, and vascular closure devices are available (Figure 10). Alternatively, the standard technique requires surgical preparation of the common femoral artery under local or general anesthesia. Major and minor postoperative vascular complications have been reported quite often in recent series (Grube *et al.*, 2006; Eltchaninoff *et al.*, 2011) and some critical events (vessel dissections, ruptures or avulsions) might be catastrophic when not promptly and adequately treated.

7.3 The trans-subclavian approach

Trans-subclavian access is an alternative retrograde pathway that has been recently explored. It requires a surgical exposure of the left subclavian artery and an adequate minimal vessel inner diameter for 18F delivery systems (Figure 11). There are some advantages in using this approach: firstly, the distance between the site of introduction and the aortic valve is short, compared with the transfemoral option, and it results in a steadier pathway. Secondly, as long as the subclavian artery is intact, the trans-subclavian procedure can be done in case of a concomitant vascular disease involving the abdominal aorta or the legs, and it does not require a thoracotomy. Unfortunately, the presence of a patent internal mammary artery, such as a diseased subclavian artery, in redo coronary surgery contraindicates this approach. However, at this moment, this interesting approach remains "off-label" and is not yet formally recommended by the industry.

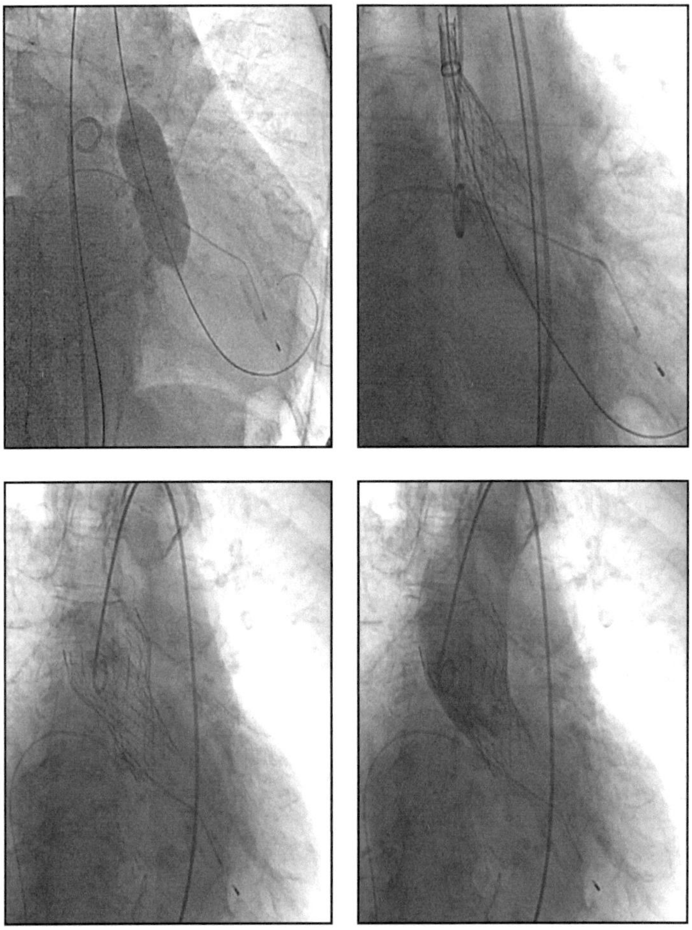

Fig. 10. TAVI using the transfemoral approach

7.4 The trans-aortic approach

In case of severe vascular disease and a concomitant contraindication to transapical procedures, an alternative, interesting, retrograde approach has been proposed: through an upper "J-shape" mini-sternotomy, the guidewire and the delivery system are inserted, retrogradely, into the ascending aorta and are secured with a double-string suture. TAVI is then done as a transfemoral procedure. The presence of "porcelain" aorta and the risk of postoperative massive bleeding limit this approach to selected patients.

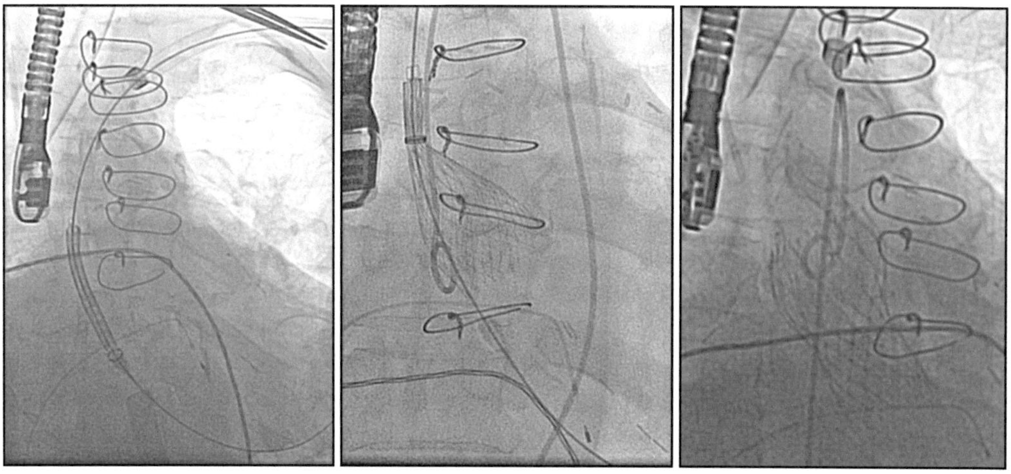

Fig. 11. TAVI using the subclavian approach

8. Results from the literature

8.1 Cribrier-Edwards valve

Cribier *et al.* (2002) did the first human implantation in 2002. The Edwards SAPIEN valve was approved for use in the European Union in November 2007 (for the transfemoral approach) and in January 2008 (for transapical delivery). In the Initial Registry of EndoVascular Implantation of Valves in Europe (I-REVIVE) trial, followed by the Registry of Endovascular Critical Aortic Stenosis Treatment (RECAST) trial, a total of 36 patients (mean (SD) EuroSCORE 12 (2)) were included (Cribrier *et al.*, 2004). Twenty-seven patients underwent successful percutaneous aortic valve implantation (23 antegrade, 4 retrograde). The 30-day mortality was 22% (6 of 27 patients), and the mean AVA increased from 0.60 ± $0.11cm^2$ to 1.70 ± $0.10cm^2$ ($p<0.001$). Importantly, this improvement in AVA was maintained up to 24 months follow-up (Cribrier *et al..*, 2006). SInce these first trials, the Cribrier-Edwards prosthesis and the Edwards SAPIEN prosthesis have been used in numerous studies. Overall, acute procedural success is achieved in 75–100% of the procedures, and 30-day mortality ranges between 8–50% in the published studies. Using the transapical technique and the Sapien valve, Walther *et al.* (2007) has reported their initial multicenter results of 59 consecutive patients, which is the largest feasibility study published thus far. Procedural success using the transapical technique was achieved in 53 patients. Thirty-day mortality was 13.6% and none of these were thought to be valve related as there was good valve function at autopsy. The overall procedural success of 1038 SAPIEN implants from 32 centers within the European SOURCE registry was 93.8%. The 30-day survival within SOURCE was 93.7% (transfemoral) and 89.7% (transapical) (Thomas, 2010). The 1-year survival of the cohort was 81.1% (transfemoral) and 72.1% (transapical), respectively. In cohort B of the PARTNER randomized trial, 179 patients receiving transfemoral SAPIEN aortic valve with 179 patients receiving standard medical therapy (including balloon aortic valvuloplasty), confirmed the superiority of transfemoral TAVI with regard to overall survival and cardiac functional status (Leon *et al.*, 2010). The Kaplan-Meier 1-year mortality from any cause was 30.7% (TAVI) versus 50.7% (standard medical therapy), corresponding to a 0.55 hazard ratio with TAVI ($p<0.001$). The fraction of surviving patients at 1-year, in New York Heart Association functional class III-IV, was lower in the TAVI group (25.2% versus 58%; $p<0.001$). Nevertheless, the TAVI group had a higher 30-day incidence of major stroke (5.0% versus 1.1%; $p=0.06$) and major vascular complications (16.2% versus 1.1%; $p<0.001$). Early and 1-year outcomes from the REVIVAL trial, which consisted of 55 patients with a mean AVA of 0.57±0.14cm2 and a mean logistic EuroSCORE of 33.5±17%, have been reported (Kodali *et al.*, 2011). TAVI was successful in 87%. Mean echocardiographic AVA improved from 0.56±14 to 1.6±0.48cm^2 after the procedure ($p<0.0001$). Thirty-day all-cause mortality and major adverse cardiac events (MACE) were 7.3% and 20%, respectively. These rates increased to 23.6% and 32.7%, respectively, at 1 year, with most late events related to underlying comorbidities. The mean NYHA functional class improved from 3.22±0.66 at baseline to 1.50±0.85 at 1-year follow-up ($p<0.001$).

8.2 CoreValve ReValving

Since the first implantation of the CoreValve prosthesis in a patient in 2005 (Grube *et al.*, 2005), a large number of patients have been treated with this device. The feasibility and safety of this valve was studied in a prospective, multicenter trial (Grube *et al.*, 2006). A total of 25 symptomatic patients with an AVA < 1cm^2 were enrolled in the study. The device was successfully implanted using the retrograde technique in 22 of 25 patients. Procedural success and aortic mean pressure gradients were markedly improved immediately following implantations with pre-procedure gradients 44.24 ± 10.79 mmHg to 12.38 ± 3.03 mmHg post-procedure, and were about the same at 30-day follow-up (11.82 ± 3.42 mm Hg). NYHA functional class improved by 1 to 2 grades in all patients. MACE, defined as death from any cause, major arrhythmia, myocardial infarction, cardiac tamponade, stroke, urgent or emergent conversion to surgery or balloon valvuloplasty, emergent percutaneous coronary intervention, cardiogenic shock, endocarditis, or aortic dissection, occurred in 8 of the 25 hospitalized patients. Recently, Grube *et al.* (2008) reported the results with the three different generations of the CoreValve Revalving system in a non-randomized, prospective study of 136 patients. Ten patients were treated with first-generation devices, 24 patients with second-generation, and 102 patients with third-generation devices. At baseline, mean AVA was 0.67cm^2 and mean logistic EuroSCORE was 23.1% in the overall study population. With the new-generation devices, the overall procedural success rate significantly increased from 70.0% and 70.8% to 91.2% for the first-, second-, and third-generation prostheses, respectively ($p = 0.003$). Interestingly, using newer devices, periprocedural mortality decreased from 10% (first-generation) to 8.3% (second-generation) to 0% (third-generation). Overall 30-day mortality for the three generations was 40%, 8.3% and 10.8%, respectively. Pooled data demonstrated a significant improvement in mean NYHA functional class (from 3.3 to 1.7, $p<0.001$), without a difference between the three generations. Importantly, NYHA functional class and mean pressure gradient remained stable up to 12 months follow-up in all three generations. In addition, the results of a multicenter registry with the third-generation CoreValve Revalving system have recently been reported (Piazza *et al.*, 2008). A total of 646 patients from 51 centers were included in the registry. It was a high-risk elderly population (mean age: 81 years) with a poor functional class (85% of the patients in NYHA class III or IV), and a high logistic EuroSCORE (mean: 23.1%). Procedural success was achieved in 628 of the 646 patients (97.2%). All-cause 30-day mortality was 8%, and the combined end point of procedural related death, stroke, or myocardial infarction was reached in 60 patients (9.3%). After successful implantation, mean pressure gradient decreased from 49 mmHg to 3 mmHg (Piazza *et al.*, 2008). The FRANCE real-world registry of 244 consecutive high-risk patients with symptomatic severe AS, enrolled from 16 centers over a period of 5 months in 2009, reported 98.3% procedural success for both Edwars SAPIEN and Medtronic CoreValve (66% transfemoral, 5% subclavian, and 29% transapical) prostheses (Eltchaninoff *et al.*, 2011). The 30-day mortality was 12.7%, and, at 1 month, 88% of patients were in NYHA class I-II. Buellesfeld *et al.* (2011) reported on a 2-year follow-up of 126 patients who underwent TAVI. Thirty-day all-cause mortality was 15.2%. At 2-years, all-cause mortality was 38.1%, with a significant difference between the moderate-risk group and the combined high-risk groups (27.8% versus 45.8%; p=0.04). This difference was attributable to an increased risk of noncardiac mortality in high-risk groups. Hemodynamic results remained unchanged during follow-up (mean gradient: 8.5±2.5mmHg at 30 days and 9.0±3.5mmHg at 2 years) without any incidence of structural valve deterioration.

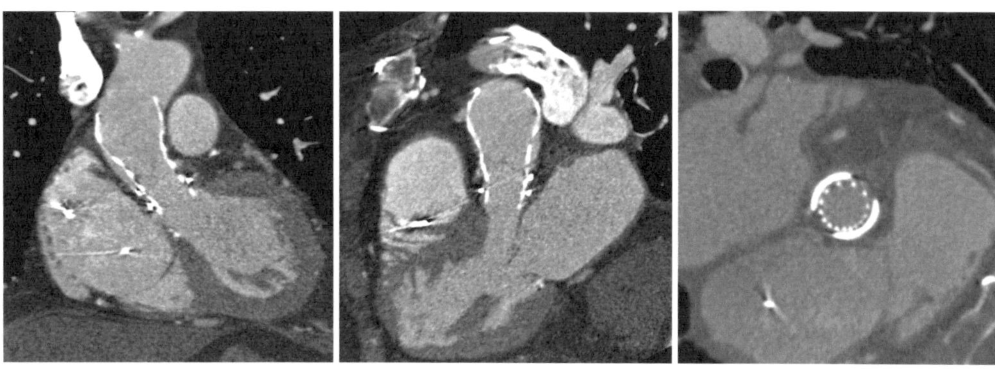

Fig. 12. TAVI in a patient with a history of AVR

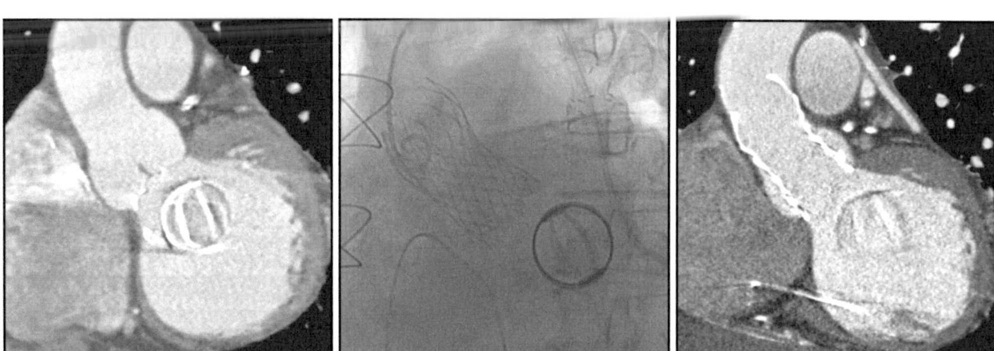

Fig. 13. TAVI in a patient with a history of mitral valve replacement

The larger CoreValve prostheses (26 and 29 mm) were the only device for annulus between 26 and 27 mm, before the currently available 29-mm SAPIEN XT valve for transapical implantation. The CoreValve prosthesis had previously been the only device suitable for transarterial implant in patients with limited iliofemoral artery access, but this has changed with the SAPIEN NovaFlex delivery system. The growing experience with the subclavian artery approach, however, allows the CoreValve prosthesis to be implanted in patients with unusable iliofemoral arteries. Because of these results, the indications for TAVI expanded (e.g. in patients with porcelain aorta, with previous cardiac surgery, etc.) (Wenaweser *et al.*, 2007) (Figure 12,13).

9. Conclusion

Transcatheter aortic valve implantation was developed to provide an alternative and less invasive method of treating aortic valve stenosis. Actually, it has been proved that the method is feasible, with results that have been reproduced by many physicians in many centers (approximately 10,000 implantations to date). Today there are at least 10 new transcatheter aortic valves that have had their first implantation in humans, many more that have reached the level of animal experiments, and even more that are still in the initial design stage. As a new treatment tool, it has to be evaluated in randomized controlled trials with long-term follow-up in order to assess safety and efficacy. Therefore, TAVI should be restricted to a limited number of high-volume centers, that have both cardiology and cardiac surgery departments as well as expertise in structural heart disease intervention and high-risk valvular surgery. Because of excellent results with surgical valve replacement, patient selection, which should be done in multidisciplinary conferences, is of utmost importance. Like other interventional procedures, there is a learning curve with significant improvements in the success rate and the clinical results after the first 25 procedures, which implies that the TAVI procedure should initially be done by and thereafter supervised by a special team (Walther *et al.*, 2009; Webb *et al.*, 2007). In addition to patient selection and intervention of TAVI, a close follow-up with assessment of clinical and objective parameters is mandatory for defining the indications of this technique.

10. References

Babaliaros V.C., Liff D., Chen E.P., *et al.* (2008). Can balloon aortic valvuloplasty help determine appropriate transcatheter aortic valve size, *JACC Intv* 1(5): 580-586.

Buellesfeld L., Gerckens U., Schuler G., *et al.* (2011). 2-year follow-up of patients undergoing transcatheter aortic valve implantation using a self-expanding valve prosthesis, *J Am Coll Cardiol* 57(16): 1650-1657.

Cribrier A., Eltchaninoff H., Bash A., *et al.* (2002). Percutaneous transcatheter implantation of an aortic valve prosthesis for calcific aortic stenosis: first human case description, *Circulation* 106(24): 3006-3008.

Cribrier A., Elchaninoff H., Tron C., *et al.* (2004). Early experience with percutaneous transcatheter implantation of heart valve prosthesis for the treatment of end-stage inoperable patients with calcific aortic stenosis, *J Am Coll Cardiol* 43(4): 698-703.

Cribrier A., Elchaninoff H., Tron C., *et al.* (2006). Treatment of calcific aortic stenosis with the percutaneous heart valve: mid-term follow-up from the initial feasibility studies: the French experience, *J Am Coll Cardiol* 47(6): 1214-1223.

De Robertis F., Asgar A., Davies S., *et al.* (2009) The left exillary arter-a new approach for transcatheter aortic valve implantation, *Eur J Cardiothorac Surg* 36(5):807-12.

Eltchaninoff H., Prat A., Gilard M., *et al.* (2011). Transcatheter aortic valve implantation: early results of the France (French Aortic National CoreValve and Edwards) registry, *Eur Heart J* 32(2): 191-197.

Grossi E.A., Schwartz C.F., Yu P.J., *et al.* (2008). High-risk aortic valve replacement: are the outcomes as bad as predicted, *Ann Thorac Surg* 85(1): 102-106.

Grube E., Laborde J.C., Zikmann B., *et al.* (2005). First report on a human percutaneous transluminal implantation of a self-expanding valve prosthesis for interventional treatment of aortic valve stenosis, *Catheter Cardiovasc Interv* 66(4): 465-469.

Grube E., Laborde J.C., Gerckens U., *et al.* (2006). Percutaneous implantation of the CoreValve self-expanding valve prosthesis in high-risk patients with aortic valve disease: Siegburg first-in-man study, *Circulation* 114(15): 1616-1624.

Grube E., Buellesfeld L., Mueller R., *et al.* (2008). Progress and current status of percutaneous aortic valve replacement: results of three device generation of the CoreValve Revalving system, *Circ Cardiovasc Intervent* 1(3): 167-175.

Iung B., Cachier A., Baron G., *et al.* (2005). Decision-making in elderly patients with sévère aortic stenosis: why are so many denied surgery, *Eur Heart J* 26(24): 2714-2720.

Kodali S.K., O'Neill W.W., Moses J.W., *et al.* (2011). Early and late (one year) outcomes following transcatheter aortic valve implantation in patients with severe aortic stenosis (from the United States REVIVAL Trial), *Am J Cardiol* 107(7): 1058-1064.

Kvidal P., Bergstrom R., Horte L.G., *et al.* (2000). Observed and relative survival after aortic valve replacement, *J Am Coll Cardiol* 35(3): 747-756.

Leon M.B., Smith C.R., Mack M., *et al.* (2010). Transcathetr aortic-valve implantation for aortic stenosis in patients who cannot undergo surgery, *N Engl J Med* 363(17): 1597-15607.

Moss R.R., Ivens E., Pasupati S., *et al.* (2008). Role of echocardiography in percutaneous aortic valve replacement, *JACC Cardiovasc Imaging* 1(1): 15-24.

Nkomo V.T., Gardin J.M., Skelton T.N., *et al.* (2006). Burden of valvular heart disease: a population-based study, *Lancet* 368(9540): 1005-1011.

Piazza N., Grube E., Gerckens U., *et al.* (2008). Procedural and 30-day outcomes following transcatheter aortic valve implantation using the third generation (18 Fr) CoreValve revalving system: results from the multicentre, expanded evaluation registry 1-year following CE mark approval, *EuroIntervention* 4(2): 242-249.

Ross J. Jr & Braunwald E. (1965). Aortic stenosis, Circulation 38(2): V61-V67.

Roques F., Nashef S.A., Michel P., *et al.* (2001). Risk factors for early mortality after valve surgery in Europe in the 1990's: lesson from the EuroSCORE pilot program, *J Heart Valve Dis* 10(5): 572-578.

Thomas M., Schymik G., Walther T., *et al.* (2010). Thirty-day results of the SAPIEN aortic Bioprosthesis Outcomes (SOURCE) Registry: A European registry of transcatheter aortic valve implantation using the Edwards SAPIEN valve, *Circulation* 122(1): 62-69.

Vahanian A., Alfieri O., Al-Attar N., *et al.* (2008). Transcatheter valve implantation for patients with aortic stenosis: a position statement from the European Association of Cardio-Thoracic Surgery (EACTS) and the European Society of Cardiology (ESC), in collaboration with the European Association of Percutaneous Cardiovascular Interventions (EAPCI), *Eur Heart J* 29(11): 1463-1470.

Varadarajan P., Kapoor N., Bansal R.C., *et al.* (2006). Clinical profile and natural history of 453 nonsurgical managed patients with severe aortic stenosis, *Ann Thorac Surg* 82(6): 2111-2115.

Walther T., Simon P., Dewey T., *et al.* (2007). Transapical minimally invasive aortic valve implantation: multicenter experience, *Circulation* 116(Suppl 11): I240-I245.

Walther T., Dewey T., Borger M.A., *et al.* (2009). Transapical aortic valve implantation: step by step, *Ann Thorac Surg* 87(1): 276-283.

Webb J.G., Pasupati S., Humphries K., *et al.* (2007). Percutaneous transarterial aortic valve replacement in selected high-risk patients with aortic stenosis, *Circulation* 116(7): 755-763.

Wenaweser P, Buellesfeld L, Gerckens U, Grube E. (2007). Percutaneous aortic valve replacement for sévère aortic régurgitation in degenerated bioprosthesis : the first valve in valve procédure using Corevlave Revalving system, *Catheter Cardiovasc Interv* 70(5) :760-764

Zegdi R., Ciobotaru V., Noghin M., *et al.* (2008). Is it reasonable to treat all calcified stenotic aortic valves with a valved stent? Results from a human anatomic study in adults, *J Am Coll Cardiol* 51(5): 579-584.

11

Transcatheter Aortic Valve Implantation: State of the Art

Alice Le Huu, Rony Atoui and Dominique Shum-Tim
Divisions of Cardiac Surgery and Surgical Research, Department of Surgery, McGill University Health Center, Montreal, Canada

1. Introduction

In the last century, medical innovation has revolutionized human lives and the management of medical diseases. Conditions which were once considered untreatable are now managed and even cured. Consequently, life expectancy has dramatically increased. The aging population brings about new challenges and pathologies that must be addressed with different approaches. As the body ages, so does the heart, bringing aortic stenosis to the forefront of valvular heart disease. It is estimated that 4.6% of patients over the age of 75 years old suffer from aortic stenosis (Nkomo et al., 2006). Traditionally, there were three modalities of treatment: conservative medical management, balloon valvuloplasty, and surgical aortic valve replacement (AVR). Long considered to be the gold-standard for aortic valve stenosis, surgical intervention provided a functional valve with acceptable mortality rates. However, the risks of surgical intervention increase dramatically depending on a patient's comorbidities. Accordingly, high-risk patients were often relegated to medical management or balloon valvuloplasty. Conservative management has yielded extremely disappointing results. Patients who underwent balloon valvuloplasty in conjunction with medical treatment had a 44-37.2% mortality rate within a year. In addition, conservative management is associated with a high rate of restenosis. Medical management alone resulted in an unacceptable 25% mortality in one year (Nkomo et al., 2006; Ben-Dor et al., 2010). Despite these staggering statistics, the Euro Heart Survey suggested that approximately 30% of patients suffering from severe aortic stenosis were not treated with surgical intervention (Lung et al., 2003). A significant portion of these patients are refused surgery because they are deemed to have elevated surgical risks. Considering the natural history of the pathology, patients who were refused for surgery suffer considerable morbidity and mortality. Even with maximum medical therapy, the future for these patients appeared bleak.

Fortunately, the advent of transcatheter aortic valve implantation (TAVI), has led to new options for non-surgical candidates. As early as 1965, an article describing a catheter-mounted valve replacement for temporary relief of aortic insufficiency in an animal (Davies H., 1965). After more than three decades of development, Cribier et al. (2002) successfully implanted a percutaneous prosthetic heart valve in a 57-year-old man. The patient, who was moribund due to numerous medical conditions, showed significant clinical and echocardiographic improvement after the valve had been implanted. Although he eventually succumbed to his multiple comorbidities, his last transesophageal echocardiography demonstrated a functional aortic valve (Webb et al., 2009). A landmark success, this intervention was followed by a flurry of developments which resulted in considerable refinement of the procedure. This would culminate in increased safety, efficiency, and physician familiarity with the intervention. It is now estimated that over 15,000 patients worldwide have undergone a TAVI procedure (Geisbusch et al., 2010).

2. Patient selection

With any medical procedure, whether it is aortic valve replacement or medical treatment, the key to a favorable outcome is appropriate patient selection. By virtue of its recent development, access to TAVI remains restricted. Presently, TAVI is offered only to patients with symptomatic, critical aortic stenosis who have been deemed unsuitable for AVR. Evaluating a patient as inoperable depends on many factors, which include patient comorbidities, the surgeon's experience, and the institution in which the surgeon practices. Subtle details may influence a physician's judgment, which renders it difficult to provide a standard definition of a non-surgical candidate. With this limitation in mind, many institutions qualify patients with a logistic EuroScore calculated ≥ 20% or an STS (Society of Thoracic Surgery) predicted mortality risk score ≥ 10% as high-risk (Bande et al., 2010). Although not included in these two scoring systems, other criteria often cited when deeming a patient high-risk include: calcified porcelain aorta, chest wall deformities, cancer, cirrhosis with portal hypertension, neurological dysfunction, perceived frailty, severe chronic obstructive disease, previous cardiac surgery, severe cerebrovascular disease, low ejection fraction, and untreatable coronary artery disease (Saia et al., 2010). Traditionally, a bicuspid valve is considered a contraindication to TAVI. Due to its elliptical rather than circular shape, TAVI may result in a morphologically distorted valve and increased incidence of perivalvular leaks. Consequently, valve durability may be compromised. Recently published experience with 11 bicuspid TAVI demonstrated decreased gradients across the valve, and increased valve area. Two patients had moderate leaks. Although interesting, these results did not address the fundamental concern of TAVI in bicuspid valves related to their durability (Wijesinghe et al., 2010).
Once patients are deemed inoperable, they must be carefully screened before proceeding to TAVI. In many centers, candidates are evaluated by a multidisciplinary committee consisting of cardiologists, cardiac surgeons, and cardiac anesthesiologists. Therefore, patients are evaluated on a case-by-case basis. Broad exclusion criteria may include dementia, life expectancy of less than 1 year, severely incapacitating neurological dysfunction, thoracic aneurysm, and a low likelihood of benefitting from the procedure (Shareghi et al., 2007). However, these selection parameters are subject to the discretion of each individual committee, and remain obscure. As TAVI becomes more prevalent, it will most certainly entail the development of specific guidelines to help orient physicians.
A patient's anatomy is crucial in the selection process. The preoperative screening tests are similar in many centers. Transthoracic echocardiography and a coronary angiogram are standard. From a purely logistic point of view, a patient with and aortic annulus diameter < 18 mm or > 26 mm may be excluded due to limited availability of valve sizes (Webb et al., 2009). However, this exclusion is likely to be attenuated in the coming years as a wider range of valve sizes are developed. Computer tomography of the thorax, abdomen, and

pelvis are done to delineate the anatomy of the patient. For technical considerations, the presence of torturous, severely diseased femoral or subclavian arteries may not be amenable to percutaneous TAVI. When available, some centers use three-dimensional reconstruction of the aortic root to detect calcifications, femoral stenosis, kinking, and aortic dissection (Geisbusch et al., 2010). While helpful, reconstructions are not essential to the screening process.

Absolute contraindications to TAVI are few, but include intolerance of anticoagulation and bleeding diathesis. There is a lack of consensus on the ideal strategy, but many centers use dual antiplatelet therapy: a loading dose of aspirin (325 mg) and clopidogrel (300-600 mg), followed by clopidogrel (75 mg) for 6 months and aspirin (81 mg) indefinitely (Gurvitch et al., 2010). Other exclusion criteria include the presence of a ventricular or atrial clot and active endocarditis.

3. Design of the device

Currently, two types of percutaneous valves dominate the market: the SAPIEN Valve manufactured by Edwards Life Sciences (Irvine, CA, USA) and the CoreValve produced by Medtronic, Inc. (Minneapolis, MN, USA). Each valve has unique properties and indications for implantation.

The SAPIEN model is a trileaflet bovine valve mounted on a cobalt-chromium stent; it is a balloon-expandable prosthesis. Designed for antegrade, retrograde, or transapical delivery, the valve is deployed by balloon expansion into a subcoronary position. The prosthetic valve uses the native calcified valve to anchor itself (Eltchaninoff et al., 2008). There are three sizes available: 23 mm, 26 mm, and 29 mm, with a 20-mm size in development (Bande et al., 2010). Presently, the SAPIEN valve employs the Novoflex delivery system, which allows the valve to be delivered via an 18F and 19F introducer sheath for a 23-mm and 26-mm valve, respectively (Lange et al., 2007).

The Medtronic CoreValve, is used worldwide but has yet to be approved in North America and Japan. The CoreValve is a trileaflet bioprosthetic porcine valve which is mounted onto a self-expanding nitinol frame. The nitinol stent has 3 portions: an upper portion which serves to anchor the device to the ascending aorta, a central component of the stent engineered to avoid obstructing the coronary ostium, and a lower portion of the stent which rests on the annulus. The CoreValve system is believed to adapt to non-circular anatomies. Two sizes are available: 22 mm and 29 mm; the valve requires an 18F introducer sheath (Bande et al., 2010). Designed for retrograde delivery, it is implanted using a transfemoral or subclavian approach; however, successful transapical implantation has been reported.

4. Methods of approach

Presently, three approaches for TAVI are used: transfemoral, transapical, and subclavian. Selecting the proper approach involves integrating patient characteristics with technical considerations. The preferred access remains the transfemoral approach. Using this access, the Novaflex delivery system requires arteries to be 6.0 to 6.5 mm in diameter. Similarly, the CoreValve requires 6.0 to 7.0 mm arteries in order to accommodate the catheter-mounted aortic valve. The size of the introducer sheath used is dictated by patient anatomy, primarily the size of the femoral artery for access and the diameter of the valve required to fit the annulus. Depending on the sheath used, surgical exposure and closure of the femoral artery may be needed. In other cases, a smaller catheter may require only a vascular closure device, and thus negate the need of a surgical team (Eltchaninoff et al., 2008). A heavily calcified arterial system with numerous tortuosities may not be amenable to access. In addition, patients who have had extensive vascular surgery are usually not suited to this approach. The transfemoral is considered to be a relatively safe method of access. However, reported complications include formation of retroperitoneal hematoma, iliac or femoral artery pseudoaneurysms, and stenosis or occlusion induced by a vascular closure device. According to Philipp et al. (2009), the majority of these complications are managed conservatively, or with endovascular intervention.

Typically, the transapical approach will be used when the iliofemoral approach is not feasible. For this approach, the SAPIEN valve is used because it is approved for antegrade delivery. The procedure is done in a hybrid suite with the guidance of transesophageal echocardiography and fluoroscopy. Under, under general anesthesia, a 6 to 8 cm anterolateral thoracotomy incision is made to expose the pericardium. Once open, temporary pacing wires are attached and a suitable puncture site in the left ventricular apex is identified. Two orthogonal U-shaped pledgeted sutures are placed in the myocardium before a needle puncture is done, followed by the insertion of a guide wire to the ascending aorta. The catheter is then increased in size to allow for balloon valvuloplasty. Once complete, the sheath size is increased to accommodate the delivery system, and the transcatheter valve is deployed. At the end of the procedure, at the discretion of the surgeon, a drain may be left in place. This method of delivery is much more invasive than the iliofemoral approach and is linked to significant complications. This may include pericarditis, tamponade, pneumothorax, and the formation of a false aneurysm at the apex of the heart (Al-Attar et al., 2009). Injury to the mitral valve using this approach is also a particular concern due to its anatomic proximity. In addition, recovery time is more extensive. Pain at the thoracotomy site is not negligible and can result in respiratory debilitation in frail and elderly patients, culminating in prolonged hospitalization.

Recently, the trans-subclavian approach has been developed as an alternative to the transapical approach. A technique described by Petronio et al. (2010) consists of surgical exposure of the subclavian artery, followed by arterial puncture between purse-string sutures. A 6F catheter is inserted, and the 18F catheter commonly used for the transfemoral approach is placed over a guide wire. It is then threaded through the subclavian artery and into the ascending aorta. Once in place, the catheter mounted valve is implanted using the same method as for the transfemoral approach. Concerns exist over the security of the trans-subclavian method. Of particular interest are patients who have had their internal mammary used in a coronary artery bypass graft. It is unclear whether this approach can safely preserve flow through the graft during implantation of the valve. By rapidly withdrawing the 18F catheter, the Petronio et al. (2010) team was able to avoid all signs of myocardial ischemia. Caution must be exercised in the interpretation of this data, as the sample size (8 patients) was quite small. Other considerations concerning the trans-subclavian approach include direct injury to the brachial plexus and damage secondary to hematoma formation. Perhaps because of its recent development, this method appears to be used less frequently than the transfemoral approach. It is usually considered a second option when the transfemoral anatomy is unsuitable for access. As the number of TAVI procedures increase, familiarity with the trans-subclavian approach will rise, and it will become more frequently employed.

Comparisons between the three methods of delivery remain in their infancy. The studies have used small sample sizes, and do not offer direct comparisons between the methods of delivery, nor were the patients randomized between the methods of approach. The trend is to favor a transfemoral approach, and, when this is not possible, to opt for a transapical approach. In theory, a transapical approach requires mechanical ventilation and general anesthesia, which renders it less desirable.

5. Outcome

Initial results from TAVI are very encouraging, albeit of a small scale. However, in recent years, large-scale studies support the assertion that TAVI is a viable treatment option for aortic stenosis. The most important study to date is the PARTNER trial, a North American multicenter trial with 2 main cohorts, run by Leon et al. (2010). Surgical candidates were randomized to TAVI or conventional aortic valve replacement (Cohort A). Patients who were deemed non-operable (358 patients) were randomized to TAVI and medical therapy (including balloon valvuloplasty: cohort B). The patients all underwent TAVI through a transfemoral approach, and were followed for up to one year post-procedure. The results of cohort B were recently published. TAVI was shown to be superior for all of the hard endpoints, including death at one year: 30.7% for TAVI compared with 71.6% for standard therapy. Patients who underwent the procedure demonstrated significantly increased freedom from symptoms associated with their valvular disease: 74.8% compared with 42.0% (Leon et al., 2010). This study is unequivocal proof that TAVI is superior to conventional medical management. The results from this randomized trial are in accordance with other studies. Gurvitch et al. (2010), sought to elucidate the long-term outcome of TAVI patients by following a cohort of 70 individuals over a period of 3 years. Survival after 1 year (excluding 11 patients that died within 30 days of the procedure and 8 patients with failed valve implantation) was 81%. Studies with mixed delivery approaches (transfemoral, transapical, and subclavian), yielded mortality rates between 5.4%-11.3% after 30 days (Gurvitch et al., 2010; Petronio et al., 2010). However, with cohort studies, it is difficult to compare the mortality rate with conventional medical treatment. Indirect comparisons can be made with published estimates of mortality, which ranges from 51%-62% in symptomatic patients after 1 year (Bach et al., 2007). The totality of the data suggests that in patients who are refused surgery, TAVI is superior to medical management.

Aside from mortality and freedom from symptoms, another important determinant of outcome is the durability of the transcatheter valves. Studies indicate that the TAVI device is quite durable. Gurvitch et al. (2010) suggests that the valve appears to be structurally normal, with very little incidence of degeneration at 3 years. Valve function appears to decrease over the years, quantified by a slight decrease in calculated valve area and an increase in valve gradient, estimated by the authors at 0.06% cm^2 per year. It is unclear whether these changes will be clinically significant. Due to its relatively recent development, the durability of the valve will be known only in the near future. It is important to note that surgically replaced aortic valves also show signs of degeneration, tearing, and calcification. The durability of surgically replaced valves compared to TAVI will only be known in years to come.

The presence of aortic insufficiency after TAVI is another important criterion of success. Unfortunately, this endpoint is exceedingly difficult to qualify because of the subjective nature of echographic findings. Notoriously operator-dependent, this issue is magnified when exams are completed by different physicians and technicians in a range of institutions. Nevertheless, the PARTNER trial found moderate or severe paravalvular aortic insufficiency in 11.8% of patients after 30 days, and 10.5% at 1 year (Leon et al., 2010). The amount of aortic regurgitation remained stable in patients after one year, did not seem to progress, and was generally well tolerated by the patients. Similarly, Gurvitch et al. (2010) determined that 6% of their patients had moderate aortic regurgitation, with no incidences of severe regurgitation. The clinical significance of these echographic findings is yet to be determined. The stability of the aortic insufficiency over time will be the key determinant of the relevance of this finding.

6. Complications

As with any other medical procedure, there are risks associated with TAVI. The most concerning complication is the risk of stroke. The culprits behind the neurological event are multifold. Atheroma in the aorta, dislodged during TAVI, may play a significant role. In addition, during TAVI many patients undergo balloon valvuloplasty, which is likely to dislodge microemboli of calcium to the cerebrovascular system. The TAVI procedure, with the self-expanding valve or manual positioning of the valve, is also traumatic to the original valve. This provides another possible source of emboli. Despite encouraging results in terms of crude outcomes such as death and freedom from repeat hospitalization, the optimism for this procedure is tempered by the risk of cerebral ischemia. The PARTNER trial found the incidence of stroke to be 5% compared with 1.1% in the medically treated group (Leon et al., 2010). Similarly, Gurvitch et al. (2010) documented a risk of 8.6% after 3 years. Even more alarming, Kahlert et al. (2010) followed 32 patients who underwent TAVI (either the SAPIEN or CoreValve), to discover the effect on their neurological status. Neurological assessment and cognitive function were assessed through the National Institute Health Stroke Scale (NIHSS) along with a Mini Mental State Examination (MMSE). In conjunction with these clinical exams, patients received preoperative and postoperative MRIs. In 84% of the patients, significant multiple and diffuse emboli were discovered on the MRIs. The investigators were unable to find a clinical correlation between the radiologic images and patients' symptoms. However, the NIHSS and the MMSE are crude methods of measuring cognitive function. Subtle changes in memory and cognitive function may be much more evident in a younger, healthier individual with fewer comorbidities. Further research must be completed on the neurological impact of TAVI before it can be offered to patients who are surgical candidates.

The need for pacemaker insertion following TAVI is also well documented. A study by Khawaja et al. (2011) quoted a rate of 33.3% requiring pacemaker insertion in the 30 days following the procedure. The study found that patients were most often susceptible to developing left bundle branch block. After studying the CoreValve, the authors reasoned that the skirt of the valve (depending on the position after the deployment) will lie in close proximity to the left bundle branch, which entails conduction abnormalities. The old valve is not excised and the placement of the CoreValve on top of the remnants may lead to compression of conduction structures.

Dislocation or migration of the valve during implantation is mentioned in several case reports. In a patient population of 212, Geisbusch et al. (2010) reported an incidence of 10%

dislocation during implantation, while Rhodes-Cabu et al. (2010) had a rate of 2%. Management of this complication primarily consists of retrieving the valve in the ascending aorta and reimplanting it. However, patients with this complication had significantly higher rates of stroke, ischemia, or renal failure than did patients whose first implantation was successful (Geisbusch et al., 2010). Although this complication is documented in other papers, this study on the CoreValve reveals it to be quite frequent. It is probable that valve dislocation is a common occurrence; however, it is not well documented in large trials as a potential source of morbidity. In addition, in cohort studies which involve databases, this information is more difficult to obtain, and is thus excluded from analysis.

Other complications include vascular-related injuries as such as dissection, perforations, ruptures, and hematomas, as well as cardiac-related issues such as aortic root rupture, mitral valve injury, tamponade, and injury to the left ventricle apex.

7. Future prospects

Preliminary data on transcatheter aortic valve implantation is very promising. It also highlights the importance of a dedicated multidisciplinary team consisting of a cardiac surgeon, interventional cardiologist, echocardiographer, cardiac anesthesiologist, perfusionist, and scrub team. As with any new technology, more research needs to be completed before its role in the management of aortic stenosis can be clearly delineated. At present, it is clearly superior to medical management, and offers non-surgical patients a viable option. However, its use in patients who are surgical candidates is likely to be tempered by several limiting factors. Of primary importance is the increased risk of cerebral ischemia during this procedure, that seems to persist overtime even after the placement of TAVI. By virtue of its delivery system and implantation mechanism, it will be very difficult to minimize thromboembolic events. In older, frail patients with many co-morbidities, TAVI may be an acceptable alternative. New generation of sutureless surgically implantable prosthetic valves are another surgical options in development (Perseval S valve by Sorin). These valves are designed to be implanted after the calcified aortic valve is surgically removed. This will theoretically diminish the potential of ongoing embolic risks that were observed in current TAVI reported by the PARTNER trial (Miller, 2011). Without the need to suture the prosthetic valve onto the aortic annulus, the valve would be quicker to implant and result in decreased cardio-pulmonary bypass time (O'Brien et al., 1998). Consequently, these sutureless valves may be more suitable for patients with intermediate risk profile, in whom a shorter cardio-pulmonary bypass time may be beneficial. Ongoing accumulation of experience and longer term follow-up are underway to assess the clinical application of this new generation of surgically implantable sutureless valve in many cardiac centers. In a younger patient, however, where mortality associated with surgical aortic valve replacement is very low, traditional surgical management is indicated.

Another area of interest is the durability of TAVI. The valve's ability to expand to fit the aortic root may be detrimental to its long-term use. It remains questionable whether this type of valve is suitable for implantation when the patient's life expectancy is beyond ten to fifteen years. Unfortunately, this data will be available only several years from now.

Currently, many questions remain unanswered. The TAVI technique is still in its infancy compared with traditional surgical and medical management of aortic stenosis, which has undergone rigorous investigation. For surgical valve replacement, there are clear indications and guidelines on the timing and management of replacement. Data on proper management of TAVI patients are lacking, including basic premises such as anticoagulation and management in conjunction with other heart pathologies. Aortic stenosis rarely exists as a single entity, and ischemic heart disease often coexists with this pathology. Initial data on the role of concomitant coronary artery disease and TAVI is conflicting. Dewey et al. (2010) reported increased mortality in patients with coronary artery disease undergoing TAVI, while Masson et al. (2010) found that this factor did not affect mortality. These are conflicting reports and illustrate that the application of TAVI in complex clinical situations remains obscure. More research must be completed to properly define the role of TAVI in the treatment of aortic stenosis.

It is undeniable that the advent of TAVI has provided physicians with an important tool for treating aortic valve disease. In non-surgical, high-risk patients, the technology may mean freedom from considerable mortality and morbidity. The therapeutic potential of this technology is astonishing; however, expectations must be tempered by caution.

8. References

Al-Attar N, Ghodbane W, Himbert D, Rau C, Raffoul R, Messika-Zeitoun D, Brochet E, Vahanian A & Nataf P. (2009) Unexpected Complications Of Transapical Aortic Valve Implantation. *Annals of Thoracic Surgery* Vol. 88, pp. 90-94, ISSN 0003-4975

Bach DS, Cimino N & Deeb MG. (2007) Unoperated Patients with Severe Aortic Stenosis. *Journal of the American College of Cardiology*. Vol. 50, pp. 2018-2019 ISSN 0735-1097

Bande M, Michev I, Sharp A, Chieffo A & Colombo A. (2010). Percutaneous Transcatheter Aortic Valve Implantation: Past Accomplishments, Present Achievements and Applications, Future Perspectives. *Cardiology in Review*. Vol. 18, pp. 111-124, ISSN 1061-5377

Dewey TM, Brown DL, Herbert MA, Culica D, Smith CR, Leon MB, Svensson LG Tuzcu M, Webb JG, Cribier A & Mack MJ. (2010). Effect Of Concomitant Coronary Artery Disease On Procedural and Late Outcomes Of Transcatheter Aortic Valve Implantation. *The Annals of Thoracic Surgery*. Vol. 89, pp. 758-767 ISSN 0003-4975

Eltchaninoff H, Zajarias A & Tron C. (2008). Transcatheter Aortic Valve Implantation: Technical Aspects, Results and Indications. *Archives Cardiovascular Disease*. Vol. 101, pp. 126-132, ISSN 1875-2136

Geisbusch S, Bleiziffer S, Mazzitelli D, Ruge H, Bauernschmitt R &Lange R. (2010). Incidence and Management of CoreValve Dislocation During Transcatheter Aortic Valve Implantation. *Circulation: Cardiovascular Intervention*. Vol. 3, pp. 531-536, ISSN 1941-7640

Gurvitch R, Wood DA, Tay EL, Leipsic J, Ye J, Lichtenstein SV, Thompson CR, Carere RG, Wijesinghe N, Nietlispach F, Boone RH, Lauck S, Cheung A & Webb JG. (2010). Transcatheter Aortic Valve Implantation: Durability of Clinical and Hemodynamic Outcomes Beyond 3 Years in a Large Patient Cohort. *Circulation*. Vol. 122, pp. 1319-1327, ISSN 0009-7322

Kahlert P, Knipp SC, Schlamann M, Thielmann M, Al-Rashid F, Weber M, Johansson U, Wendt D, Jakob HG, Forsting M, Sack S, Erbel R & Eggebrecht H. (2010). Silent and Apparent Cerebral Ischemia After Percutaneous Transfemoral Aortic Valve Implantation: A Diffuse-Weighted Magnetic Resonance Imaging Study. *Circulation*. Vol. 121, pp. 870-878 ISSN 0009-7322

Khawaja MZ, Rajani R, Cook A, Khavandi A, Moynagh A, Chowdhary S, Spence SM, Brown S, Khan SQ, Walker N, Trivedi U, Hutchinson N, De Belder AJ, Moat N, Blackman DJ, Levy RD, Manoharan G, Roberts D, Khogali SS, Crean P, Brecker SJ, Baumbach A, Mullen M, Laborde JC & Hildick-Smith D. (2011). Permanent Pacemaker Insertion After CoreValve Transcatheter Aortic Valve Implantation: Incidence and Contributing Factors (the UK CoreValve Collaborative). *Circulation.* Vol. 123, pp. 951-960 ISSN 0009-7322

Lange R, Schreiber C, Gotz W, Hettich I, Will A, Libera P, Laborde JC & Beurnschmitt R. (2007). First Successful Transapical Aortic Valve Implantation With the CoreValve Revalving System: A Case Report. *Heart Surgery Forum.* Vol. 10, E478-E479 ISSN 1522-6662

Leon MB, Smith CR, Mack M, Miller DC, Moses JW, Svensson LG, Tuzcu EM, Webb JG, Fontana GP, Makkar RR, Brown DL, Block PC, Guyton RA, Pichard AD, Bavaria JE, Herrmann HC, Douglas PS, Petersen JL, Akin JJ, Anderson WN, Wang D & Pocock S; PARTNER Trial Investigators. (2010). Transcatheter Aortic-Valve Implantation For Aortic Stenosis In Patients Who Cannot Undergo Surgery. *New England Journal of Medicine.* Vol. 17, pp. 1597-607 ISSN 0028-4793

Masson JB, Lee M, Boone RH, Al Ali A, Bugami SA, Hamburger J, Mancini J, Ye J, Cheung A, Humphries KH, Wood J, Nietlispach F & Webb JG. (2010). Impact Of Coronary Artery Disease On Outcomes After Transcatheter Aortic Valve Implantation. *Catheterization and Cardiovascular Intervention.* Vol. 76, pp. 165-173 ISSN 1522-1946

Miller, C. (2011). "Late-breaking Clinical Trial: Frequency and Severity of Neurologic Events after Aortic Valve Replacement or Transcatheter Aortic Valve Implantation in High Surgical Risk Patients with Aortic Stenosis: The PARTNER Trial Stroke Substudy," American Association for Thoracic Surgery 91st Annual Meeting, Philadelphia, Pennsylvania

O'Brien MF, Gardner MA, Garlick RB, Davison MB, Thomson HL, Burstow DJ. (1998). The Cryolife-O'Brien stentless aortic porcine xenograft valve. *Journal of Cardiac Surgery* Vol. 13, pp. 376–385 ISSN 0886-0440

Petronio AS, De Carlo M, Bodogoni F, Marzocchi A, Klugmann S, Maisano F, Ramondo A, Ussia GP, Ettori F, Poli A, Brambilla N, Saia F, De Marco F & Colombo A. (2010). Safety and Efficacy of the Subclavian Approach For the Transcatheter Aortic Valve Implantation with the CoreValve Revalving System. *Circulation: Cardiovascular Intervention.* Vol. 3, pp. 359-366 ISSN 1941-7640

Philipp K, Al-Rashid F, Weber M, Wendt D, Heine T, Kottenberg E, Thielmann M, Kühl H, Peters J & Heinz JG. (2009). Vascular Access Site Complications After Percutaneous Transfemoral Aortic Valve Implantation. *Herz.* Vol. 5, pp. 398-408, ISSN 0340-9937

Saia F, Marrozzini C, Dall'Ara G, Russo V, Martin-Suarez S, Ortolani P, Palmerini T, Taglieri N, Bordoni B, Pilato E, Di Bartolomeo R, Branzi A & Marzocchi A. (2010). How Many Patients With Severe Symptomatic Aortic Stenosis Excluded For Cardiac Surgery Are Eligible For Transcatheter Heart Valve Implantation? *Journal of Cardiovascular Medicine (Hagerstown).* Vol. 10, 727-732 ISSN 1558-2027

Shareghi S, Rasouli L, Shavelle DM, Burstein S & Matthews RV. (2007). Current Results Of Balloon Aortic Valvuloplasty In High Risk Patients. *Journal of Invasive Cardiology.* Vol. 19, pp. S37-S42 ISSN 1042-3931

Webb J, Altwegg L, Boone RH, Cheung A, Ye J, Lichenstein S, Lee M, Masson JB, Thompson C, Moss R, Carere R, Munt B, Nietlispach F & Humphries K. (2009). Transcatheter Aortic Valve Implantation: Impact On Clinical and Valve-Related Outcome. *Circulation*. Vol. 119, pp. 3009-3016 ISSN 0009-7322

Wijesinghe N, Ye J, Rodés-Cabau J, Cheung A, Velianou JL, Natarajan MK, Dumont E, Nietlispach F, Gurvitch R, Wood DA, Tay E, Webb JG. (2010). Journal American College Cardiology: Cardiovascular Interventions. Volume 3, 1122-1125 ISSN: 1936-8798

12

Transcatheter Aortic Valve Implantation

Hunaid A. Vohra, Robert N. Whistance and Sunil K. Ohri
Wessex Cardiac Centre,
Southampton University Hospitals Trust
UK

1. Introduction

Calcific aortic stenosis (AS) is the most common form of degenerative heart valve disease in developed countries. AS predominantly affects the elderly with a prevalence of 4% in people over the age of 80 years. With increasing longevity and an ageing population the absolute number of people afflicted with AS is set to rise. The clinical course of the disease is insidious at first (Ross & Braunwald, 1968), but is followed by rapid progression once symptoms of congestive cardiac failure, angina and syncope develop (Cheitlin *et al.*, 1979; Otto *et al.*, 1989; Davies *et al.*, 1991; Peter *et al.*, 1993). If left untreated mortality exceeds 50% at two years (Kelly *et al.*, 1988; Turina *et al.*, 1987) and AS is, therefore, set to become a major public health problem in the ensuing decades.

Aortic valve replacement (AVR) has been the gold standard intervention for AS for more than 40 years (Charlson *et al.*, 2006) and over 60,000 procedures are performed annually in the European Union. However, one third of patients are denied access to surgery, often due to their advanced age (Iung *et al.*, 2003, 2005). Percutaneous balloon valvuloplasty was heralded initially as a promising breakthrough for high-risk symptomatic patients with AS (Cribier *et al.*, 1986). However, long-term follow-up has yielded unacceptable rates of restenosis and poor event-free survival (Otto *et al.*, 1994; Lieberman *et al.*, 1995). Balloon valvuloplasty is now recommended only as a bridge to emergency AVR or in the palliation of symptoms in the frailest of patients (Ussia *et al.*, 2010; Zahn *et al.*, 2011).

Transcatheter aortic valve implantation (TAVI) has recently emerged as an effective therapeutic alternative to conventional AVR for high-risk AS patients. TAVI was developed initially in porcine models (Anderson *et al.*, 1992), but it took a decade for this technology to be translated to humans (Cribier *et al.*, 2002). Initially, an antegrade transseptal approach was used, but this has now been superseded by transapical (Ye *et al.*, 2006; Webb *et al.*, 2007) and retrograde percutaneous techniques (transarterial or transaxillary) (Webb *et al.*, 2006). The range of different approaches has increased the feasibility of TAVI in patients with relative contraindications, such as extensive peripheral vascular disease, porcelain aorta and thoracic radiotherapy. TAVI is also less invasive than open AVR and permits replacement of the native diseased valve in the beating heart without the need for sternotomy and cardiopulmonary bypass. Consequently, TAVI may be less influenced by a patient's comorbidities and may facilitate faster recovery.

A multidisciplinary team consisting of interventional cardiologists, cardiothoracic surgeons, cardiac anesthetists and imaging specialists is best suited to make decisions between open

AVR, TAVI and medical management. This ensures apt patient selection and prompt delivery of care. There has been a rapid expansion in the number of studies investigating TAVI in the last five years and these have demonstrated promising results in terms of feasibility, safety and efficacy. Doubts remain, however, about the long-term durability of TAVI implants and their disposition to valvular dysfunction and about the need for reoperation. This chapter discusses the selection of patients for TAVI, techniques of implantation, clinical and patient-reported outcomes and future directions of research and development.

2. Patient selection

Clinical decision-making in patients with AS is complex and from the outset requires a patient-centered approach and the involvement of a multidisciplinary team. Open AVR is associated with excellent clinical and functional outcomes in large modern series (Brown *et al.*, 2009; Malaisrie *et al.*, 2010) and, at present, is the gold standard intervention for patients with severe, symptomatic AS (Bonow *et al.*, 2006). However, patient selection is controversial. Central to the controversy is a belief that elderly patients, especially those with major comorbidities or with complications of AS (e.g. left ventricular dysfunction) present too great an operative risk or lack sufficient life expectancy to justify surgical AVR (Asimakopoulos *et al.*, 1997; Connolly *et al.*, 2000; Elayda *et al.*, 1993; Monin *et al.*, 2003). AVR is highly invasive and requires sternotomy, cardiopulmonary bypass, hypothermic cardioplegic arrest and cardiotomy. These factors expose patients to certain deleterious effects on end-organs, including ischemia, reperfusion injury, systematic inflammatory response, surgical trauma and oxidative stress (Anselmi *et al.*, 2004). In 2003, the Euro Heart Survey on Valvular Heart Disease reported that approximately one third of patients with severe, symptomatic AS are denied potentially life-saving surgery because of concerns over age, comorbidities and likely longevity (Iung *et al.*, 2003, 2005). This is in spite of some recent series demonstrating promising safe and efficacious outcomes for AVR in octogenarians (Melby *et al.*, 2007; Florath *et al.*, 2010; Leontyev *et al.*, 2009).

TAVI is a novel approach to AS in high-risk patients and provides an alternative management option that negates invasive surgery. TAVI is still in its infancy in terms of the operator learning curve, the level of technological development of the implants and the evidence base required to determine which patients are most likely to benefit. At present, TAVI is recommended only for patients not considered suitable for open AVR and who have a life expectancy of greater than one year (Vahanian *et al.*, 2008). This section will describe some of the available patient risk stratification tools used for clinical decision-making in AS, the current indications and contraindications to TAVI, and possible diversification in the use of minimally invasive aortic valve interventions.

2.1 Risk stratification tools

The choice between treatment options in AS should ideally be based upon a shared decision between the fully informed patient and a multidisciplinary team who guide the patient to the required information. Part of this process includes an assessment by physicians of the likely risk of mortality and serious morbidity of undergoing open AVR. A range of scoring systems have been developed that are designed to assist surgeons in such risk stratification (Ambler *et al.*, 2005; Edwards *et al.*, 2001; Florath *et al.*, 2003; Hattler *et al.*, 1994; Higgins *et al.*,

1992; Nashef *et al.*, 1999; Nowicki et al, 2004; O'Brien *et al.*, 2009; Parsonnet *et al.*, 1989; Pons *et al.*, 1997; Roques *et al.*, 1995; Roques *et al.*, 1999; Tremblay *et al.*, 1993; Tu *et al.*, 1995). These systems are usually derived from multivariate analyses of preoperative and operative variables believed to influence outcomes in large cohorts of cardiothoracic patients. Risk stratification tools may be either generic for all open cardiothoracic procedures or specific to heart-valve interventions. The focus of this subsection is to discuss some of the widely used risk stratification tools.

The Parsonnet score was one of the first mortality indicators developed to calculate average risk estimates of death in adult cardiothoracic patients (Parsonnet *et al.*, 1989). The model allocates "additive" points for 14 risk factors associated with perioperative mortality, which are subsequently used to assign a percentage probability of death. The factors include female gender, obesity, diabetes, hypertension, low ejection fraction, increased age, first or second reoperation, preoperative intra-aortic balloon pump, emergency presentation from the cardiac catheter laboratory, dialysis dependency, catastrophic clinical state, valve surgery and combined valve surgery and coronary artery bypass grafts (CABG). In addition to overestimating mortality in high-risk cases, the Parsonnet score has been criticized for being subjective and including some factors that are now known not to be linked to early postoperative death (Gabrielle *et al.*, 1997). The Parsonnet score also omits other potentially important factors, such as the urgency of surgery, which is widely considered to be strongly associated with perioperative outcome (Wynne-Jones *et al.*, 2000).

The Parsonnet score has been superseded by the European System for Cardiac Operative Risk Evaluation (EuroSCORE). The EuroSCORE was developed by analyzing survival outcomes for 19,030 cardiac surgical patients in eight European countries (Roques *et al.*, 1999). Logistic regression was used to reduce a list of 97 potential postoperative mortality risk factors to 18 independent variables with odds ratios of >1 predictive of death. It bears many similarities to the Parsonnet system and involves calculation of percentage predicted mortality by addition of points ascribed to various risk factors to produce an "additive" mortality score (Table 1). For AVR, the EuroSCORE study reported an overall procedural mortality of 6% and mortality in the absence of risk factors of 1.1%. The precision and accuracy of the EuroSCORE has been demonstrated in numerous studies (Kobayashi et al, 2009; Wendt *et al.*, 2010), but it has several limitations that compromise its validity in sufferers of severe, symptomatic AS. First, the data is derived from patients undergoing cardiac surgery for heterogeneous indications, including a high percentage of cases of isolated coronary artery bypass grafts (63.9%). Risk factors are, therefore, not specific to AVR. Secondly, there is evidence that the EuroSCORE overestimates mortality in high-risk patients or is inaccurate in those with unusual combinations of risk factors (Brown *et al.*, 2008; Dewey *et al.*, 2008). This can exaggerate mortality estimates and may mean that patients are not offered AVR, even if they are potential surgical candidates. The "logistic" EuroSCORE has since been introduced for use in high-risk individuals because of its greater accuracy (Roques *et al.*, 2003). Nonetheless, it still suffers from problems with clinical relevance. Consequently, the "additive" and "logistic" algorithms have been combined to form the "modified" EuroSCORE (Nissinen *et al.*, 2009). Further problems with the EuroSCORE relate to the fact that it does not take into account local institutional outcomes (Vahanian *et al.*, 2008) or characteristics unique to certain AS patients (e.g. previous CABG with patent grafts, porcelain aorta or thoracic radiotherapy). These factors may confer additional risks that can alter the choice of intervention at the institutional level (Robes-Cabau *et al.*, 2010).

Variable	Odds ratio ± Standard error	P-value	Additional % mortality
Age per 5 years after 60 years	1.1 ± 0.007	0.001	1
Female gender	1.4 ± 0.128	0.001	1
Preoperative creatinine > 200 μmol/L	1.9 ± 0.256	0.001	2
Extracardiac arteriopathy	1.9 ± 0.376	0.001	2
Pulmonary disease	1.6 ± 0.284	0.006	1
Neurological dysfunction	2.3 ± 0.584	0.001	2
Previous cardiac surgery	2.6 ± 0.324	0.001	3
Recent myocardial infarction	1.6 ± 0.208	0.001	2
LVEF 30-50%	1.5 ± 0.138	0.001	1
LVEF < 30%	2.5 ± 0.340	0.001	3
Pulmonary hypertension (> 60 mmHg)	2.0 ± 0.423	0.001	2
Active endocarditis	2.5 ± 0.678	0.001	3
Unstable angina	1.5 ± 0.202	0.001	2
Emergency operation	2.8 ± 0.440	0.001	2
Critical perioperative condition	2.2 ± 0.319	0.001	3
Ventricular septal rupture	3.8 ± 1.735	0.002	4
Noncoronary surgery	1.6 ± 0.170	0.001	2
Thoracic aortic surgery	3.2 ± 0.650	0.001	3

Table 1. Risk factors for mortality in patients undergoing cardiac surgery based on the EuroSCORE dataset (reproduced from Roques *et al.*, 1999; LVEF = left ventricular ejection fraction)

Recently, emphasis has been placed on developing risk stratification tools with greater reliability and validity in patients with valvular heart disease. The Ambler score was published in 2005 after it had been field-tested in 32,839 consecutive patients undergoing heart valve surgery in the UK (Ambler *et al.*, 2005). It identified 14 risk factors associated with in-hospital mortality (operative priority, age, renal failure, operation sequence, ejection fraction, concomitant tricuspid valve surgery, type of valve surgery, concomitant CABG, body mass index, preoperative arrhythmia, diabetes, gender, and hypertension). Its development involved robust methodology in a large cohort of patients, but it has not been widely adopted, perhaps because of concerns over external validity in non-UK populations. The Society of Thoracic Surgeons has since built on the advantages of the Ambler score by producing a tool that assists in predicting nine different postoperative variables (STS-PROM; O'Brien *et al.*, 2009). These are mortality, permanent stroke, renal failure, prolonged ventilation, deep sternal wound infection, reoperation, a composite endpoint of mortality and major morbidity, and short and prolonged postoperative stay. In addition to extending predictive models to several causes of major morbidity, the STS-PROM has been shown to be more reliable than the EuroSCORE in estimating mortality in high-risk patients (Dewey *et al.*, 2008). At present, most major studies involving the selection of patients for TAVI use the EuroSCORE and STS-PROM.

2.2 Indications and assessment of suitability for TAVI

TAVI is recommended for use only in patients with calcified pure or predominant AS, and not in cases where aortic regurgitation is the primary pathology. In 2008, the European

Association of Cardiothoracic Surgery (EACTS), the European Society of Cardiology (ECS), and the European Association of Percutaneous Cardiovascular Intervention (EAPCI) issued a joint statement describing a four-stage assessment procedure to be undertaken to differentiate between treatment options in AS and to confirm suitability for TAVI (Vahanian *et al.*, 2008). The first stage involves echocardiography to confirm the diagnosis and severity of AS, and to exclude significant aortic regurgitation. TAVI is presently restricted to cases of severe AS because of the proven effectiveness of AVR. The inclusion criteria of well-designed trials offer some insight into the definition of the severity of AS at echocardiography. In THE PARTNER TRIAL: Placement of AoRTic TraNscathetER Valve Trial, patients were randomized to interventions (AVR, TAVI, or medical management) only if proved to have an aortic valve area (AVA) of < 0.8 cm^2 (or an indexed AVA of < 0.6 cm^2) or a peak aortic valve gradient of > 40 mmHg (or a peak velocity of > 4.0 m/s) (Leon *et al.*, 2010). Analogous values should be used when deciding whether TAVI is appropriate for particular individuals, and many studies have used similar cut-offs to assign patients to treatment with TAVI (Clavel *et al.*, 2010; Malaisrie *et al.*, 2011; Zahn *et al.*, 2011). In certain circumstances, low-dose dobutamine echocardiography may also be of value to distinguish between severe AS and the rare "pseudo-severe" AS, especially in patients with a low left ventricular (LV) ejection fraction and a low aortic transvalvular gradient (Bonow *et al.*, 2006; Vahanian *et al.*, 2007).

The second stage in TAVI assessment involves an accurate evaluation of the presenting symptoms and clinical findings. Current guidelines recommend that TAVI should be undertaken only when symptoms are directly attributable to AS (Vahanian *et al.*, 2008). Several concurrent diseases may mimic the symptom profile of AS, such as chronic obstructive pulmonary disease or pulmonary hypertension. A clear history and chronology of the symptoms of dyspnea, chest pain, and syncope are, therefore, required, and when the diagnosis is uncertain, biomarkers of increased myocardial mechanical load, such as beta-type natriuretic peptide (BNP), may be of value (Vahanian *et al.*, 2010). Clinical confirmation of the diagnosis is necessary because of concerns over the long-term durability of TAVI devices.

Arguably, the most complex stage when assessing patients with AS is deciding between AVR, TAVI, and conservative management. This requires multidisciplinary team evaluation of the possible risks of open AVR and TAVI, predicted life expectancy, and quality of life. To evaluate the risk of operative mortality and serious morbidity, it is recommended that clinical judgment be combined with the scores from two risk stratification tools (Vahanian *et al.*, 2008). This combination allows for an objective risk assessment, while ensuring that additional factors not included in risk stratification tools (e.g. porcelain aorta, previous CABG with patent grafts, previous thoracic radiotherapy, or liver cirrhosis) are taken into account. Typically, mortality > 20% calculated using the logistic EuroSCORE or > 10% using the STS-PROM are seen as high-risk indicators that would preclude open AVR in most cases (Leon *et al.*, 2010; Vahanian *et al.*, 2008; Vahanian *et al.*, 2010). However, scoring systems should not necessarily be viewed as a substitute for experienced clinical judgment or informed patient choice. As part of the multidisciplinary approach, it is recommended that patient-reported outcomes, such as health-related quality of life (HRQL), be considered. The use of validated HRQL tools should be combined with clinical parameters to assist in the shared decision-making process (Lee *et al.*, 2006; Vahanian *et al.*, 2008).

The final stage before TAVI insertion in high-risk patients with severe, symptomatic AS includes an assessment of the feasibility and contraindications to TAVI. The first-line investigation is coronary angiography to identify occlusive lesions in need of revascularization. Lesions amenable to percutaneous angioplasty and stenting can be treated either before, during, or after TAVI. The decision on the timing of revascularization is complex and should be tailored to individual cases. Patients with proximal coronary stenoses may not be appropriate candidates for TAVI (Vahanian *et al.*, 2008) because of concerns over occlusion of the coronary ostia by the device (Gogas *et al.*, 2011; Gurvitch *et al.*, 2011). If coronary stenoses can be managed only surgically, then a choice must be made between high-risk AVR and the poor outcomes associated with medical management and balloon valvuloplasty.

Determining the diameter of the aortic annulus is a prerequisite to TAVI operational planning and ensures that an appropriately sized implant is deployed. This can be accomplished using either invasive techniques (e.g. aortography as part of balloon valvuloplasty) or noninvasive imaging modalities (e.g. echocardiography, multislice high resolution computed tomography, or magnetic resonance imaging) (Tops *et al.*, 2008; Vahanian *et al.*, 2008). Transthoracic echocardiography has been shown to underestimate the size of the aortic annulus, and should be supplemented with transesophageal echocardiography when borderline sizes result in doubt over the feasibility of the procedure (Moss *et al.*, 2008). Accurate sizing prior to TAVI is necessary to prevent paravalvular leak and rupture of the aortic annulus. The peripheral vasculature must also be imaged, in particular the aortic arch, descending aorta, and iliac vessels. This can be achieved with either formal or computed tomography angiography. Gadolinium magnetic resonance angiography is an alternative in patients with impaired renal function. Both the size and tortuosity of the vessels are important because they affect access and help to decide between the transarterial and transapical approaches.

2.3 Contraindications to TAVI

For technical reasons, TAVI is not possible in all high-risk patients with AS, but using different access ports has increased the number of patients who can be successfully treated. General contraindications to TAVI include:

- Aortic annulus diameter < 18 mm or > 25 mm for balloon expandable implants, and < 20 mm or > 27 mm for self-expandable devices.
- Bicuspid aortic valves that may lead to incomplete deployment of the device and paravalvular leak (Zegdi *et al.*, 2008).
- Heavy asymmetrical aortic valve calcification because of concerns over occlusion of the coronary ostia (Webb *et al.*, 2006).
- Low position of the coronary ostia (< 8 mm from the aortic annulus).
- Aortic root diameter of > 45 mm at the aorto-tubular junction for self-expandable devices.
- Severe organic mitral regurgitation.
- LV thrombus.

There are a number of contraindications specific to the type of approach. For the transfemoral approach, these are:

- Severely calcified or tortuous iliac arteries.
- Iliac artery diameter of < 6 mm to < 9 mm, depending on the type of device used.
- Previous aorto-femoral bypass grafts.
- Severely angulated aorta or atherosclerotic aortic arch.

- Transverse ascending arch (for balloon expandable devices).
- Aortic aneurysm with extensive mural thrombus.
- Coarctation of the aorta.

For the transapical approach, contraindications are:

- Previous surgical patch of the left ventricle (e.g. Dor procedure).
- Calcified pericardium.
- Severely impaired respiratory function.
- Inability to access the apex of the left ventricle due to anatomical constraints (e.g. chest deformity).

2.4 Expanding the role of TAVI

Implants used in open AVR are either mechanical or bioprosthetic. Mechanical valves have the advantage of long-term durability, but require life-long anticoagulation with the associated risk of major hemorrhage. Patients fitted with bioprosthetic valves do not need to take anticoagulants, but the chance of valvular degeneration increases with time. Mechanical valves are, therefore, usually restricted to younger patients, while bioprosthetic implants are used more frequently in the elderly population, in which the chance of surviving to revision surgery is low. Nonetheless, valvular degeneration occurs in a proportion of patients, and treatment typically necessitates revision AVR, which is inherently high-risk.

In 2008 the first case of valve-in-valve (VIV) TAVI was reported in an 82-year-old patient with valvular degeneration of a Carpentier-Edwards Perimount aortic valve (Walther *et al.*, 2008a). This pioneering procedure was performed off-pump using a transapical approach. VIV is an attractive technique that involves placing the implant within the previous prosthetic valve, abutting the degenerated valve leaflets up against the aortic annulus. Typically, transapical access is preferred for VIV procedures, although reports have recently emerged describing the transaxillary (Sharp *et al.*, 2010) and trans-subclavian approaches (Olsen *et al.*, 2010). The Edwards SAPIEN valve may be better suited to VIV implantation (Kempfert *et al.*, 2010), although the Medtronic CoreValve system has been successfully used (Khawaja *et al.*, 2010).

There are promising early results for VIV, although reports tend to be anecdotal or restricted to small case series, and no large comparative studies are currently available (Ferrari *et al.*, 2010; Kempfert *et al.*, 2010; Khawaja *et al.*, 2010; Olsen *et al.*, 2010; Sharp *et al.*, 2010). Transvalvular gradients post-procedure are usually satisfactory (Ferrari *et al.*, 2010; Kempfert *et al.*, 2010; Walther *et al.*, 2008a), while residual aortic regurgitation tends to be minimal (Kempfert *et al.*, 2010). Severe paravalvular leak is a feared complication of TAVI, but several authors have described its successful treatment with rescue VIV (Rodes-Cabau *et al.*, 2009; Taramasso *et al.*, 2010). Concerns exist over excessive transvalvular gradients of VIV implants in patients fitted previously with small-diameter prostheses (e.g. < 23 mm in diameter) (Ferrari *et al.*, 2010). For TAVI, the diameter of the device is typically oversized by 10-20% in relation to the aortic annulus, but for VIV undersizing is preferred, which is currently not feasible in some patients with small annuli because of the size of available implants. At present, VIV is off-label in many countries, including the United States.

TAVI is minimally invasive and has consistently demonstrated promising outcomes in high-risk patients (see Section 4). In the future, it is likely that the indications for TAVI will be expanded to include younger patients at low operative risk. However, caution is advised for several reasons. Despite the lack of randomized clinical trial (RCT) data to support the use of open surgery, AVR has shown excellent long-term clinical, hemodynamic and functional outcomes in low-risk AS patients (Hammermeister *et al.*, 1993; Myken *et al.*, 1995; Peterseim *et al.*, 1999). Modern RCT's comparing AVR to medical management would be unethical because of a lack of clinical equipoise, leading to appropriate patients being denied access to a treatment with proven long-term effectiveness. The durability of TAVI implants is still a concern due to the technique's relative age. More work to characterize the long-term outcomes of TAVI is necessary before it is offered routinely to low-risk patients.

3. Devices and techniques

The technology that underpins TAVI has evolved dramatically in the last two decades since its inception in animal models (Anderson *et al.*, 1992) and later realization in humans (Cribier *et al.*, 2002). At present, there are two major producers of TAVI devices that are used routinely in clinical practice (Edwards Lifesciences, Irvine, CA, USA & Medtronic Inc., Minneapolis, MN, USA). Technological development of both implants is on-going, and each has its advantages and disadvantages in different clinical situations. There are a variety of access sites through which TAVI can be performed, including directly through the left ventricular apex as well as the femoral, axillary and subclavian arteries. This section will describe the features of current and future implants and the techniques required for their implantation.

3.1 TAVI devices

The prototypic Cribier-Edwards TAVI device was one of the earliest deployed in humans. It has now been replaced by newer Edwards Lifesciences designs, including the SAPIEN transcatheter heart valve (THV) (Figure 1) and, more recently, by the SAPIEN XT. The SAPIEN devices are constructed from bovine pericardial leaflets mounted on a cobalt-chromium frame. The device is balloon expandable and manufactured in 23-mm and 26-mm sizes, which allows it to be used in patients with aortic annulus diameters of between 18 mm and 25 mm. As the implant is deployed (Figure 2), it fixes within the aortic annulus without the need for stabilization in the ascending aorta (Webb and Cribier, 2010). Early devices required large-caliber delivery systems; however, the latest versions can be deployed through vessels with a minimum diameter of 6 mm. Transapical and percutaneous approaches can both be used with the SAPIEN system.

The Medtronic CoreValve consists of a porcine pericardial valve mounted on a nitinol self-expandable metal frame. It is considerably longer than SAPIEN devices (53-55 mm versus 15-17 mm) and anchors distally in both the ascending aorta and supracoronary region. The CoreValve can be deployed through an access channel with a minimum diameter of 6 mm and can be used in patients with an aortic annulus diameter of between 20 mm and 27 mm. The device is not licensed for transapical use, but when used via a peripheral access vessel, it is associated with greater hemodynamic stability during deployment, more forgiving positioning and can be retrieved if sited incorrectly (Webb and Cribier, 2010). Despite this, the CoreValve suffers from a high incidence of post-procedural heart block, which requires prolonged cardiac monitoring, and pacemaker insertion is necessary in up to 40% of cases.

A number of next generation TAVI devices are currently undergoing clinical testing (Falk *et al.*, 2009; Low *et al.*, 2008; Schofer at al., 2008; Treede *et al.*, 2010). These are based generally on the self-expandable CoreValve system and allow for smaller caliber delivery systems,

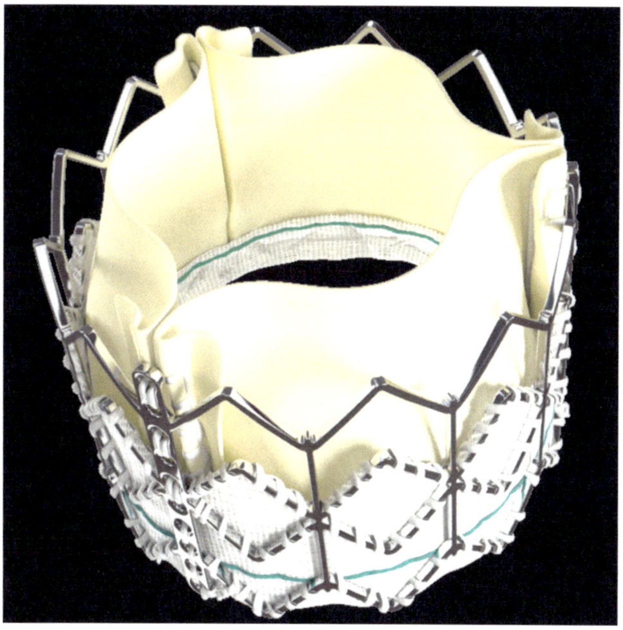

Fig. 1. The Edwards SAPIEN Transcatheter aortic valve (Photo courtesy of Edwards Lifesciences)

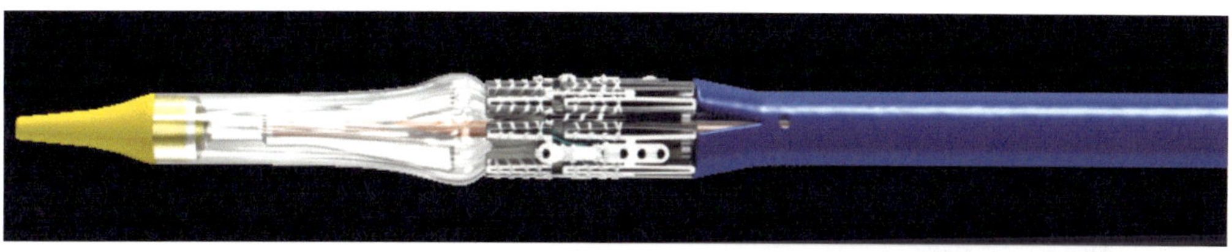

Fig. 2. Transcatheter aortic valve crimped onto the introducing catheter (Photo courtesy of Edwards Lifesciences)

retrieval and greater accuracy when deployed. Examples include the DirectFlow (Direct Medical Flow Inc., Santa Rosa, CA, USA), Lotus (Boston Scientific Inc., Natick, MA, USA) and HLT (Heart Leaflet Technologies Inc., Maple Grove, MN, USA). Other systems incorporate features that allow fixation in the supracoronary aorta (Accurate, Symentis Inc., Lausanne, Switzerland; St Jude, St Jude Medical Inc., St. Paul, MN, USA) and anatomical guides to demonstrate the position of the native valve and coronary arteries, thus facilitating deployment (Engager, Medtronic Inc., USA; JenaClip, JenaValve Inc., Munich, Germany). At present, little is known about these novel valves in terms of their efficacy, safety, feasibility, and long-term durability. Further work is required to characterize their outcomes before they can be recommended for use in routine clinical practice.

3.2 Percutaneous access

Initial reports of TAVI used a transseptal approach with access via the venous system (Cribier *et al.*, 2002). This route was technically challenging and not reproducible. Retrograde arterial approaches are now much more widely used. Access is gained typically through the femoral artery (Webb *et al.*, 2006). The axillary, subclavian, and retroperitoneal iliac arteries, as well as the ascending aorta, have also been successfully used (Webb and Cribier, 2010). Cut-down to expose the arteries is sometimes done: this improves the ease of cannulation of the vessels and ensures safe closure. In such cases, the patient is usually anesthetized, which confers additional risks in this frail population. Percutaneous arterial puncture and suture closure is now the standard of care and can be completed safely under sedation (De Jaegere *et al.*, 2007; Vavuranakis *et al.*, 2010). After arterial puncture, aortography is done to characterize the coronary vessels, diseased valve, and aorta. Balloon valvuloplasty is then used to dilate the native valve under rapid ventricular pacing, which decreases cardiac output while the balloon is inflated. Between periods of rapid pacing, the blood pressure must be allowed to normalize. Intraoperative imaging, including aortography, transesophageal echocardiography, and fluoroscopy, is used to identify the optimal position for the new valve. Once this has been determined, the valve is deployed. Rapid ventricular pacing is required for balloon expandable devices (Figure 3), but not for self-expandable systems. Post-procedural echocardiography and aortography are done to check the position and function of the implant, the patency of the coronary vessels, and the presence of early complications (e.g. aortic regurgitation, paravalvular leak, aortic dissection, hemopericardium). It is recommended that patients are nursed postoperatively in the cardiac intensive care unit with invasive monitoring.

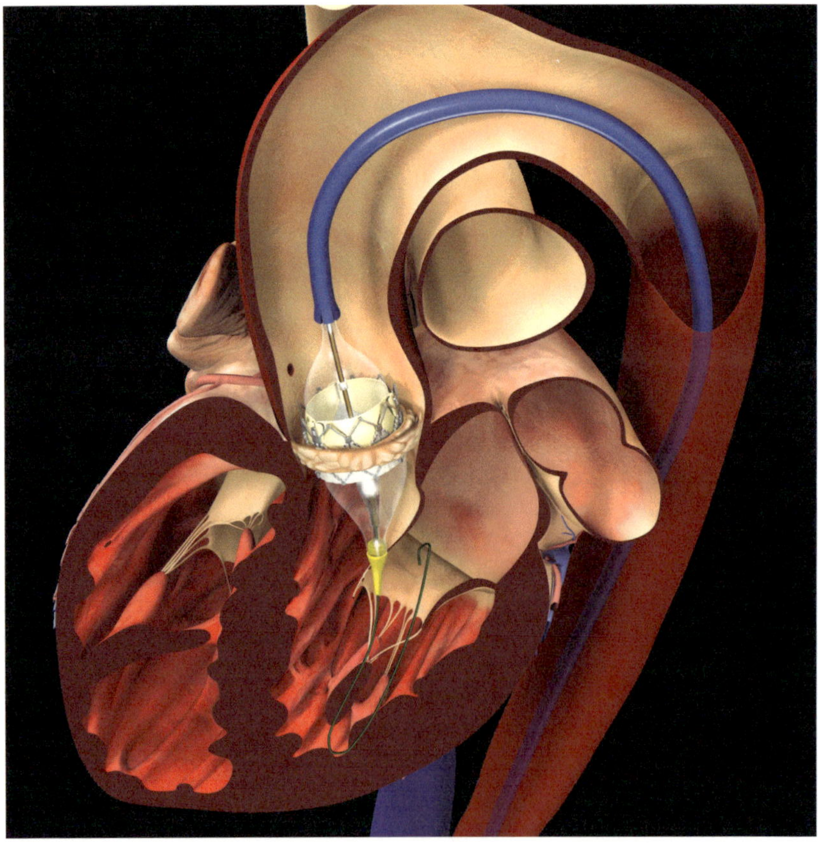

Fig. 3. Showing the retrograde approach and balloon inflation (black arrow) of the trans-catheter aortic valve (white arrow) (Photo courtesy of Edwards Lifesciences)

3.3 Transapical approach

Transapical TAVI involves inserting the valve device in an antegrade fashion through the anterolateral chest wall and apex of the left ventricle (Figure 4). This is done under general anesthesia with cardiopulmonary bypass (CPB) on standby. CPB is usually established through the femoral vessels if required. The site of the incision is determined by transthoracic echocardiography. After the chest cavity has been entered, the pericardium is opened and secured to the thoracic wall. Pacing wires are then attached to the myocardium to facilitate rapid ventricular pacing. Two purse-string sutures are inserted into the apex, and an introducer sheath is passed between them into the left ventricle. Guided by imaging, the implant is positioned across the native valve and then deployed using balloon inflation and rapid ventricular pacing. Postoperatively, the patient should be nursed in an intensive care unit for at least 24 hours. Transapical TAVI involves a thoracotomy, and for this reason is not recommended for patients with severe respiratory disease that precludes one-lung ventilation. In rare instances, a mini-sternotomy has been combined with retrograde transaortic TAVI, where the device is inserted via the ascending aorta (Latsios *et al.*, 2010). This technique is reserved for patients with no other access sites.

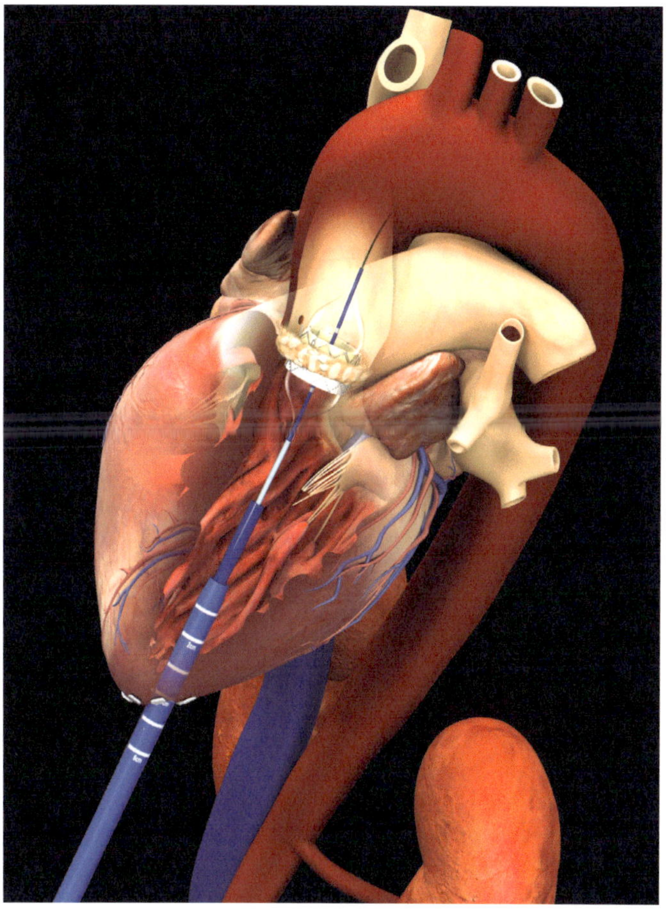

Fig. 4. Trocar being antegradely introduced through the apex of the left ventricle (Photo courtesy of Edwards Lifesciences)

3.4 Service structure

The performance of TAVI should be restricted to a small number of high-volume centers with readily available input from specialist cardiothoracic surgeons, interventional cardiologists, cardiac anesthetists, intensivists and perfusionists. The center must be proficient in dealing with both open and percutaneous valvular interventions in high-risk populations. Familiarity with the procedure and multidisciplinary management are likely to improve the rate of successful implantation and limit the number of complications. Furthermore, if complications do occur, they can be managed without the delay associated with transferring patients to another institution. Interventional cardiologists should have experience of a range of percutaneous valvular interventions, large-bore peripheral cannulation, and percutaneous suture closure. Cardiac surgeons should routinely perform complex open valvular procedures and be able to offer rescue or salvage surgery when complications arise. Bleeding from damaged peripheral vessels is not infrequent following TAVI, so it is also advantageous to also have onsite access to vascular surgeons and radiologists trained in either open or endovascular arterial repair.

4. Outcomes

Outcomes are events that are either present or absent in study participants at specific time points after an intervention or exposure. They can be clinical, patient-reported, healthcare economic, composite, or surrogate. Studies investigating outcomes of interventions for aortic valve pathology concentrate on the safety, feasibility, efficacy, and durability of treatment options. Safety is typically assessed with clinical measures, such as operative morbidity and mortality. Feasibility describes whether the procedure can be accomplished successfully without recourse to alternative treatment. Efficacy is defined as whether an intervention works in those who receive it. For aortic valve therapies, it is usually based on echocardiographic findings and functional outcomes, such as the New York Heart Association (NYHA) classification and HRQL tools. Durability includes long-term outcomes such as prosthesis failure, reoperation, and survival. High quality studies, including randomized controlled trials (RCTs), are required to evaluate these outcomes in patients with severe AS and to inform treatment choices between open AVR, TAVI, balloon valvuloplasty, and medical management. This section will summarize outcomes from studies that have investigated the use of TAVI.

4.1 Evidence from the PARTNER Trial

RCTs are the gold standard study design for assessing surgical innovation. However, there is a paucity of well-designed surgical RCTs, which is in part due to specific methodological difficulties. Surgery is a complex intervention and is comprised of multiple events that interact together to affect outcomes. For example, perioperative mortality may be affected by patient factors (e.g. comorbidities), surgeon factors (e.g. skill and technique), anesthetic factors (e.g. quality of postoperative care) and service factors (e.g. number of nursing staff, rehabilitation services). If these factors are poorly controlled in an RCT, then confounding variables may result in bias. It is important that trials clearly predefine all aspects of the intervention in the study protocol and report protocol deviations in subsequent publications. The timing of surgical RCTs is also critical. RCTs undertaken too early in the development of a novel intervention may underestimate treatment effect magnitude as a consequence of operator learning-curve effects. RCTs undertaken too late after the introduction of a procedure can be unethical because of a loss of equipoise. It is difficult to blind participants and clinicians in surgical RCTs due to differences in outward appearances of wounds, and because the surgeon will always know which procedure has been performed. This problem can be overcome by blinding outcome assessors and data analysts to the allocation sequence. Another problem with surgical RCTs relates to the fact that they are often costly to undertake, and follow-up needs to be long-term to identify late and rare events.

The PARTNER Trial was the first RCT to compare outcomes between TAVI and other interventions for severe AS (Leon *et al.*, 2010). The study consisted of two parallel, prospective, multicenter, randomized trials. The first of these (Cohort A) randomized to either TAVI or open AVR participants with severe AS who were considered high-risk for surgery (STS-PROM > 10% mortality risk or > 15% predicted 30-day mortality). In Cohort B, patients with severe AS and considered unsuitable for surgery (> 50% predicted 30-day mortality or a serious irreversible condition) were allocated to either TAVI or medical management, which included balloon valvuloplasty. The primary outcome measure in Cohort A was survival at one year. In Cohort B, the primary endpoint was initially survival for the duration of the study, although this was supplemented partway through the trial with a composite co-primary outcome of survival and time to first rehospitalization. Secondary outcome measures included: functional improvement in NYHA classification; freedom from major adverse cardiovascular and cerebrovascular events (MACCE); evidence of prosthetic valve dysfunction (hemolysis, infection, thrombosis, severe paravalvular leak, or migration); a six-minute walk test; length of hospital stay; total hospital days from the index procedure to one year postoperatively; HRQL at 30 days, six months, and one year; improvement in aortic valve area; and a composite of survival, recurrent hospitalization, and NYHA class. The eligibility criteria for the PARTNER Trial are listed in Table 2.

To date only results from Cohort B have been published, with the findings of Cohort A expected in late 2011. Between May 2007 and March 2009, 358 consecutive patients with severe AS who were considered unsuitable for surgery (Cohort B) were enrolled at 21 centers. Randomization allocated 179 patients to receive TAVI (Edwards SAPIEN device using the transfemoral approach) and 179 to be treated with medical management. Participants were followed-up for at least one year. The rate of death from any cause at one year post-randomization (primary endpoint) was 30.7% in those treated with TAVI and 50.7% in those treated with medical care alone (hazard ratio: 0.55; 95% confidence interval: 0.40 to 0.76; $p < 0.001$). The cardiovascular mortality rate one year after randomization was also lower in the TAVI group (20.5% vs. 44.6%; hazard ratio: 0.39; 95% confidence interval: 0.27 to 0.56; $p < 0.001$). Furthermore, the composite endpoint of rate of death from any cause and rehospitalization at one year (co-primary endpoint) was 42.7% with TAVI compared with 71.6% with medical care alone (hazard ratio: 0.46; 95% confidence interval: 0.35 to 0.59; $p < 0.001$).

Complications were observed more frequently in the TAVI arm of the trial. There was a greater incidence of cerebrovascular events after TAVI at both 30 days after randomization (6.7% vs. 1.7%, $p = 0.03$) and at one year (10.6% vs. 4.5%, $p = 0.04$). Patients who received TAVI were also more likely to suffer major bleeding or vascular complications. Despite this, 30-day mortality was similar between groups. Patients treated with TAVI demonstrated marked improvements in functional outcomes: 74.8% of patients alive at one year in the TAVI arm were asymptomatic or had only mild symptoms (NYHA classes I or II), compared with 42.0% of surviving participants in the medical care alone group ($p < 0.001$). In addition,

Inclusion criteria for the PARTNER Trial:

- Patients must have comorbidities such that the surgeon and cardiologist Co-Principle Investigators concur that the predicted risk of operative mortality is ≥ 15% and/ or a minimum STS-PROM score of 10.
- Patient has senile degenerative aortic valve stenosis with echocardiographically derived criteria: mean gradient > 40 mmHg or jet velocity greater than 4.0 m/s or an initial aortic valve area of < 0.8 cm^2.
- Patient is symptomatic from his/her aortic valve stenosis, as demonstrated by NYHA Functional Class II or greater.
- The patient or the patient's legal representative has been informed of the nature of the study, agrees to its provisions, and has provided written informed consent as approved by the IRB of the respective clinical site.
- The patient and the treating physician agree that the patient will return for all required post-procedure follow-up visits.

Cohort B All candidates for Cohort B in this study must meet #2, 3, 4, 5 of the above criteria and:

- The patient, after formal consults by a cardiologist and two cardiovascular surgeons, agrees that medical factors preclude operation, based on a conclusion that the probability of death or serious, irreversible morbidity exceeds the probability of meaningful improvement. Specifically, the probability of death or serious, irreversible morbidity should exceed 50%.

Exclusion Criteria for the PARTNER Trial:

- Evidence of an acute myocardial infarction ≤ 1 month before the intended treatment (defined as Q wave MI, or non-Q wave MI with total CK elevation ≥ twice normal in the presence of CK-MB elevation or troponin level elevation (WHO definition).
- Aortic valve was a congenital unicuspid or congenital bicuspid valve, or was noncalcified.
- Mixed aortic valve disease (aortic stenosis and aortic regurgitation with predominant aortic regurgitation > 3+).
- Any therapeutic invasive cardiac procedure performed within 30 days of the index procedure, (or 6 months if the procedure was a drug eluting coronary stent implantation).
- Pre-existing prosthetic heart valve in any position, prosthetic ring, severe mitral annular calcification, or severe (greater than 3+) mitral regurgitation.
- Blood dyscrasias as defined: leukopenia (WBC < 3000 mm^3); acute anemia (Hb < 9 mg%); thrombocytopenia (platelet count < 50,000 cells/mm^3); history of bleeding diathesis or coagulopathy.
- Untreated clinically significant coronary artery disease requiring revascularization.
- Hemodynamic instability requiring inotropic therapy or mechanical hemodynamic support devices.
- Need for emergency surgery for any reason.
- Hypertrophic cardiomyopathy with or without obstruction.
- Severe ventricular dysfunction with LVEF < 20%.
- Echocardiographic evidence of intracardiac mass, thrombus or vegetation.
- Active peptic ulcer or upper gastrointestinal bleeding within the prior 3 months.
- A known hypersensitivity or contraindication to aspirin, heparin, ticlopidine (Ticlid),

or clopidogrel (Plavix), or sensitivity to contrast media, which cannot be adequately premedicated. • Native aortic annulus size < 18 mm or > 25 mm as measured by echocardiogram. • Recent (within 6 months) cerebrovascular accident or transient ischemic attack. • Renal insufficiency (creatinine > 3.0 mg/dL) or end-stage renal disease requiring chronic dialysis. • Life expectancy < 12 months due to noncardiac comorbid conditions. • Significant abdominal or thoracic aorta disease, including aneurysm (defined as maximal luminal diameter 5 cm or greater), marked tortuosity (hyperacute bend), aortic arch atheroma (especially if thick [> 5 mm], protruding, or ulcerated), narrowing of the abdominal aorta (especially with calcification and surface irregularities), or severe "unfolding" and tortuosity of the thoracic aorta. • Iliofemoral vessel characteristics that would preclude safe placement of 22F or 24F introducer sheath, such as severe calcification, severe tortuosity or vessels size diameter < 7 mm for 22F sheath or < 8 mm for 24F sheath.

Table 2. Eligibility criteria for participants included in the PARTNER Trial (Leon *et al.*, 2010)

there was a significant improvement in the six-minute walk test in patients treated with TAVI, but not in those who received medical care alone. Echocardiography demonstrated a significant reduction in aortic valve area and transvalvular gradient at 30 days in patients receiving TAVI. Moreover, these findings were maintained at one year, which suggested that TAVI devices are durable at least into the medium term.

Leon *et al.* (2010) concluded that medical care alone did not alter the course of severe AS in patients who were not candidates for surgery. Transfemoral TAVI was markedly superior to medical care alone in this high-risk cohort of patients, and TAVI improved the rates of all-cause and cardiovascular mortality. This is emphasized by the fact that only five patients needed to be treated with TAVI to prevent one death in the first year of follow-up. The safety of TAVI was highlighted by the similar 30-day mortality rate to medical care alone, despite a greater risk of vascular damage and bleeding, which were attributed to the large bore femoral access sheaths required in early versions of the Edwards SAPIEN heart-valve system. It is likely that future use of lower profile sheaths will reduce the incidence of vascular damage. Stroke rates were greater with TAVI and are the likely consequence of atherosclerotic emboli released during deployment of the valve. Less traumatic TAVI systems and novel cerebrovascular protection devices may help limit the incidence of stroke. It is noteworthy that increased survival was associated with improved function: patients treated with TAVI not only lived longer but also had fewer symptoms. Transfemoral TAVI is the current standard of care in patients who are not considered candidates for open AVR.

The PARTNER Trial provides the best evidence yet to support the use of TAVI, although it is important to interpret the findings of Cohort B in the light of several limitations. The first of these relates to external validity: the PARTNER Trial was predominantly explanatory rather than pragmatic and had strict eligibility criteria (Table 2). Consequently, the results should not be extrapolated to patients with characteristics different from those enrolled in the trial, such as patients with peripheral vascular disease or severe LV dysfunction and those requiring coronary artery bypass grafts. Furthermore, the trial investigated only the transfemoral approach with a single device (Edwards SAPIEN), which has now been superseded by newer prostheses. Methodologically the trial is limited by poor reporting of randomization, allocation concealment, and blinding, while there is evidence of selective reporting of outcomes and the introduction of a co-primary outcome during the conduct of the trial. One final observation is that the trial offers only limited information on the long-term durability of TAVI prostheses. Additional long-term randomized controlled trials are warranted, the results of which, together with the results of Cohort A, will offer some insight into the relative efficacy of TAVI and open AVR in high-risk patients.

Since the first report of TAVI almost a decade ago, there has been an explosion in the number of related publications. Most of these are retrospective case series or comparative studies contrasting different approaches (transapical vs. transfemoral) or devices (Medtronic CoreValve vs. Edwards SAPIEN). Although the publications do not provide the same level of evidence as RCTs and are open to selection and recall bias, it is worth considering their findings because of their number. The next section summarizes the support or otherwise for TAVI from nonrandomized studies in terms of feasibility, safety, efficacy, and durability.

4.2 Feasibility of TAVI

The feasibility of TAVI can be assessed by considering the procedural success rate, defined as whether the implant was successfully deployed without immediate complications or the need to convert to open surgery. Early reports of procedural success rates are likely to have been affected by operator learning-curve effects. Cribier *et al.* (2002) reported that, using the antegrade transvenous approach, 22 out of 26 implants (84.6%) were successfully deployed, with four failures due to technical complications. Failures occurred as a consequence of valve migration immediately after the procedure (n = 2) and poor tolerance of the guide wire across the mitral valve (n = 2). This high rate of technical achievement could not be replicated by other researchers using transvenous access due to the complexity of passing the guide wire through the interventricular septum and mitral valve.

The introduction of retrograde methods for accessing the diseased aortic valve has led to greater procedure reproducibility. Webb *et al.* (2007) initially reported outcomes for transfemoral TAVI using the Edwards prosthesis in 50 patients. The procedural success rate in this cohort was 86% (43 out of 50 patients), with failure associated with inability to pass the catheter through the iliac artery (n = 1) or across the aortic valve (n = 3), device malpositioning (n = 2), or malfunction of the delivery system (n = 1). Other authors have demonstrated similar success rates for the transfemoral approach using the Edwards Lifesciences devices. Rodes-Cabau *et al.* (2008) successfully implanted TAVI prostheses in 91% of their patients, with failure occurring as a result of severely calcified iliac disease (n = 1) and intra-operative death secondary to myocardial ischaemia (n = 1). Similarly, Descoutures *et al.* (2008) reported success in 10 out of 12 patients (83%). In this series, procedural failure was the consequence of an inability to cannulate the iliac vessels (n = 1) and of fatal hemopericardium due to left ventricular perforation by the guide wire (n = 1).

Only Edwards Lifesciences devices are currently licensed for use using the transapical approach. Ye *et al.* (2009) and Zierer *et al.* (2008) both reported success rates of 100% in small case series using transapical access. In larger studies the success rates are similarly impressive. In a study by Walther *et al.* (2008) successful implantation was accomplished in 47 out of 50 patients (94%), with three patients requiring conversion to open AVR. In another multicentre study by Walther *et al*, 55 out of 59 implants were deployed successfully with four patients requiring urgent sternotomy and AVR due to device malposition (Walther *et al.*, 2007). In an article by Svensson *et al.* (2008), procedural success was 88% in 40 patients undergoing transapical TAVI. Of the five patients in whom TAVI was deemed to have failed, the etiological factors were valve embolization (n = 3), valve migration (n = 1), and paravalvular leak (n = 1).

The Medtronic CoreValve system is licensed for use using only retrograde percutaneous methods, typically transfemoral. The feasibility outcomes for this device are excellent, with several studies reporting 100% success rates (Behan *et al.*, 2008; Berry *et al.*, 2007; De Jaegere *et al.*, 2008). In a large prospective registry of 646 patients by Piazza *et al.* (2008), the procedural success rate was 97%. The authors did not present reasons for failure of implantation of the CoreValve device. In a small study, Grube *et al.* (2006) achieved successful implantation of TAVI prostheses in 21 out of 25 patients (84%). Reasons for procedural failure included paravalvular leak (n = 2), inability to cross a heavily calcified aortic valve (n = 1), and sudden death during balloon valvuloplasty (n = 1). In a second multicenter study by Grube et al. (2007), the procedural success rate was comparatively low (74%), which appears to be the consequence of malpositioning of a significant number of implants. Tamburino *et al.* (2009) reported outcomes for 30 patients treated with CoreValve TAVI. The procedural success rate was 93%, with one incident of pericardial tamponade and one of malpositioning of the TAVI device necessitating VIV implantation. It can be concluded from these reports that TAVI is a feasible procedure and that success rates are likely to improve with greater operator experience and more advanced devices.

4.3 Safety of TAVI

The assessment of safety in cardiothoracic surgery is made through reporting 30-day major adverse cardiovascular and cerebrovascular events (MACCE). Thirty-day mortality is conventionally defined as the occurrence of death from any cause within 30 days of a procedure. However, definitions are sometimes heterogeneous and must be considered carefully when outcomes from multiple studies are combined. In the case of TAVI, 30-day mortality is generally favorable and ranges from 0% to 25% (Behan *et al.*, 2008; Berry *et al.*, 2007; Cribier *et al.*, 2002; De Jaegere *et al.*, 2008; Descoutures *et al.*, 2008; Grube *et al.*, 2006; Grube *et al.*, 2007; Piazza *et al.*, 2008; Rodes-Cabau *et al.*, 2008; Spargias *et al.*, 2008; Svensson *et al.*, 2008; Tamburino *et al.*, 2009; Walther *et al.*, 2007; Walther *et al.*, 2008; Webb *et al.*, 2007; Ye *et al.*, 2009; Zierer *et al.*, 2008). Thirty-day mortality rates appear to be similar between the different devices and between transapical and transfemoral access routes.

Vascular complications are one of the major concerns with percutaneous approaches. Vascular injury has been shown to occur in up to 18% of TAVI procedures and can lead to hemorrhage, limb ischemia, and amputation (Behan *et al.*, 2008; Descoutures *et al.*, 2008; Leon *et al.*, 2010; Piazza *et al.*, 2008; Rodes-Cabau *et al.*, 2008; Spargias *et al.*, 2008; Tamburino *et al.*, 2009; Thomas *et al.*, 2010; Webb *et al.*, 2007; Zierer *et al.*, 2008). The etiology of vascular damage is often attributed to the large-caliber sheaths used with early TAVI devices. It is envisaged that the introduction of low-profile introducers and greater operator experience will reduce vascular complications. In addition, percutaneous vessel closure devices for transfemoral access are now widely available and will contribute further to the reduction in periprocedural major hemorrhage. Onsite access to vascular surgeons and interventional radiologists with experience of open and endovascular repair of damaged vessels is encouraged. The team should be familiar with the use of crossover femoral cannulation, covered stents and balloon tamponade to control bleeding vessels.

Stroke and transient ischemic attacks (TIAs) are common sequelae of TAVI deployment (range: 0% to 10%) and are believed to be the consequence of atheromatous emboli from the ascending aorta and diseased aortic valve (Berry *et al.*, 2007; Cribier *et al.*, 2002; Descoutures *et al.*, 2008; Grube *et al.*, 2006; Grube *et al.*, 2007; Leon *et al.*, 2010; Piazza *et al.*, 2008; Rodes-Cabau *et al.*, 2008; Svensson *et al.*, 2008; Tamburino *et al.*, 2009; Thomas *et al.*, 2010; Walther *et al.*, 2007; Webb *et al.*, 2007, Ye *et al.*, 2009; Zierer *et al.*, 2008). The risk of cerebrovascular events is increased in TAVI patients with atrial fibrillation and in those in whom valve thrombosis has occurred. Diffusion-weighted magnetic resonance imaging has demonstrated new cerebral lesions in up to 91% of patients undergoing TAVI (Ghanem *et al.*, 2010; Kahlert *et al.*, 2010). Fortunately, these radiological images do not correlate with clinically observed neurological deficits, which suggests that ischemic brain injury is predominantly subclinical (Lefevre *et al.*, 2011; Webb *et al.*, 2009a). The introduction of less traumatic delivery devices may help to reduce the incidence of cerebrovascular events, while novel catheters that are designed to capture or deflect emboli are under evaluation (Nietlispach *et al.*, 2010).

Occlusion of the left main coronary ostium is a potentially fatal complication of TAVI insertion. The usual mechanism involves upward displacement of the native aortic valve leaflet such that it completely covers the coronary ostia. Rarely, the device itself can abut against the coronary ostia, which reduces blood flow to the myocardium. Low coronary origin (less than 12 mm superior to the aortic annulus on computed tomography) or shallow coronary sinuses are thought to predispose to left main coronary artery occlusion (Tops *et al.*, 2008; Webb, 2009b). The Medtronic CoreValve has a tampered proximal end, which is designed to prevent coronary occlusion.

Bradycardia requiring a permanent pacemaker is a frequent problem following TAVI. It results from pressure effects on the conduction pathways that pass through the membranous interventricular septum beneath the aortic valve. This is particularly common in patients with a pre-existing bundle branch or atrioventricular block. Several additional factors are believed to predispose to pacemaker insertion: advanced age, oversizing of the implant, and the depth of the implant within the LV outflow tract (Willson & Webb, 2011). The Medtronic CoreValve is considerably longer than the Edwards SAPIEN and is in contact with a larger area of the interventricular septum. The CoreValve device is associated with considerably higher rates of pacemaker insertion (range: 20% to 38%) (Elchaninoff *et al.*, 2011; Jilaihawi *et al.*, 2010; Piazza *et al.*, 2010; Zahn *et al.*, 2011) compared to the Edwards SAPIEN (range 3% to 10%) (Elchaninoff *et al.*, 2011; Thomas *et al.*, 2010; Webb *et al.*, 2009a).

Although valvular aortic regurgitation is rare after TAVI, paravalvular leak occurs more commonly and is moderate or severe in up to 15% of patients (Leon *et al.*, 2010; Sherif *et al.*, 2010; Webb *et al.*, 2009a; Zahn *et al.*, 2011). Leak occurs when there is an inadequate seal between the outer surface of the device and the aortic annulus, which allows blood to flow around the periphery of the prosthesis. This may occur if the implant is deployed either too proximally or too distally in relation to the plane of the aortic annulus; when the chosen device is undersized in relation to the aortic annulus; or if the prosthesis fails to expand completely. Acute paravalvular leak can be treated with balloon valvuloplasty, retrieval of the device (if possible), or VIV techniques. TAVI has been shown to be associated with a higher incidence of paravalvular leak than open AVR (12% vs. 1%) (Leon *et al.*, 2010).

Acute renal impairment, defined as a glomerular filtration rate reduction of greater than 25%, is associated with a four-fold increase in 30-day mortality following TAVI (Willson & Webb, 2011). Acute renal impairment and renal replacement therapy occur in 11% and 1.4% of TAVI patients, respectively, with risk factors including chronic kidney disease, blood transfusion, hypertension, chronic obstructive pulmonary disease, and transapical access (Bagur *et al.*, 2010). In patients with chronic kidney disease, the incidence of acute renal impairment is lower in those treated with TAVI than with open AVR (9% vs. 26%, $p < 0.001$) (Bagur *et al.*, 2010), which perhaps reflects the deleterious effects of cardiopulmonary bypass, hypotension, and ischemia associated with open surgery. TAVI may therefore be a safer therapeutic option for AS patients with a history of chronic renal impairment.

Open AVR in the presence of severe LV dysfunction is high-risk, and TAVI may be an appropriate alternative in this situation. A recent nonrandomized study (Clavel *et al.*, 2010) compared TAVI ($n = 83$) to open AVR ($n = 200$). Despite a higher STS-PROM score in patients who received TAVI, the authors reported that TAVI was associated with a greater improvement in ejection fraction than open AVR (14% vs. 7%; $p < 0.001$) and better hemodynamics at one year. Evidence from randomized trials is required to assess whether TAVI results in better recovery of LV function than does AVR.

Other complications associated with TAVI include: supraventricular tachyarrhythmia (range: 5% to 31%); ventricular tachyarrhythmia (range: 0% to 4%); myocardial infarction (range: 0% to 15%); cardiac tamponade (range: 2% to 10%); conversion to open surgery (range: 0% to 8%); conversion to valvuloplasty (range: 0% to 4%); emergency valve-in-valve procedure (range: 2% to 12%); and aortic dissection or rupture (range: 0% to 4%) (Behan *et al.*, 2008; Berry *et al.*, 2007; Cribier *et al.*, 2002; De Jaegere *et al.*, 2008; Descoutures *et al.*, 2008; Grube *et al.*, 2006; Grube *et al.*, 2007; Piazza *et al.*, 2008; Rodes-Cabau *et al.*, 2008; Spargias *et al.*, 2008; Svensson *et al.*, 2008; Tamburino *et al.*, 2009; Walther *et al.*, 2007; Walther *et al.*, 2008; Webb *et al.*, 2007; Ye *et al.*, 2009; Zierer *et al.*, 2008). The overall 30-day MACCE ranges from 3% to 35% (Behan *et al.*, 2008; Berry *et al.*, 2007; Cribier *et al.*, 2002; De Jaegere *et al.*, 2008; Descoutures *et al.*, 2008; Grube *et al.*, 2006; Grube *et al.*, 2007; Piazza *et al.*, 2008; Rodes-Cabau *et al.*, 2008; Spargias *et al.*, 2008; Svensson *et al.*, 2008; Tamburino *et al.*, 2009; Walther *et al.*, 2007; Walther *et al.*, 2008; Webb *et al.*, 2007; Ye *et al.*, 2009; Zierer *et al.*, 2008).

4.4 Efficacy of TAVI

The efficacy of valvular procedures can be determined by whether they improve echocardiographic measurements of hemodynamic performance and by the effect of treatment on patient function and quality of life. The main pathological findings at echocardiography in patients with severe AS are reduced AVA, raised peak and mean pressure gradients across the aortic valve, reduced LV ejection fraction, and LV dysfunction. Numerous studies have investigated the echocardiographic outcomes of TAVI and have consistently demonstrated statistically significant ($p < 0.05$) improvements in AVA, mean and peak aortic valve pressure gradients, and LV ejection fraction between preoperative and early postoperative values (Behan *et al.*, 2008; Berry *et al.*, 2007; Clavel *et al.*, 2009; Cribier *et al.*, 2002; De Jaegere *et al.*, 2008; Descoutures *et al.*, 2008; Figulla *et al.*, 2011; Grube *et al.*, 2006; Grube *et al.*, 2007; Piazza *et al.*, 2008; Rodes-Cabau *et al.*, 2008; Spargias *et al.*, 2008; Svensson *et al.*, 2008; Tamburino *et al.*, 2009; Walther *et al.*, 2007; Walther *et al.*, 2008; Webb *et al.*, 2007; Ye *et al.*, 2009; Zierer *et al.*, 2008). Furthermore, there is no deterioration in echocardiographic outcomes in patients followed-up for at least a year, which suggests that TAVI produces longer-lasting effects than balloon valvuloplasty alone (Cribier *et al.*, 2002; Figulla *et al.*, 2011; Webb *et al.*, 2007; Ye *et al.*, 2009).

It is imperative that improvements in hemodynamics translate into tangible benefits to patient function and health status. In studies of cardiothoracic surgery, patient function and the severity of symptoms are most commonly assessed through changes in NYHA classification. This clinician-reported outcome assigns patients to one of four categories, ranging from no symptoms or limitations on ordinary physical activity (Class I) to severe symptoms at rest necessitating continuous bed rest (Class IV). TAVI has been shown consistently to improve NYHA classification, with between 50% and 100% of patients demonstrating an improvement of at least one grade in NYHA classification at one-month post-procedure (Cribier *et al.*, 2002; Gotzmann *et al.*, 2010; Grube *et al.*, 2006; Grube *et al.*, 2007; Rodes-Cabau *et al.*, 2008; Spargias *et al.*, 2008; Svensson *et al.*, 2008; Webb *et al.*, 2007; Ye *et al.*, 2009). The short duration of follow-up of most studies means that it is difficult to determine whether these benefits are sustained, but some publications have reported that functional improvements last at least a year (Leon *et al.*, 2010; Webb *et al.*, 2009a). NYHA classification is also correlated with performance in the 6-minute walk test (Demers *et al.*, 2001; Gotzmann *et al.*, 2010).

Patient-reported outcomes (PROs), including health-related quality of life, provide unbiased assessments of health status from the patient's perspective. Instruments (most often questionnaires) designed to capture these issues are called HRQL tools and are multidimensional, encompassing perceptions of physical, emotional, and social function, as well as assessing specific symptoms caused by the disease and treatment (Fayers & Hays., 2005). The development of symptoms of congestive cardiac failure confers a poor prognosis on patients with severe AS and is likely to significantly affect HRQL. It is important to determine whether TAVI has a beneficial effect on HRQL and symptom palliation, in addition to increasing survival. Several studies have reported HRQL outcomes in patients treated with TAVI. Gotzmann *et al.*, (2010) reported that HRQL (assessed using the Minnesota Living with Heart Failure Questionnaire [MLHFQ]) was significantly better 30 days after TAVI when compared to baseline. This correlated with observed improvements in the 6-minute walk test and a reduction in serum beta-natriuretic peptide. Krane *et al.* (2010) measured HRQL with the Medical Outcomes Study Short Form-36 (SF-36) in a cohort of 99 patients treated with TAVI. Physical functioning, bodily pain, general health, and vitality all improved significantly from baseline at the three-month follow-up. Scores for social functioning and mental health remained static, while only role-emotional functioning deteriorated after TAVI. Ussia *et al.* (2009) used the SF-12 to compare HRQL in patients before and after TAVI with aged matched population reference values. Preprocedural AS patients had markedly worse HRQL than the general population for both physical and mental function. Five months after TAVI, HRQL had improved dramatically and was similar to that in the general population. This suggests that recovery following TAVI does occur, but takes several months. In the REVIVAL II feasibility study, HRQL was measured using the SF-12 and the Kansas City Cardiomyopathy Questionnaire (KCCQ) at 30 days and 6 months after TAVI insertion in 75 patients (Reynolds *et al.*, 2008). At 30 days, a significant improvement in KCCQ score was observed, but not in the physical or mental functioning scales of the SF-12. However, by the 6-month follow-up, improvements in all facets of HRQL were evident. Taken together, these results provide strong evidence that TAVI improves HRQL in patients with severe AS, although it takes up to 6 months for HRQL to match that in the general population.

4.5 Durability of TAVI

TAVI is a relatively new intervention, and long-term outcome data is scarce beyond one year of follow-up. A recent systematic review (Figulla *et al.*, 2011) incorporating pooled data from multiple studies reported that mean one-year survival after TAVI was 75.9% (range: 64.1% to 87.0%) (Al-Attar *et al.*, 2009; Grube *et al.*, 2008; Himbert *et al.*, 2009; Kapadia *et al.*, 2009; Otten *et al.*, 2009; Rajani *et al.*, 2010; Rodes-Cabau *et al.*, 2010; Thielmann *et al.*, 2009; Walther *et al.*, 2010; Webb *et al.*, 2009a; Ye *et al.*, 2009). In contrast the mean one-year survival rate for patients treated with medical care alone was 62.4% (range: 40.0% to 84.8%; $p < 0.01$ vs. TAVI), revealing a 13.5% survival advantage in favor of TAVI at one year. This is in agreement with the PARTNER Trial, which reported a 20% survival advantage for TAVI (Leon *et al.*, 2010). Gurvitch *et al.* (2010) are one of the few groups to report outcomes for TAVI beyond one year of follow-up: In a cohort of 70 patients undergoing TAVI, they reported one-, two-, and three-year survival rates of 81%, 74%, and 61%, respectively, although patients who died within 30-days or in whom TAVI failed were excluded from the analysis. During the follow-up period, there were 30 late deaths, of which three were valve-related: two patients died from intracerebral hemorrhage secondary to supratherapeutic anticoagulation, and sudden death occurred in another patient who was found postmortem to have an overgrowth of fibrous connective tissue around the prosthesis. No deaths were directly related to valvular dysfunction, which is in agreement with other studies reporting outcomes up to one year (Grube *et al.*, 2008; Rodes-Cabau., 2010; Webb *et al.*, 2009a).

In the review by Figulla *et al.* (2011), one-year survival following transfemoral TAVI (79.2%, range: 68.1% to 87.0%) was superior to transapical access (73.6%, range 60.0% to 78.0%, $p = 0.04$). Reduced survival in patients receiving transapical TAVI may be explained by the need for general anesthesia, thoracotomy, and cannulation of the left ventricular apex. It is important to note that most studies included in Figulla *et al.* were retrospective and nonrandomized, and consequently at risk of bias. RCTs are required to determine which method of gaining access to the diseased aortic valve is the most efficacious when undertaking TAVI.

Very little is known about the risk of valvular degeneration with TAVI devices. *In vitro* testing of the latest generation of Edwards SAPIEN/XT and Medtronic CoreValve devices suggests that durability in excess of 10 years can be expected (Willson & Webb., 2010). Because of the proven efficacy of open AVR, without long-term *in vivo* data, it is very unlikely that TAVI devices will be licensed for use in younger patients without comorbidities. Indeed, freedom from reoperation for valvular degeneration is greater than 95% with modern surgical bioprostheses (Jamieson *et al.*, 1995). The results of long-term follow-up will be required to answer this clinical question, but it is unlikely that TAVI will replace open AVR for the management of uncomplicated, severe AS.

5. Future directions

The evidence base for TAVI is rapidly evolving, and there has been a significant rise in the number of new publications over the last five years. Most eagerly awaited are the findings of Cohort A of the PARTNER Trial. This will provide insight into the comparative efficacy of TAVI and open AVR in high-risk patients with severe symptomatic AS. The results of this trial will have important implications for healthcare policy implementation and may mean greater financial provision for TAVI in high-risk patients. In addition, the two main techniques for accessing the aortic valve (transfemoral and transapical) will need to be compared in an RCT, especially given that pooled data suggests one-year survival is worse after transapical TAVI (Figulla *et al.*, 2011). If this is proved to be the case, then the transapical approach may be restricted to patients in whom the transfemoral route is contraindicated.

Using TAVI in moderate- or low-risk patients is not currently justified, because it would be unethical to withhold access to open AVR with its proven efficacy. The results of long-term follow-ups (> 10 years) of high-risk patients will be necessary to assess the durability of TAVI implants and to inform decisions about their use in younger, fitter patients. Given the short life expectancy of patients denied open surgery, it is unlikely that sufficient data will be available in the foreseeable future to determine whether TAVI is appropriate in low-risk candidates. It is also worth noting that a number of new prostheses will undoubtedly emerge in the next decade and that they will require appropriate evaluation against existing gold standards. An RCT using the Medtronic CoreValve system is also anticipated to publish its findings in 2013. Once the feasibility, safety, efficacy, and durability of TAVI devices have been established, the onus will shift towards healthcare economic evaluation to identify the most cost-effective means of treating severe AS. It is certainly conceivable that minimally invasive techniques, such as TAVI, will prove cost-effective in the long-term.

6. Conclusions

Severe aortic stenosis has a poor prognosis once symptoms of congestive cardiac failure and angina develop. It is conventional wisdom that surgical AVR offers the best hope of symptom palliation and long-term survival. However, approximately one-third of patients with severe symptomatic AS are denied access to surgery because of comorbidities and high operative risk. The last decade has witnessed the introduction of transcatheter aortic valve implantation, a surgical innovation that permits percutaneous replacement of the diseased aortic valve without sternotomy and a cardiopulmonary bypass. TAVI remains in its infancy, yet it has demonstrated superior medium-term survival, fewer symptoms, and a better quality of life than medical care alone. Doubts persist over the durability of the implants, long-terms outcomes, and the relative efficacy compared with surgical AVR in high-risk patients. However, TAVI is set to continue to revolutionize the management of severe symptomatic aortic stenosis.

7. References

Al-Attar, N., Himbert, D., Descoutures, F., *et al.* (2009). Transcatheter aortic valve implantation: selection strategy is crucial for outcome, *Ann Thorac Surg* 87(6): 1757–1762.

Ambler, G., Omar, R. Z., Royston, P., Kinsman, R., Keogh, B. E., & Taylor, K. M. (2005). Generic, simple risk stratification model for heart valve surgery, *Circulation* 112: 224–231.

Anderson, H. R., Knudsen, L. L., & Hasenkam, J. M. (1992). Transluminal implantation of artificial heart valves. Description of a new expandable aortic valve and initial results with implantation by catheter technique in closed chest pigs, *Eur Heart J* 13: 704-708.

Anselmi, A., Abbate, A., Girola, F., *et al.* (2004). Myocardial ischaemia, stunning, inflammation, and apoptosis during cardiac surgery: a review of evidence, *Eur J Cardiothorac Surg* 25: 304-311.

Asimakopoulos, G., Edwards, M. B., & Taylor, K. M. (1997). Aortic valve replacement in patients 80 years of age and older: survival and cause of death based on 1100 cases: collective results from the UK Heart Valve Registry, *Circulation* 96: 3403-3408.

Bagur, R., Webb, JG., Nietlispach, F., *et al.* (2010). Acute kidney injury following transcatheter aortic valve implantation: predictive factors, prognostic value, and comparison with surgical aortic valve replacement, *Eur Heart J* 31: 865–874.

Behan, M., Haworth, P., Hutchinson, N., Trivedi, U., Laborde, JC., & Hildick-Smith, D (2008). Percutaneous aortic valve implants under sedation: our initial experience, *Catheter Cardiovasc Interv* 72: 1012-1015.

Berry, C., Asgar, A., Lamarche, Y., *et al.* (2007). Novel therapeutic aspects of percutaneous aortic valve replacement with the 21F CoreValve Revalving system, *Catheter Cardiovasc Interv* 70: 610-616.

Bonow, R. W., Carabello, B. A., Kanu, C., *et al.* (2006). ACC/AHA 2006 guidelines for the management of patients with valvular heart disease: a report of the American College of Cardiology/American Heart Association Task Force on Practice Guidelines, *Circulation* 114: e84-e231.

Brown, M. L., Schaff, H. V., Sarano, M. E., *et al.* (2008). Is the European System for cardiac Operative Risk Evaluation model valid for estimating operative risk of patients considered for percutaneous aortic valve replacement? *J Thorac Cardiovasc Surg* 136: 566-571.

Brown, J. M., O'Brien, S. M., Wu, C., Sikora, J. A., Griffith, B. P., & Gammie, J. S. (2009). Isolated aortic valve replacement in North America comprising 108,687 patients in 10 years: changes in risks, valve types, and outcomes in the Society of Thoracic Surgeons National Database, *J Thorac Cardiovasc Surg* 137: 82-90.

Charlson, E., Legedza, A. T. R., & Hamel, M. B. (2006). Decision-making and outcomes in severe symptomatic aortic stenosis, *J Heart Valve Dis* 15: 312-321.

Cheitlin, M. D., Gertz, E. W., Brundage, B. H., Carlson, C. J., Quash, J. A., & Bode, R. S. Jr (1979). Rate of progression of severity of valvular aortic stenosis in the adult, *Am Heart J* 98: 689-700.

Clavel, M. A., Webb, J. G., Rodés-Cabau, J., *et al.* (2010). Comparison between transcatheter and surgical prosthetic valve implantation in patients with severe aortic stenosis and reduced left ventricular ejection fraction, *Circulation* 122: 1928-1936.

Clavel, MA., Webb, JG., Pibarot, P., *et al.* (2009). Comparison of the hemodynamic performance of percutaneous and surgical bioprostheses for the treatment of severe aortic stenosis, *J Am Coll Cardiol* 53: 1883–1891.

Connolly, H. M., Oh, J. K., Schaff, H. V., *et al.* (2000). Severe aortic stenosis with low transvalvular gradient and severe left ventricular dysfunction: result of aortic valve replacement in 52 patients, *Circulation* 101: 1940-1946.

Cribier, A., Savin, T., Saoudi, N., Rocha, P., Berland, J., & Letac, B (1986). Percutaneous transluminal valvuloplasty of acquired aortic stenosis in elderly patients: an alternative to valve replacement? *Lancet* 1: 63-67.

Cribier, A., Eltchaninoff, H., Bash, A., *et al.* (2002). Percutaneous transcatheter implantation of an aortic valve prosthesis for calcific aortic stenosis: first human case description, *Circulation* 106: 3006-3008.

Davies, S. W., Gershlick, A. H., & Balcon, R. (1991). Progression of valvular aortic stenosis: a long-term retrospective study, *Eur Heart J* 12: 10-14.

De Jaegere, P., Van Dijk, L. C., Laborde, J. C., *et al.* (2007). True percutaneous implantation of the CoreValve aortic valve prosthesis by the combined use of ultrasound guided vascular access, Prostar XL and the TandemHeart, *EuroIntervention* 2: 500–505.

De Jaegere, P. P., Piazza, N., Galema, T. W., *et al.* (2008). Early echocardiographic evaluation following percutaneous implantation with the self-expanding CoreValve Revalving System aortic valve bioprosthesis, *Eurointervention* 4: 351-357.

Demers, C., McKelvie, RS., Negassa, A., & Yusuf, S. (2001). Reliability, validity, and responsiveness of the six- minute walk test in patients with heart failure, *Am Heart J* 142: 698-703.

Descoutures, F., Himbert, D., Lepage, L., *et al.* (2008). Contemporary surgical or percutaneous management of severe aortic stenosis in the elderly, *Eur Heart J* 29: 1410-1417.

Dewey, T. M., Brown, D., Ryan, W. H., Herbert, M. A., Prince, S. L., & Mack, M. J. (2008). Reliability of risk algorithms in predicting early and late operative outcomes in high-risk patients undergoing aortic valve replacement, *J Thorac Cardiovasc Surg* 135: 180-187.

Edwards, F. H., Peterson, E. D., Coombs, L. P., *et al.* (2001). Prediction of operative mortality after valve replacement surgery, *J Am Coll Cardiol* 37: 885–892.

Elayda, MA., Hall, RJ., Reul, RM., *et al.* (1993). Aortic valve replacement in patients 80 years and older, operative risks and long-term results, *Circulation* 88: 11-16.

Eltchaninoff, H., Prat, A., Gilard, M., *et al.* (2011). Transcatheter aortic valve implantation: early results of the FRANCE (FRench Aortic National CoreValve and Edwards) registry, *Eur Heart J* 32(2): 191–197.

Falk, V., Schwammenthal, E. E., Kempfert, J., *et al.* (2009). New anatomically oriented transapical aortic valve implantation, *Ann Thorac Surg* 87: 925-926.

Fayers, P., & Hays, R. (2005). Assessing quality of life in clinical trials. 2nd ed. Oxford: Oxford University Press.

Ferrari, E., Marcucci, C., Sulzer, C., & von Segesser, LK (2010). Which available transapical transcatheter valve fits into degenerated bioprostheses? *Interact Cardiovasc Thorac Surg* 11: 83-85.

Figulla, L., Neumann, A., Figulla, H. R., Kahlert, P., Erbel, R., & Neumann, T (2011). Transcatheter aortic valve implantation: evidence on safety and efficacy compared with medical therapy. A systematic review of current literature, *Clin Res Cardiol* 100: 265-276.

Florath, I., Rosendahl, U. P., Mortasawi, A., *et al.* (2003). Current determinants of operative mortality in 1400 patients requiring aortic valve replacement, *Ann Thorac Surg* 76: 75-83.

Florath, I., Albert, A., Boening, A., Ennker, I. C., & Ennker, J., (2010). Aortic valve replacement in octogenarians: identification of high-risk patients, *Eur J Cardiothorac Surg* 37: 1304-1310.

Gabrielle, F., Roques, F., Michel, P., *et al.* (1997). Is the Parsonnet's score a good predictive score of mortality in adult cardiac surgery? Assessment by a French multicentre study, Eur J Cardiothoracic Surg 11: 400–411.

Ghanem, A., Muller, A., Nahle, C. P., *et al.* (2010). Risk and fate of cerebral embolism after transfemoral aortic valve implantation: a prospective pilot study with diffusion-weighted magnetic resonance imaging, *J Am Coll Cardiol* 55: 1427–1432.

Gogas, B. D., Zacharoulis, A. A., & Antoniadis, A. G. (2011). Acute coronary occlusion following TAVI, *Catheter Cardiovasc Interv* 77: 435-438.

Gotzmann, M., Hehen, T., Germing, A., *et al.* (2010). Short-term effects of transcatheter aortic valve implantation on neurohormonal activation, quality of life and 6-minute walk test in severe and symptomatic aortic stenosis, *Heart* 96: 1102-1106.

Grube, E., Laborde, J. C., Gerckens, U., *et al.* (2006). Percutaneous implantation of the CoreValve self-expanding valve prosthesis in high-risk patients with aortic valve disease: the Siegburg first-in-man study, Circulation 114: 1616-24.

Grube, E., Schuler, G., Buellesfeld, L., *et al.* (2007). Percutaneous aortic valve replacement for severe aortic stenosis in high-risk patients using the second- and current third-generation self expanding CoreValve prosthesis. Device success and 30-day clinical outcome, *J Am Coll Cardiol* 50: 69-76.

Grube, E., Buellesfeld, L., Mueller, R., *et al.* (2008). Progress and current status of percutaneous aortic valve replacement: results of three device generations of the CoreValve Revalving System, *Circ Cardiovasc Interv* 1(3): 167–175.

Gurvitch, R., Wood, D. A., Tay, E. L., *et al.* (2010). Transcatheter aortic valve implantation: durability of clinical and hemodynamic outcomes beyond 3 years in a large patient cohort, *Circulation* 122: 1319–1327.

Gurvitch, R., Cheung, A., Bedogni, F., & Webb, J. G. (2011). Coronary obstruction following transcatheter aortic valve-in-valve implantation for failed surgical bioprostheses, *Catheter Cardiovasc Interv* 77: 439-444.

Hammermeister, K. E., Sethi, G. K., Henderson, W. G., Oprian, C., Kim, T., & Rahimtoola, S. (1993). A comparison of outcomes in men 11 years after heart-valve replacement with a mechanical or bioprosthesis, *N Engl J Med* 328: 1289-1296.

Hattler, B. G., Madia, C., Johnson, C., *et al.* (1994). Risk stratification using the Society of Thoracic Surgeons program, *Ann Thorac Surg* 52: 1348-1352.

Higgins, T. L., Estafanous, F. G., Loop, F. D., Beck, G. J., Blum, J. M., & Paranandi, L. (1992). Stratification of morbidity and mortality outcome by preoperative risk factors in coronary artery bypass patients, *J Am Med Assoc* 267: 2344-2348.

Himbert, D., Descoutures, F., Al-Attar, N., *et al.* (2009). Results of transfemoral or transapical aortic valve implantation following a uniform assessment in high-risk patients with aortic stenosis, *J Am Coll Cardiol* 54(4): 303–311.

Iung, B., Baron, G., Butchart, E. G., *et al.* (2003). A prospective survey of patients with valvular heart disease in Europe: The Euro Heart Survery on Valvular Heart Disease, *Eur Heart J* 24: 1231-1243.

Iung, B., Cachier, A., Baron, G., *et al.* (2005). Decision-making in elderly patients with severe aortic stenosis: why are so many denied surgery? *Eur Heart J* 26: 2714-2720.

Jamieson, W. R., Burr, L. H., Tyers, G. F., *et al.* (1995). Carpentier-Edwards supraannular porcine bioprosthesis: clinical performance to twelve years, *Ann Thorac Surg* 60: S235–S240.

Jilaihawi, H., Chin, D., Spyt, T., *et al.* (2010). Prosthesis-patient mismatch after transcatheter aortic valve implantation with the Medtronic-Corevalve bioprosthesis, *Eur Heart J* 31:857–864.

Kahlert, P., Knipp, S. C., Schlamann, M., *et al.* (2010). Silent and apparent cerebral ischemia after percutaneous transfemoral aortic valve implantation: a diffusion-weighted magnetic resonance imaging study, *Circulation* 121: 870–878.

Kapadia, S. R., Goel, S. S., Svensson, L. G., *et al.* (2009). Characterization and outcome of patients with severe symptomatic aortic stenosis referred for percutaneous aortic valve replacement, *J Thorac Cardiovasc Surg* 137(6): 1430– 1435.

Kelly, T. A., Rothbart, R. M., Cooper, C. M., Kaiser, D. L., Smucker, M. L., & Gibson, R. S. (1988). Comparison of outcome of asymptomatic to symptomatic patients older than 20 years of age with valvular aortic stenosis, *Am J Cardiol* 61: 123-130.

Kempfert, J., Van Linden, A., Linke, A., *et al.* (2010). Transapical off-pump valve-in-valve implantation in patients with degenerated aortic xenografts, *Ann Thorac Surg* 89: 1934-1941.

Khawaja, M. Z., Haworth, P., Ghuran, A., *et al.* (2010). Transcatheter aortic valve implantation for stenosed and regurgitant aortic valve bioprostheses CoreValve for failed bioprosthetic aortic valve replacements, *J Am Coll Cardiol* 55: 97-101.

Kobayashi, K. J., Williams, J. A., Nwakanma, L. U., *et al.* (2009). EuroSCORE predicts short- and mid-term mortality in combined aortic valve replacement and coronary artery bypass patients, *J Card Surg* 24: 637-643.

Krane, M., Deutsch, M. A., Bleizffer, S., *et al.* (2010). Quality of life among patients undergoing transcatheter aortic valve implantation, *Am Heart J* 160: 451-457.

Latsios, G., Gerckens, U., & Grube, E (2010). Transaortic transcatheter aortic valve implantation: a novel approach for the truly "no-access option" patients, *Catheter Cardiovasc Interv* 75: 1129-1136.

Lee, S. J., Lindquist, K., Segal, M. R., & Covinsky, K. E (2006). Development and validation of a prognostic index for 4-year mortality in older adults, *JAMA* 295 : 801-808.

Lefevre, T., Kappetein, A. P., Wolner, E., *et al.* (2011). One year follow-up of the multi-centre European PARTNER transcatheter heart valve study, *Eur Heart J* 32(2):148–157.

Leon, M. B., Smith, C. R., Mack, M., *et al.* for the PARTNER Trial Investigators (2010). Transcatheter aortic-valve implantation in patients who cannot undergo surgery, *N Eng J Med* 363: 1578-1607.

Leontyev, S., Walther, T., Borger, MA., *et al.* (2009). Aortic valve replacement in octogenarians: utility of risk stratification with EuroSCORE, *Ann Thorac Surg* 87: 1440-1445.

Lieberman, E. B., Bashore, T. M., Hermiller, J. B., *et al.* (1995). Balloon aortic valvuloplasty in adults: failure of procedure to improve long-term survival, *J Am Coll Cardiol* 26: 1522-1528.

Low, R. I., Bolling, S. F., Yeo, K. K., & Ebner, A. (2008). Direct flow medical percutaneous aortic valve: Proof of concept, *EuroInterv* 4: 256–261.

Malaisrie, S. C., McCarthy, P. M., McGee, E. C., *et al.* (2010). Contemporary perioperative results of isolated aortic valve replacement for aortic stenosis, *Ann Thorac Surg* 89: 751-756.

Malaisrie, S. C., Tuday, E., Lapin, B., *et al.* (2011). Transcatheter valve implantation decreases the rate of unoperated aortic stenosis, *Eur J Cardiothorac Surg* 40(1): 43-48.

Melby, S. J., Zierer, A., Kaiser, S. P., *et al.* (2007). Aortic valve replacement in octogenarians: risk factors for early and late mortality, *Ann Thorc Surg* 83: 1651-1657.

Monin, J. L., Quere, J. P., Monchi, M., *et al.* (2003). Low-gradient aortic stenosis: operative risk stratification and predictors for long-term outcome: a multicenter study using dobutamine stress hemodynamics, *Circulation* 108: 319-324.

Moss, R. R., Ivens, E., Pasupati, S., *et al.* (2008). Role of echocardiography in percutaneous aortic valve implantation, *J Am Coll Cardiol Imaging* 1:15–24.

Myken, P. S. U., Caidahl, K., Larsson, P., Larsson, S., Wallentin, I., & Berggren, H. E. (1995). Mechanical versus biological valve prosthesis: a ten-year comparison regarding function and quality of life, *Ann Thorac Surg* 60: S447-S452.

Nashef, S. A. M., Roques, F., Michel, P., Gauducheau, E., Lemeshow, S., & Salamon, R. (1999). European system for cardiac operative risk evaluation (EuroSCORE), *Eur J Cardiothorac Surg* 16: 9-13.

Nietlispach, F., Wijesinghe, N., Gurvitch, R., *et al.* (2010). An embolic deflection device for aortic valve interventions, *JACC Cardiovasc Interv* 3: 1133–1138.

Nissinen, J., Biancari, F., Wistbacka, J. O., *et al.* (2009). Is it possible to improve the accuracy of the EuroSCORE? *Eur J Cardiothorac Surg* 36: 799-804.

Nowicki, ER., Birkmeyer, NJO., Weintraub, RW., *et al.* (2004). Multivariable prediction of in-hospital mortality associated with aortic and mitral valve surgery in northern New England, *Ann Thorac Surg* 77: 1966-1977.

O'Brien, SM., Shahian, DM., Filardo, G., *et al.* (2009). The Society of Thoracic Surgeons 2008 cardiac risk models: part 2 - isolated valve surgery, *Ann Thorac Surg* 88: S23-S42.

Olsen, L. K., Engstrøm, T., & Søndergaard, L (2010). Transcatheter valve-in-valve implantation due to severe aortic regurgitation in a degenerated aortic homograft, J Invasive Cardiol 21:E197-E200.

Otten, A. M., van Domburg, R. T., van Gameren, M., *et al.* (2008). Population characteristics, treatment assignment and survival of patients with aortic stenosis referred for percutaneous valve replacement, *EuroIntervention* 4(2): 250–255.

Otto, C. M., Pearlman, A. S., & Gardner, C. L. (1989). Hemodynamic progression of aortic stenosis in adults assessed by Doppler echocardiography, *J Am Coll Cardiol* 13: 545-550.

Otto, C. M., Mickel, M. C., Kennedy, J. W., *et al.* (1994). Three-year outcome after balloon aortic valvuloplasty. Insights into prognosis of valvular aortic stenosis, *Circulation* 89: 642-650.

Parsonnet, V., Dean, D., & Bernstein, A. D. (1989). A method of uniform stratification of risk for evaluating the results of surgery in acquired adult heart disease, *Circulation* 79: I3-I12.

Peter M, Hoffmann A, Parker C, Lüscher T, Burckhardt D (1993). Progression of aortic stenosis: role of age and concomitant coronary artery disease, *Chest* 103: 1715-1719.

Peterseim, D. S., Cen, Y. Y., Cheruvu, S., *et al.* (1999). Long-term outcome after biologic versus mechanical aortic valve replacement in 841 patients, *J Thorac Cardiovasc Surg* 117: 890-897.

Piazza, N., Grube, E., Gerckens, U., *et al.* (2008). Procedural and 30-day outcomes following transcatheter aortic valve implantation using the third generation (18 Fr) CoreValve revalving system: results from the multicentre, expanded evaluation registry 1-year following CE mark approval, *Eurointervention* 4: 242-249.

Piazza, N., Nuis, R. J., Tzikas, A., *et al.* (2010). Persistent conduction abnormalities and requirements for pacemaking six months after transcatheter aortic valve implantation. *EuroIntervention*, 6, pp. 475–484.

Pons, J. M. V., Granados, A., Espinas, J. A., Borras, J. M., Martin, I., & Moreno, V. (1997). Assessing open heart surgery mortality in Catalonia (Spain) through a predictive risk model, *Eur J Cardiothorac Surg* 11: 415-423.

Rajani, R., Buxton, W., Haworth, P., *et al.* (2010). Prognostic benefit of transcatheter aortic valve implantation compared with medical therapy in patients with inoperable aortic stenosis, *Catheter Cardiovasc Interv* 75(7): 1121–1126.

Reynolds, M. R., Moses, J. W., Svensson, L. G., *et al.* (2008). For the REVIVAL II Investigators. Quality of life improvements following transcatheter aortic valve replacement: results from the REVIVAL II feasibility study, *J Am Coll Cardiol* 51: B1-B122.

Rodes-Cabau, J., Dumont, E., De La Rochelliere, R., *et al.* (2008). Feasibility and initial results of percutaneous aortic valve implantation including selection of the transfemoral or transapical approach in patients with severe aortic stenosis, *Am J Cardiol* 102 : 1240-1246.

Rodes-Cabau, J., Dumont, E., & Doyle, D. (2009). "Valve-in-valve" for the treatment of paravalvular leaks fol- lowing transcatheter aortic valve implantation, *Catheter Cardiovasc Interv* 74: 1116-1119.

Rodes-Cabau, J., Webb, J. G., Cheung, A., *et al.* (2010). Transcatheter aortic valve implantation for the treatment of severe symptomatic aortic stenosis in patients at very high or prohibitive surgical risk acute and late outcomes of the multicenter Canadian experience, *J Am Coll Cardiol* 50: 69-76.

Roques, F., Gabrielle, F., Michel, P., de Vincentiis, C., David, M., & Baudet, E. (1995). Quality of care in adult heart surgery: proposal for a self-assessment approach based on a French multicenter study, *Eur J Cardiothorac Surg* 9: 433-440.

Roques, F., Nashef, S. A., Michel, P., *et al.* (1999). Risk factors and outcome in European cardiac surgery: an analysis of the EuroSCORE multinational database of 19030 patients, *Eur J Cardiothorac Surg* 15: 816-823.

Ross, J. Jr., & Braunwald, E. (1968). Aortic stenosis, *Circulation* 38: 61-67.

Schofer, J., Schluter, M., Treede, H., *et al.* (2008). Retrograde transarterial implantation of a nonmetallic aortic valve prosthesis in high-surgical-risk patients with severe aortic stenosis. A first-in-man feasibility and safety study, *Circ Cardiovasc Intervent* 1:126-133.

Sharp, A. S., Michex, I., & Colombo, A. (2010). First transaxillary implantation of Edwards Sapien valve to treat incompetent aortic bioprosthesis, Catheter Cardiovasc Interv 75: 507-510.

Sherif, MA., Abdel-Wahab, M., Stocker, B., *et al.* (2010). Anatomic and procedural predictors of paravalvular aortic regurgitation after implantation of the Medtronic CoreValve bioprosthesis, *J Am Coll Cardiol* 56: 1623–1629.

Spargias, K., Manginas, A., Pavlides, G., Khoury, M., Stavridis, G., & Rellia, P. (2008). Transcatheter aortic valve implantation: first Greek experience, *Hellenic J Cardiol* 49: 397-407.

Svensson, L. G., Dewey, T., Kapadia, S., *et al.* (2008). United States feasibility study of transcatheter insertion of a stented aortic valve by the left ventricular apex, *Ann Thorac Surg* 86: 46-55.

Tamburino, C., Capodanno, D., Mul, E. M., *et al.* (2009). Procedural success and 30-day clinical outcomes after percutaneous aortic valve replacement using current third-generation self-expanding CoreValve prosthesis. *J Invasive Cardiol*, 21: 99-100.

Taramasso, M., Sharp, A. S., & Maisano, F. (2010). First-in-man case report of the use of an Edwards Sapien valve to treat regurgitant CoreValve aortic valve prosthesis, *Catheter Cardiovasc Interv* 75: 51- 55.

Thielmann, M., Wendt, D., Eggebrecht, H., *et al.* (2009). Transcatheter aortic valve implantation in patients with very high risk for conventional aortic valve replacement, *Ann Thorac Surg* 88(5): 1468– 1474.

Thomas, M., Schymik, G., Walther, T., *et al.* (2010). Thirty-day results of the SAPIEN aortic bioprosthesis European outcome (SOURCE) registry: a European registry of transcatheter aortic valve implantation using the Edwards SAPIEN valve, *Circulation* 122: 62–69.

Tops, L. F., Wood, D. A., Delgado, V., *et al.* (2008). Noninvasive evaluation of the aortic root with multislice computed tomography: implications for transcatheter aortic valve replacement, *J Am Coll Cardiol Imaging* 1: 321-330.

Treede, H., Tubler, T., Reichenspurner, H., *et al.* (2010). Six-month results of a repositionable and retrievable pericardial valve for transcatheter aortic valve replacement: The direct flow medical aortic valve, *J Thorac Cardiovasc Surg* 140: 897-903.

Tremblay, N. A., Hardy, J. F., Perault, J., & Carrier, M. (1993). A simple classification of the risk in cardiac surgery: the first decade, *Can J Anaesth* 40: 103-111.

Tu, J. V., Jaglal, S. B., & Naylor, C. D. (1995). Multicenter validation of a risk index for mortality, intensive care unit stay, and overall hospital length of stay after cardiac surgery, *Circulation* 91: 677-684.

Turina, J., Hess, O., Sepulcri, F., & Krayenbuehl, H. P. (1987). Spontaneous course of aortic valve disease, *Eur Heart J* 8: 471-483.

Ussia, G. P., Mule, M., Barbanti, M., *et al.* (2009). Quality of life assessment after percutaneous aortic valve implantation, *Eur Heart J* 30: 1790-1796.

Ussia, G. P., Capodanno, D., Brbanti, M., *et al.* (2010). Balloon aortic valvuloplasty for severe aortic stenosis as a bridge to high-risk transcatheter aortic valve implantation, *J Invasive Cardiol* 22: 161-166.

Vahanian, A., Baumgartner, H., Bax, J., *et al.* (2007). Task Force on the Management of Valvular Heart Disease of the European Society of Cardiology; ESC Committee for Practice Guidelines. Guidelines on the management of valvular heart disease: The Task Force on the Management of Valvular Heart Disease of the European Society of Cardiology, *Eur Heart J* 28: 230-268.

Vahanian, A., Alfieri, O. R., Al-Attar, N., *et al.* (2008). Transcatheter valve implantation for patients with aortic stenosis: a position statement from the European association of Cardio-Thoracic Surgery (EACTS) and the European Society for Cardiology (ESC) in collaboration with the European Association of Percutaneous Cardiovascular Interventions (EAPCI), *Eur Heart J* 29: 1463-1470.

Vahanian, A., Himbert, D., & Brochet, E. (2010). Transcatheter valve implantation for patients with severe aortic stenosis, *Heart* 96: 1849-1856.

Vavuranakis, M., Voudris, V., Vrachatic, D. A., *et al.* (2010). Transcatheter aortc valve implantation, patient selection process and procedure: two centres' experience of the intervention without general anaesthesia, *Hellenic J Cardiol* 51: 492-500.

Walther, T., Simon, P., Dewey, T., *et al.* (2007). Transapical minimally invasive aortic valve implantation: multicenter experience, *Circulation* 116: I240-I245.

Walther, T., Kempfert, J., Borger, M. A., *et al.* (2008a). Human minimally invasive off-pump valve-in-a-valve implantation, *Ann Thorac Surg* 85: 1072-1073.

Walther, T., Falk, V., Kempfert, J., *et al.* (2008b). Transapical minimally invasive aortic valve implantation; the initial 50 patients, *Eur J Cardiothorac Surg* 33: 983-988.

Walther, T., Schuler, G., Borger, M. A., *et al.* (2010). Transapical aortic valve implantation in 100 consecutive patients: comparison to propensity-matched conventional aortic valve replacement, *Eur Heart J* 31(11): 1398–1403.

Webb, J. G., Chandavimol, M., Thompson, C. R., *et al.* (2006). Percutaneous aortic valve implantation retrograde from the femoral artery, *Circulation* 113: 842-850.

Webb, J. G., Pasupati, S., Humphries, K., *et al.* (2007). Percutaneous transarterial aortic valve replacement in selected high-risk patients with aortic stenosis, *Circulation* 116: 755-763.

Webb, J. G., Altwegg, L., Boone, R. H., *et al.* (2009a). Transcatheter aortic valve implantation: impact on clinical and valve-related outcomes, *Circulation* 119: 3009–3016.

Webb, J. G. (2009b). Coronary obstruction due to transcatheter valve implantation, *Catheter Cardiovasc Interv* 73: 973.

Webb, J. G., & Cribier, A. (2010). Percutaneous transarterial aortic valve implantations: what do we know? *Eur Heart J* 32(2): 140-147.

Wendt, D., Osswald, B., Thielmann, M., *et al.* (2010). The EuroSCORE - still helpful in patients undergoing isolated aortic valve replacement? *Interact Cardiovasc Thorac Surg* 10: 239-244.

Willson, A., & Webb, J. G. (2011). Transcatheter treatment approaches for aortic valve disease, *Int J Cardiovasc Imaging* epub ahead of print 24th February 2011.

Wynne-Jones, K., Jackson, M., Grotte, G., & Bridgewater, B, on behalf of the North West Regional Cardiac Surgery Audit Steering Group (2000). Limitations of the Parsonnet score for measuring risk stratification in the north west of England, *Heart*, 84: 71-78.

Ye, J., Cheung, A., Lichtenstein, S. V., *et al.* (2006). Transapical aortic valve implantation in humans, *J Thorac Cardiovasc Surg* 131: 1194-1196.

Ye, J., Cheung, A., Lichtenstein, SV., *et al.* (2009). Transapical transcatheter aortic valve implantation: 1-year outcome in 26 patients, *J Thorac Cardiovasc Surg* 137: 167-173.

Zahn, R., Gerckens, U., Grube, E., *et al.* on behalf of the German Transcatheter Aortic Valve Interventions-Registry Investigators (2011). Transcatheter aortic valve implantation: first results from a multi-centre real-world registry, *Eur Heart J* 32: 198-204.

Zegdi, R., Ciobotaru, V., Noghin, M., *et al.* (2008). Is it reasonable to treat all calcified stenotic aortic valves with a valved stent? Results form a human anatomic study in adults, *J Am Coll Cardiol* 51: 579-584.

Zierer, A., Wimmer-Greinecker, G., Martens, S., Moritz, A., & Doss, M (2008). The transapical approach for aortic valve implantation, *J Thorac Cardiovasc Surg* 136: 948-953.

Zierer, A., Wimmer-Greinecker, G., Martens, S., Moritz, A., & Doss, M (2009). Is transapical aortic valve implantation really less invasive than minimally invasive aortic valve replacement? *J Thorac Cardiovasc Surg* 138(5): 1067–1072.

13

Image-Guided Transcatheter Aortic Valve Implantation Assistance System

Mohamed Esmail Karar[1], David Holzhey[2], Matthias John[3], Ardawan Rastan[2], Friedrich-Wilhelm Mohr[2] and Oliver Burgert[1]
[1]*Innovation Center Computer Assisted Surgery (ICCAS), University of Leipzig*
[2]*Department of Cardiac Surgery, Heart Center, University of Leipzig*
[3]*Siemens AG, Healthcare Sector, Forchheim*
Germany

1. Introduction

Transcatheter aortic valve implantation (TAVI) is a recently developed surgical technique to treat symptomatic aortic valve stenosis in elderly and high-risk patients (Eltchaninoff et al., 2008; Ferrari & von Segesser, 2010). Compared to the standard aortic valve replacement surgery, the TAVI limits the surgical access to either a small minithoracotomy (transapical TAVI) or femoral approach (transfemoral TAVI) causing minimal tissue trauma. Independently of the TAVI approach it can be performed on the beating heart without cardiopulmonary bypass support (Walther et al., 2009). Recovery time may be reduced and the patient can eventually return to normal activity more quickly. More than 70,000 transcatheter valve implantations have been performed worldwide (Valle-Fernández et al., 2010).

The TAVI is done via a retrograde (transfemoral, transaxillary) or antegrade (transapical) approach (Singh et al., 2008). The main advantage of the transapical TAVI technique is the direct access to the aortic valve which eliminates the need for a large peripheral vascular access in patients with peripheral vascular disease, small tortuous vasculature, a history of major vascular complications, or previous vascular interventions (Singh et al., 2008).

In transapical TAVI (Walther et al., 2009), a stented valve bioprosthesis that is temporarily crimped upon a balloon catheter, is inserted through the apex into the aortic root via a left anterolateral minithoracotomy. For that the apex of the left ventricle is punctured with a needle, and after balloon valvuloplasty the aortic valve prosthesis (AVP) is positioned within the stenotic aortic valve using guide wire techniques. After reaching the correct position, the stented AVP is deployed by an inflatable balloon to reach its final diameter, thus fixing the prosthesis to the aortic annulus (Fig. 1a).

The Edwards SAPIEN™ prosthesis (Edwards Lifesciences Inc, Irvine, CA, USA) is the most commonly used prosthesis for TAVI in several European countries and the only one approved for transapical approach so far (Thomas et al., 2010). Thus the Edwards SAPIEN™ prosthesis has been used in this study. It consists of three bovine pericardial cusps mounted into a stainless-steel balloon-expandable stent (Fig. 1b).

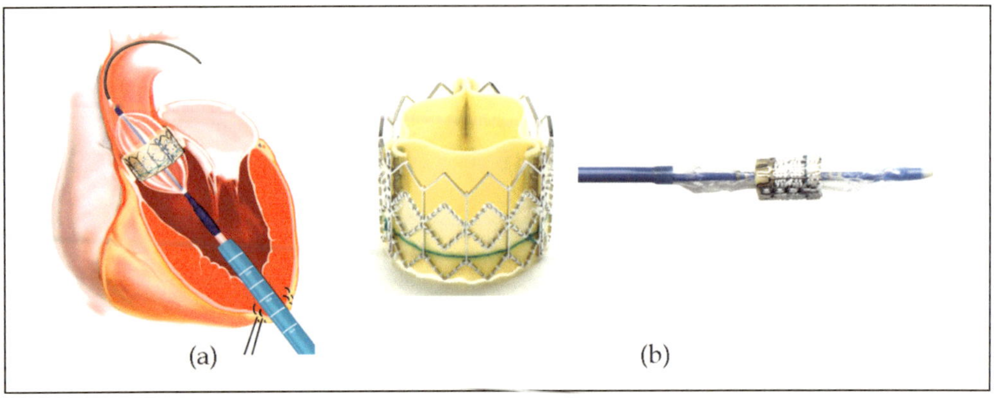

Fig. 1. Transcathete aortic valve implantation. (a) Schematic view of the transapical approach. (b) Edwards SPAIEN™ prosthesis and the balloon-based delivery system

Medical imaging technology, including computed tomography (CT), X-ray fluoroscopy, magnet resonance imaging (MRI), and echocardiography, is needed to provide accurate information on the stenotic valve and to choose the appropriate prosthetic valve size for TAVI procedures (Kaleschke et al., 2010; Van de Veire, 2010). Live two-dimensional (2D) X-ray fluoroscopy guidance is mostly used during the intervention, in order to determine proper valve positioning and the plane of alignment of the aortic valve cusps with supplemental echocardiography confirmation (Walther et al., 2009).

X-ray angiography and fluoroscopy C-arm imaging system (Siemens AG, Healthcare Sector, Forchheim, Germany) is recently used to capture both intraoperative three-dimensional (3D) C-arm CT images and live 2D fluoroscopic image sequences (Kempfert et al., 2009). At the begin of the surgical procedure, the physician uses the interventional C-arm imaging system to reconstruct a 3D CT image of the aortic root under a short episode of rapid ventricular pacing (RVP) from acquired rotational 2D image sequences by applying 75 ml diluted contrast agent of 200° over 5 seconds (Fig. 2).

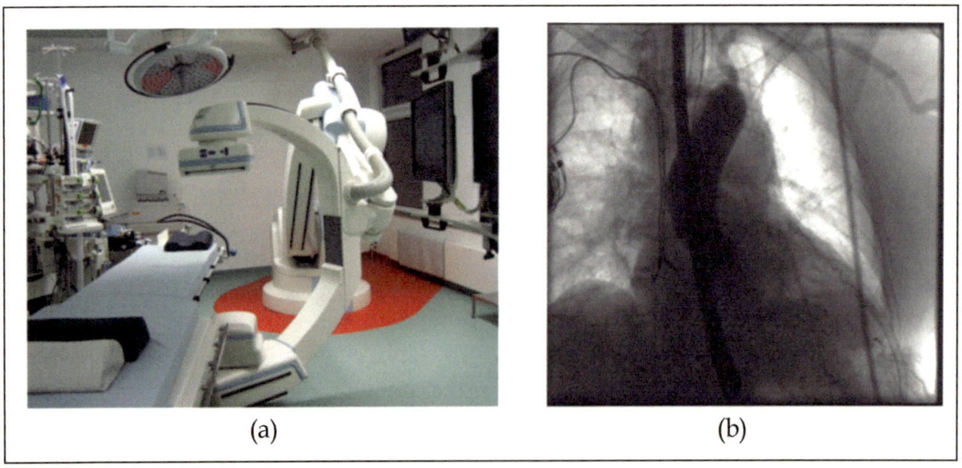

Fig. 2. (a) Angiography and fluoroscopy C-arm system (Artis Zeego, Siemens AG, Healthcare Sector, Forchheim, Germany). (b) Rotational angiographic scan such that 75 ml diluted contrast agent is injected into the aortic root, followed by 5 seconds run under rapid ventricular pacing

In the presence of contrast agent, different fluoroscopic projections are used to visualize the aortic root and the aortic annulus in a perpendicular view (Fig. 3a). The ventricular-aortic angle can only be estimated in the right anterior oblique (RAO) view, because the left anterior oblique (LAO) view looks at this angulation en face. The annular plane is sometimes visible depending on the amount of annular calcification, but often only indirect clues are provided by the position of a pigtail catheter. The pigtail catheter should be placed at the bottom of a coronary sinus. Information from planning CT or intraoperative C-arm CT images can be used to calculate the best possible fluoroscopic view for a coaxial implantation and automatically adjust the angulation of the C-arm without giving additional contrast agent. However, the following valve adjustment in the aortic annulus requires additional contrast injections and radiation exposure. When valve positioning is considered correct, the balloon-expandable prosthesis is released to replace the diseased valve under RVP as shown in Fig. 3b. After the implantation, the assessment of implanted AVP is also done using fluoroscopy guidance (Fig. 3c).

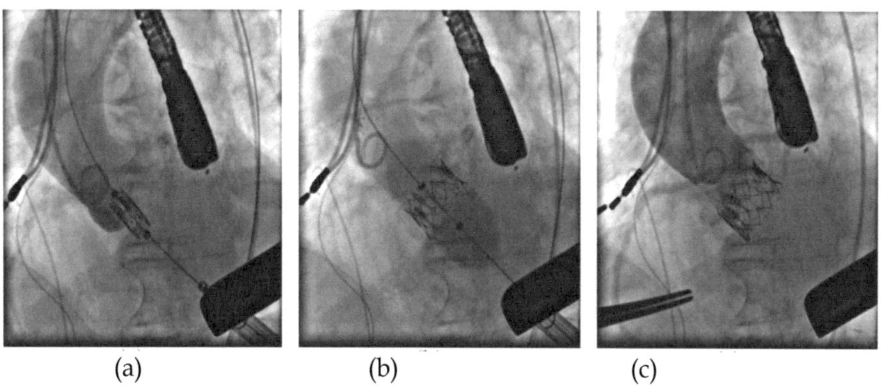

Fig. 3. 2D Fluoroscopy guidance during the transapical TAVI. (a) Valve positioning. (b) Valve implantation. (c) Final assessment after valve implantation

Exact valve placement is crucial during the intervention, because complications can arise from a misplaced valve, which are difficult to manage and requires different bailout strategies. These complications have been reported (Yan et al., 2010) such as high-degree atrioventricular (AV) block (10-30%), paravalvular leak (4-35%), coronary ostia occlusion (0.5-1%), aortic dissection (0-4%), cardiac tamponade (1-9%). A malposition of the prosthesis rarely occurs, however, 5.3% incidence (9/170) patients was reported (Al Ali et al., 2008). The 30-day mortality of the TAVI in Europe is 5-10 % (Thomas et al., 2010; Walther et al., 2010). Also, the contrast of fluoroscopic images is generally limited to minimize the radiation exposure for the patient and the physician. The contrast agent is injected to visualize the aortic root, valve annulus, and coronary ostia in few seconds. The amount of contrast injections must be minimized to avoid renal insufficiencies in high-risk elderly patients.

Only few previous studies deal with image-guided planning and intraoperative support of the TAVI procedure. Our research group has previously proposed a guidance system including a planning system (Gessat et al., 2009) and tracking the AVP in fluoroscopic image sequences (Karar et al., 2009, 2010). Siemens has prototypically equipped the interventional

C-arm with a system for automatic segmentation and overlay of aortic root volume and landmarks on 2D fluoroscopic images, but without motion correction (John et al., 2010). Robotic systems have been developed for the TAVI using intraoperative MRI guidance (Li et al., 2008, 2011). Real-time 3D transesophageal (TEE) is recently presented for guiding the TAVI (Siegel et al., 2011).

In order to potentially overcome the current difficulties associated with the TAVI under 2D fluoroscopy guidance, we present a new system that integrates a 3D aortic mesh model and landmarks form intraoperative C-arm CT images with tracking the prosthesis in live fluoroscopic images. The developed system is mainly based on image processing and visualization techniques, avoiding the use of additional implanted radiopaque markers or external tracking systems which may complicate the surgical workflow. Moreover, our system determines automatically a target area of implantation to allow the physician to identify the optimal position of the AVP without further contrast injections.

2. System overview

To assist the TAVI, our image-guided system is connected with the fluoroscopy C-arm system as depicted in Fig. 4. 2D fluoroscopic image sequences and a 3D geometrical mesh

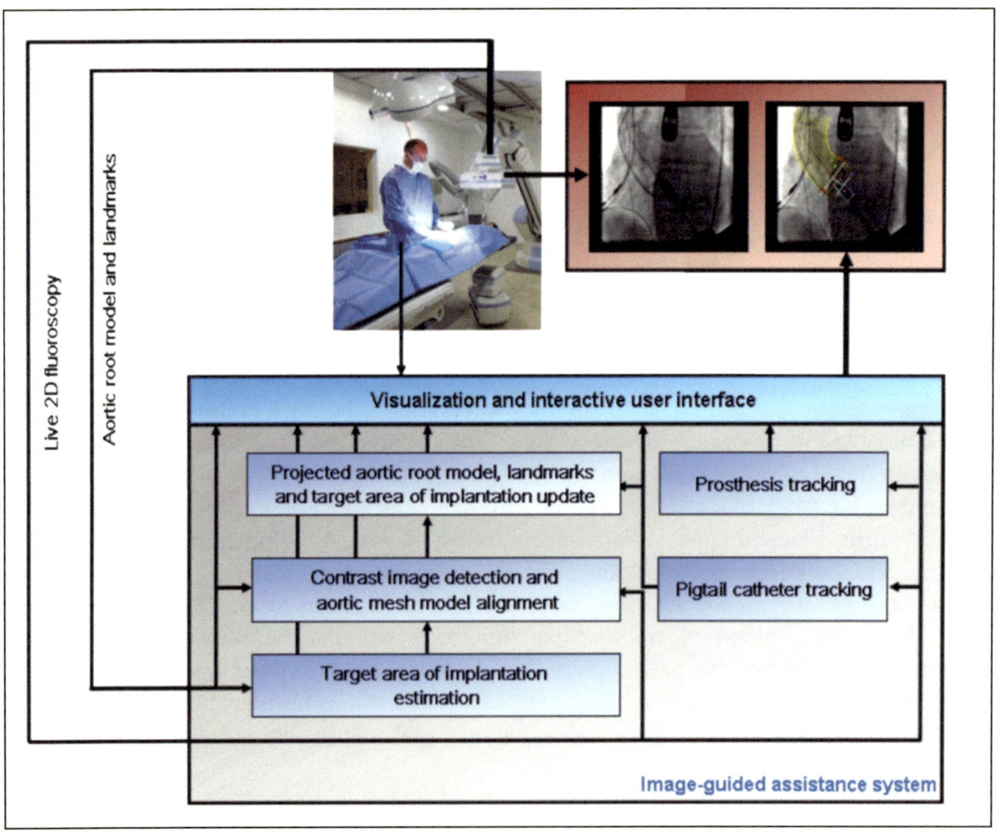

Fig. 4. Block diagram of the developed assistance system connected with the interventional C-arm imaging system for guiding the TAVI

model of the aortic root together with valve landmarks are acquired from the interventional C-arm system. A target area of valve implantation is automatically estimated inside the 3D mesh model based on the best experience and knowledge of the physician. The overlaid aortic mesh model, landmarks, and estimated target area of implantation are updated onto 2D fluoroscopic images by approximating the translational motion of the aortic root without contrast injections from the pigtail catheter motion. In parallel, the prosthesis is also tracked to assist the positioning of AVP within the clinical accepted margins.

2.1 Target area of implantation estimation

The 3D geometrical mesh model of the aortic root and eight anatomical landmarks of the stenotic valve are generated based on an automatic segmentation of the aortic root in intraoperative C-arm CT images (Zheng et al., 2010). The eight landmark points are the two points of coronary ostia [left and right], the three points of commissures [left, right, and non-coronary], and the three lowest points (hinge points) of each leaflet cusp [left, right, and non-coronary]

The correct position of the AVP should be 1/3 to 1/2 of its length above and perpendicular to the aortic annulus (Walther et al., 2009). In this study, the target area of valve implantation is automatically defined by two embedded circles of the annulus and ostia planes with the normal center line to the annulus (Gessat et al., 2009). Fig. 5a shows the aortic mesh model, landmarks and estimated target area of implantation.

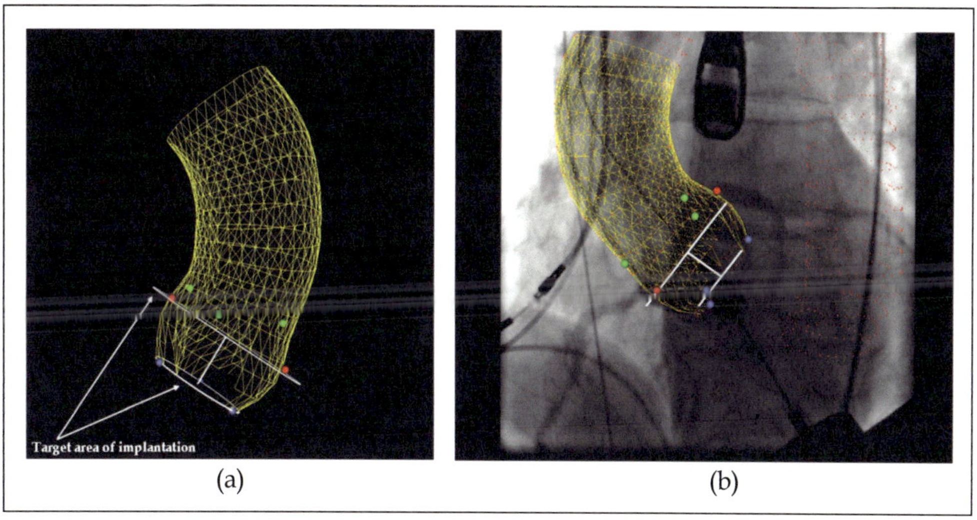

Fig. 5. (a) 3D model of the aortic root (yellow meshes) and valve landmarks as colored points; namely coronary ostia (red), commissures (green) and lowest points of the leaflets cusps (blue) and estimated target area of the valve implantation (white). (b) Alignment of the projected model and landmarks with a contrast image

2.2 Contrast image detection and aortic mesh model alignment

Automatic detection of contrast agent in a fluoroscopic image is used to initialize the synchronized mesh model tracking with aortic root motion in interventional image sequences. Enhanced contrasted aortic root shows up dark pixels in the entire aorta roadmap if the contrast agent is injected. By analyzing the histogram and using the 98-percentile as a

threshold measure of contrast agent, the enhanced contrast image is automatically detected after learning histogram feature curve of the first 20 images of sequence without contrast agent (Condurache et al., 2004).
The aortic mesh model, valve landmarks and target area of implantation are projected to the fluoroscopic image plane using the transformation matrix of interventional C-arm imaging system. They are manually aligned to the contrast image as shown in Fig. 5b.

2.3 Pigtail catheter tracking for approximating aortic root motion

Fluoroscopic images are pre-processed using a 2-D Gabor filter (Kong et al., 2003), in order to reduce the image noise and adjust intensities within the sequence while preserving the important pigtail features.
The position of the pigtail catheter is detected in all image sequences using the template matching approach (Briechle & Hanebeck, 2001). The template image of the pigtail catheter t is manually defined on the first image of sequence. A region of interest (ROI) of the image is defined to reduce the processing time and increase the algorithm robustness. In practice, the size of the ROI is 2.5 times the size of the template image and is constant for all images of each sequence.
In this approach, I(x,y) denotes the intensity of a preprocessed ROI image of the size $S_x \times S_y$ at point (x, y), $x \in \{0, ..., S_x\text{-}1\}$, $y \in \{0, ..., S_y\text{-}1\}$ and the template image t of the size $s_x \times s_y$. The position of catheter is determined by a pixelwise comparison of the ROI image with the target window based on the computing of fast normalized cross correlation coefficient γ at each point (u, v) for ROI and template images. Eq. 1 gives the definition of γ. $\bar{i}_{u,v}$ and $\bar{t}$ are the mean brightness values within the ROI and the template image respectively. The normalized maximal value γ_{max} at the point (u, v) in the current ROI image defines the best matching location of the template.

$$\gamma(u,v) = \frac{\sum_{x,y}[I(x,y) - \bar{i}_{u,v}][t(x-u,y-v) - \bar{t}]}{\sqrt{\sum_{x,y}[I(x,y) - \bar{i}_{u,v}]^2 \sum_{x,y}[t(x-u,y-v) - \bar{t}]^2}} \quad (1)$$

The global translational motion of aortic mesh model is then updated during the intervention by calculating the updated displacement of pigtail catheter between two frames such that the difference between the matching locations of template in one frame and the corresponding template position in the other frame defines the 2D displacement of the pigtail catheter.
We assumed that the tracking of the aortic mesh model could be automatically stopped in the images with or without contrast injections if the best matching value of γ_{max} is less than 50%, avoiding the failure of template-based tracking algorithm.

2.4 Prosthesis tracking

Real-time tracking of the AVP is performed by using template matching approach to estimate the position of the AVP and a shape model of the prosthesis to extract the corner points of the AVP in fluoroscopic image sequences (Karar et al., 2010). To start the AVP tracking procedure, an initialization step is performed by manually defining the corner points of the prosthesis in the first image of sequence to provide the required algorithm parameters which are prosthesis model parameters and a target window including the template image of the AVP.

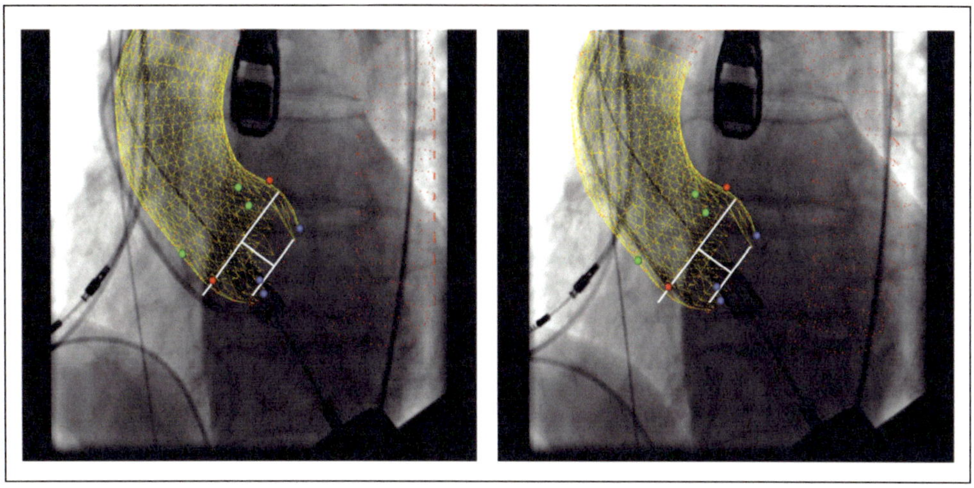

Fig. 6. Overlay of aortic mesh model, landmarks and target area of implantation onto a fluoroscopic image of sequence without updating (a) and with updating via pigtail catheter tracking (b)

The geometrical parameters of the model of the prosthesis are estimated. Fig. 7a shows the AVP model which is defined as a semi-rectangle with the height h. The upper and lower widths are w_1 and w_2 respectively. Corner points are noted p_1, p_2, p_3, and p_4. The prosthesis's angle φ is defined between the two segments (p_1-p_2) and (p_1-p_4). The angle θ between (p_c-p_1) and the horizontal line represents the orientation of the prosthesis in the current image. The measures h, w_1, w_2 and φ are assumed to be constant for all images in the sequence and just before inflating the balloon to reach the prosthesis's final diameter.
The target window of the prosthesis image is automatically defined around AVP corner points such that the height and the width of the target window are $|p_{4y} - p_{2y}|$ and $|p_{3x} - p_{1x}|$ with one pixel offset to get the complete image of AVP respectively.
Similar to template-based tracking algorithm of pigtail catheter, the prosthesis template image is detected within all images of the sequence. We proposed using the prosthesis model (Fig. 7a) to perform AVP corner points localization as follows: The target window always shows the corner point p_1 of the prosthesis at the maximum x-coordinate value in the image plane which is detected by Canny filter edge detection (Canny, 1986).
In Fig. 7a, the angle θ in the current image i is determined between (p_c-p_1) line and the horizontal line. The prosthesis center p_c is obtained using template matching. The orientation difference $\Delta\theta_i$ represents the rotation angle of the prosthesis, calculated between the current orientation in a processed image θ_i and the initial orientation in the first image of sequence θ_1. The initial AVP orientation θ_1 is used as a reference orientation angle to minimize the distance errors of prosthesis tracking in the image sequences as follows:

$$\Delta\theta_i = \theta_i - \theta_1, \quad i = 2 \ldots n \tag{2}$$

Then the new positions of three corner points namely p_2, p_3 and p_4 are obtained by rotating the position of AVP model in the first image with $\Delta\theta_i$. Finally, the tracked prosthesis is displayed linking the four corner points on the current image of sequence (Fig. 7b).

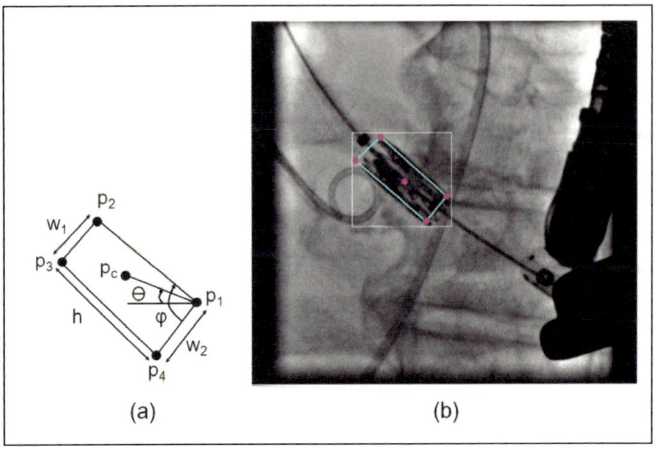

Fig. 7. (a) Prosthesis shape model. (b) Tracked prosthesis inside the target window onto a fluoroscopic image

2.5 Visualization and interactive user interface

An interactive graphical user interface (GUI) has been implemented to be integrated with the proposed method based on visual C++ programming language. Different views of projected mesh model, landmarks and target area of implantation are separately visualized to allow the physician to display only the required information for the prosthesis deployment (Fig. 8). Using the developed GUI, the localization errors of model projection as well as tracking of aortic mesh model and AVP can be also manually minimized if occur.

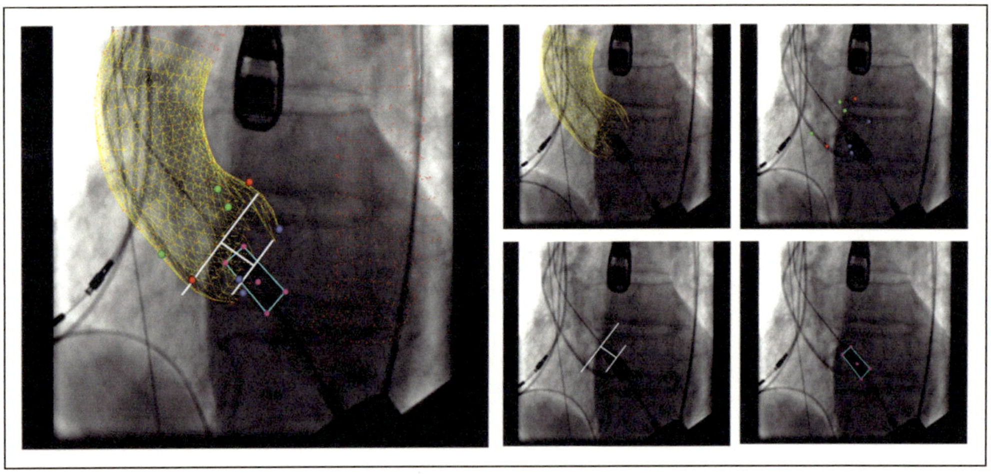

Fig. 8. Different visualization views of the projected aortic mesh model, landmarks, target area of implantation and tracked prosthesis onto a fluoroscopic image

The parameter values needed to compute the 3D-2D transformation matrix of the C-arm imaging system are imported from a fluoroscopic DICOM (Digital Imaging and Communications in medicine) file or given by the user. A template image of pigtail catheter and alignment of projected mesh model to the contrast image are manually defined before tracking of the catheter.

3. Experiments and evaluation

3.1 Experimental setup

We have tested the image-guided assistance system in a hybrid operating room at the Heart Center, University of Leipzig, Germany (Fig. 9). The hybrid operating room is a special operating room equipped with angiography and fluoroscopy C-arm system (Artis Zeego, Siemens AG, Healthcare Sector, Forchheim, Germany) and offering all surgical prerequisites such as sterile valve preparation before implantation, anaesthetic equipment, appropriate lighting, and the heart-lung machine as a backup to perform a safe TAVI procedure (Nollert & Wich, 2009; Pasic et al., 2010).
The assistance system is a PC (Intel® Core™ Quad CPU 2.4 GHz, 3.25 GB RAM) equipped with our guidance software that is able to capture live fluoroscopy video images via the Matrox Helios eA/XA frame grabber card. The Siemens C-arm system sends fluoroscopy images to our assistance system workstation over multi-mode optical fiber cables, DVI-D/VGA adapter, and a video-switcher. The captured fluoroscopic images are 1280x1024 pixels.
To start the experiment, 3D aortic mesh model and valve landmarks are reconstructed on a Siemens Workstation from the corresponding 3D DynaCT images and saved on an USB-stick as SEG (Society of Exploration Geophysicists) files to be read by the image-guided assistance system.

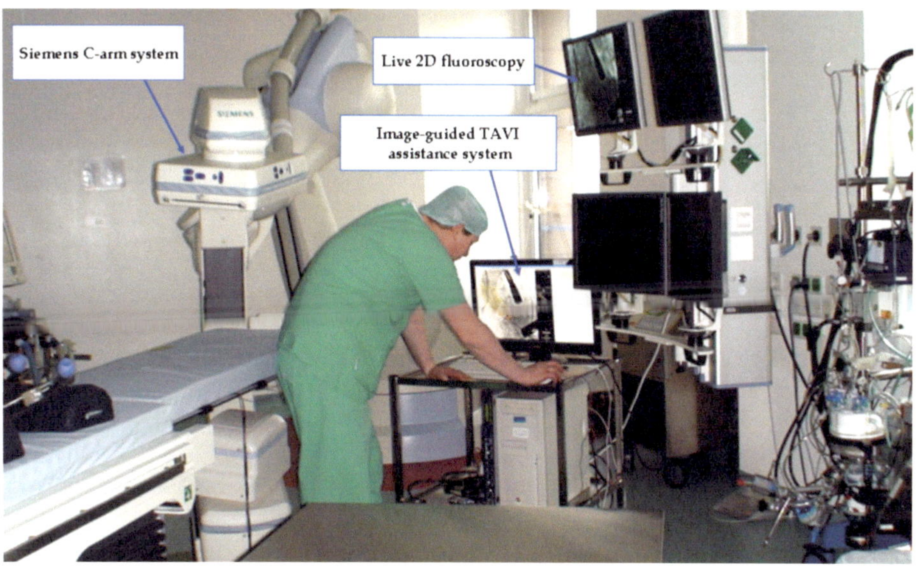

Fig. 9. Integration of image-guided TAVI assistance system in the hybrid operating room

3.2 Patient datasets and results

Experiments were retrospectively performed on ten patient datasets from clinical routine of the TAVI. Each patient dataset include a fluoroscopic image sequence and the related aortic mesh model with valve landmarks. The fluoroscopic sequences include 70-100 images per sequence with 512 × 512 to 1024 × 1024 pixels. The pixel size was approximately 0.2 mm. Fig. 10 shows assistance system results for a sample of three different datasets.

The initialization step for defining a template image of pigtail catheter, template image of the AVP, importing 3D aortic mesh model with landmarks including estimated target area of implantation and its alignment with detected contrast image varied between three to five minutes. The total computation time for fluoroscopic image processing algorithms was approximately 100 milliseconds per frame.

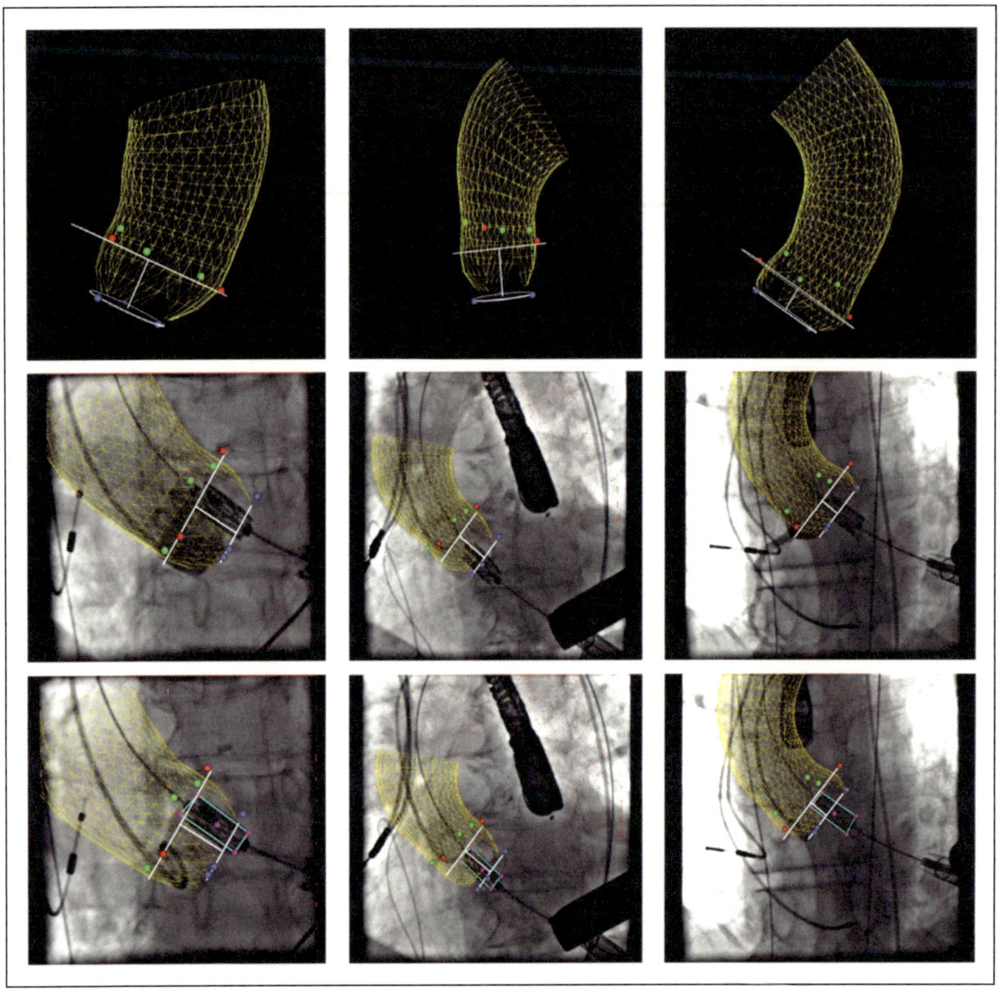

Fig. 10. Examples of the developed system results. First row: aortic mesh models with landmarks and estimated target area of implantation. Second row: Alignment of projected aortic mesh models with detected contrast images. Third row: Updating of visualized models based on tracked aortic pigtail catheter without contrast injections

3.3 Evaluation

3.3.1 Methods

The developed assistance system's guidance accuracy was determined by the tracking accuracy of both the pigtail catheter and the AVP. In each image of all tested datasets, the tracking accuracy was assessed by computing the absolute displacement errors between the automatically and manually located pigtail's template and two upper corner points of the prosthesis p_2 and p_3, because the upper side of prosthesis (p_2-p_3) must be positioned below the coronary ostia. For each image *i* of the sequence, the automatic localization target point (x_i^A, y_i^A) and manual localization target point (x_i^M, y_i^M) are used to compute the displacement error d_i. The absolute mean error d_{mean} ± standard deviation (SD) and maximum error d_{max} are also computed over n images of the sequence as:

$$d_i = \sqrt{(x_i^A - x_i^{M})^2 + (y_i^A - y_i^M)^2} \tag{3}$$

$$d_{mean} = \frac{\left(\sum_{i=1}^{n} d_i\right)}{n} \tag{4}$$

$$d_{max} = \max_i |d_i| \tag{5}$$

3.3.2 Results

Figure 11 shows the evaluation results of the tracked pigtail catheter for ten fluoroscopic image sequences, excluding the images with high dose contrast injections (3-10 images per each sequence) which temporarily switch off the tracking procedure of the pigtail catheter. Seq . 1 shows relatively high displacement errors d_{mean} = 1.73 ± 0.86 mm and d_{max} = 4.37 mm because the pigtail catheter had been slightly repositioned by the physician, Seq. 7 and Seq. 8 present the highest maximum displacement errors 4.65 mm and 4.84 mm respectively. However, all tested fluoroscopic images showed that the maximum and mean displacement errors of the pigtail tracking were less than 5.0 mm for one to three images per each sequence only and less than 2.0 mm respectively. These error values remain within the clinical accepted range.

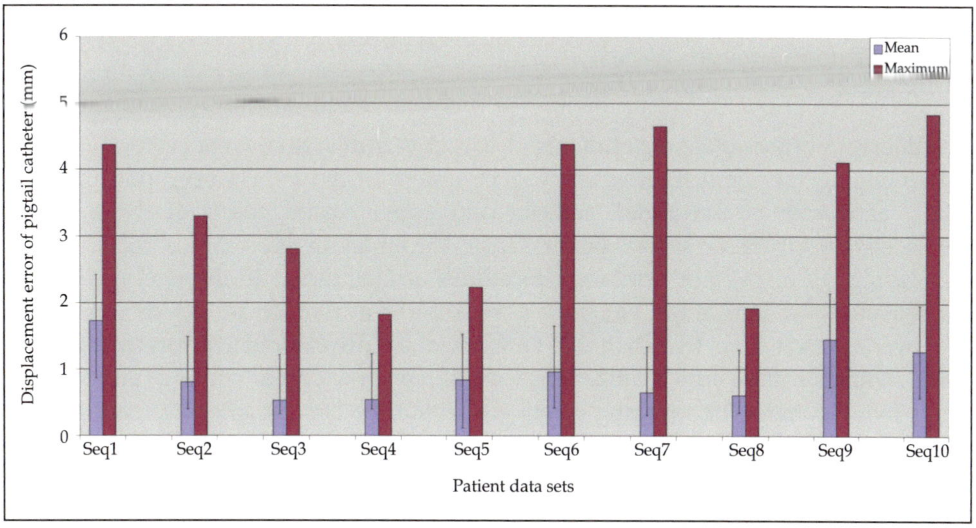

Fig. 11. Evaluation tracking results of the pigtail catheter for ten fluoroscopic image sequences. The maximum errors are less than 5.0 mm only for one to three images per sequence, while the absolute mean errors are less than 2.0 mm for all tested fluoroscopic images

The displacement errors of the prosthesis corner points p_2 and p_3 are depicted in Fig. 12. The mean errors of p_2 and p_3 were approximately similar and varied from 0.26 ± 0.05 to 0.42 ± 0.06 mm. Because the images of Seq. 1 and Seq. 7 have been captured at low contrast agent doses in the images, the lowest localization errors were obtained ($d_{max} \leq 0.3$ mm). The maximum localization error of p_2 and p_3 was less than 0.5 mm in all tested image sequences.

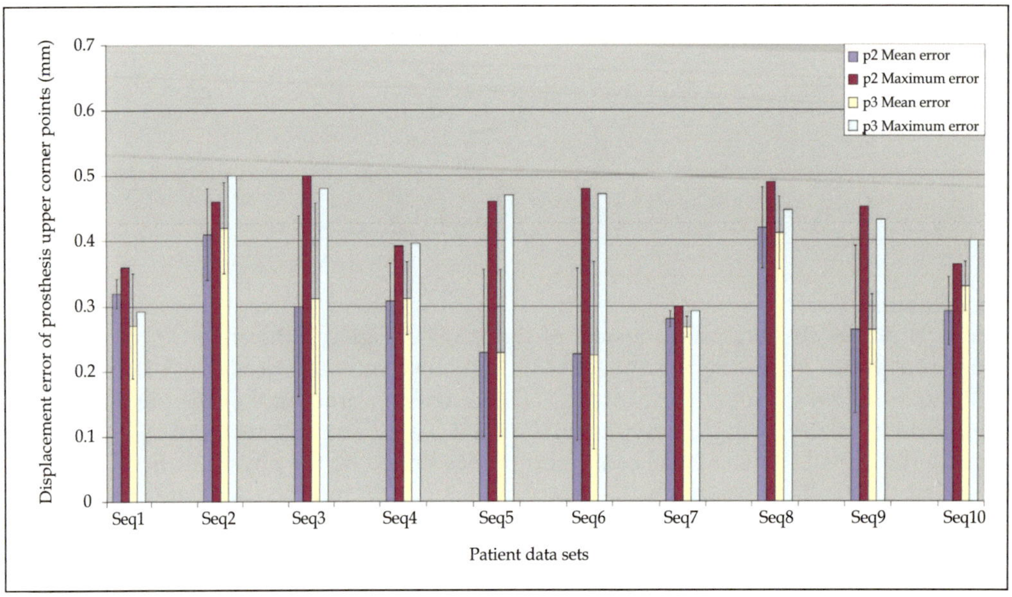

Fig. 12. Evaluation tracking results of two upper corner points of the prosthesis p_2 and p_3. The maximum displacement errors of two corner points p_2 and p_3 are less than 0.5 mm in all tested fluoroscopic images

4. Discussion

For validation purposes, the experiments of our assistance system were performed using a Siemens angiography and fluoroscopy C-arm system in the hybrid operating room. The tracking accuracies of the pigtail catheter and upper corner points of the AVP were determined to evaluate the system performance. The failure in one image of sequence could occur during template-based tracking procedures and corrected in the next image of the same sequence. As depicted in Fig. 11 and Fig. 12, the evaluation results showed that the mean overlay errors are less than 2.0 mm based on displacement errors of the pigtail catheter, while the maximum localization errors of the upper corner points p_2 and p_3 of AVP are less than 0.5 mm. The resulting errors are within the clinical accepted margins for all tested fluoroscopic images.

We demonstrated that a fast approach to track successfully the pigtail catheter without contrast agent injection and the prosthesis with using a shape model, see Fig. 7. The pigtail catheter tracking is only stopped during the contrast injection, because the overlay is not required and should be switch off if the contrast agent appears in fluoroscopic images (Condurache et al., 2004). For the AVP tracking, the prosthesis detection can be affected by

possible rotation of the prosthesis ($\Delta\theta_i$) and the presence of contrast agent. But the template matching algorithm is still robust enough in finding the correct position of AVP in all tested fluoroscopic images.
In summary, our image-guided TAVI assistance system has been developed to assist the positioning of the AVP under live 2D fluoroscopy guidance. To allow continuous visualization of diseased valve without further contrast injections, the projected 3D aortic root mesh model and landmarks from intraoperative C-arm CT images are overlaid and updated onto fluoroscopic images according to the aortic root motion via tracking the pigtail catheter. Moreover, the AVP is tracked to align with the estimated target area of implantation. Interactive user interface is integrated with the image-guided TAVI assistance system to ensure the safe guidance procedures of the TAVI.

5. Conclusion

The developed fluoroscopy-guided TAVI assistance system aims to guide the physician to accurately define the exact position of the AVP. Only a minimal user-interaction is required for initializing the image processing algorithms and visually correcting possible displacement errors of projected aortic shape model and AVP during the intervention if needed. In addition to the transapical TAVI discussed here, the assistance system can be also applied for the transfemoral approach. Now, the developed assistance system is undergoing evaluation during real-time TAVI intervention.

6. Acknowledgement

The authors would like to thank Alois Nöttling and Stefan Ammon for the technical support to obtain the experimental imaging data. The authors also thank Petra Bergmann, Frank Wüst, and Michael Heinze from Edwards Lifesciences Inc. for providing the images of Edwards-SPAIEN prosthesis for this study. We gratefully thank Prof. Volkmar Falk from University Hospital Zurich and Dr. Claire Chalopin from Innovation Ceneter Computer Assisted Surgery (ICCAS) for their comments and fruitful discussions. This work is supported by German Academic Exchange Service (DAAD) in cooperation with the Egyptian Supreme Council of Universities (ESCU) under scholarship number A0690520. This work is partially funded by Siemens Healthcare AG, Forchheim, Germany.

7. References

Al Ali, A. M., Altwegg, L., Horlick, E. M., Feindel, C., Thompson, C. R., Cheung, A., Carere, R. G., Humphries, K., Ye, J., Masson, J. B. & Webb, J. G. (2008). Prevention and Management of Transcatheter Balloon-Expandable Aortic Valve Malposition. *Catheter Cardiovasc Interv*, Vol.72, No.4, (October 2008), pp. 573-578, DOI 10.1002/ccd.21667

Briechle, K. & Hanebeck, U. D (2001). Template Matching Using Fast Normalized Cross Correlation. *Proceedings of SPIE 2001 International Conference on Optical Pattern Recognition XII*, Vol.4387, pp. 95-102, DOI 10.1117/12.421129, Orlando, Florida, USA, 19 April, 2001

Canny, J. (1986). A Computational Approach to Edge Detection. *IEEE Trans. Pattern Anal. Mach. Intell.*, Vol.8, No.6, (November 1986), pp. 679-698, ISSN 0162-8828

Condurache, A. P., Aach, T., Eck, K. & Bredno, J. (2004). Fast Detection and Processing of Arbitrary Contrast Agent Injections in Coronary Angiography and Fluoroscopy. *Presented at Bildverarbeitung für die Medizin 2004 (Algorithmen, Systeme, Anwendungen)*, pp. 5-9, ISBN 978-3-540-21059-7, Berlin, Germany, March 29-30, 2004

Eltchaninoff, H., Zajarias, A., Tron, C., Litzler, P. Y., Baala, B., Godin, M., Bessou, J. P. & Cribier, A. (2008). Transcatheter Aortic Valve Implantation: Technical Aspects, Results and Indications. *Arch Cardiovasc Dis*, Vol.101, No.2, (February 2008), pp. 126-132, ISSN 1875-2136

Ferrari, E. & von Segesser, L. K. (2010). Transcatheter Aortic Valve Implantation (TAVI): State of the Art Techniques and Future Perspectives. *Swiss Med Wkly*, Vol. 140, (December 2010), pp. w13127, ISSN 0036-7672

Gessat, M., Merk, D. R., Falk, V., Walther, T., Jacobs, S., Nottling, A. & Burgert, O. (2009). A Planning System for Transapical Aortic Valve Implantation. *Proceedings of SPIE Medical Imaging 2009: Visualization, Image-Guided Procedures, and Modeling*, Vol.7261, pp. 72611E, DOI 10.1117/12.810270, Orlando, Florida, USA, February 8, 2009

John, M., Liao, R., Zheng, Y., Nottling, A., Boese, J., Kirschstein, U., Kempfert, J. & Walther, T. (2010). System to Guide Transcatheter Aortic Valve Implantations Based on Interventional C-arm CT Imaging. *Med Image Comput Comput Assist Interv*, Vol. 13, No. Pt 1, (2010), pp. 375-382, DOI 10.1007/978-3-642-15705-9_46

Kaleschke, G., Seifarth, H., Kerckhoff, G., Reinecke, H. & Baumgartner, H. (2010). Imaging Decision-Making for Transfemoral or Transapical Approach of Transcatheter Aortic Valve Implantation. *EuroIntervention : journal of EuroPCR in collaboration with the Working Group on Interventional Cardiology of the European Society of Cardiology*, Vo. 6, Suppl. G, (June 2010), pp. G20-27, ISSN 1774-024X

Karar, M. E., Gessat, M., Walther, T., Falk, V. & Burgert, O. (2009). Towards A New Image Guidance System for Assisting Transapical Minimally Invasive Aortic Valve Implantation. *Conf Proc IEEE Eng Med Biol Soc* 2009, pp. 3645-3648, Minneapolis, Minnesota, USA, Septemper 3-6, 2009, ISSN 1557-170X

Karar, M. E., Merk, D. R., Chalopin, C., Walther, T., Falk, V. & Burgert, O. (2010). Aortic Valve Prosthesis Tracking for Transapical Aortic Valve Implantation. *Int J Comput Assist Radiol Surg*. (September 2010), pp. 1-8, ISSN 1861-6410

Kempfert, J., Falk, V., Schuler, G., Linke, A., Merk, D., Mohr, F. W. & Walther, T. (2009). Dyna-CT During Minimally Invasive Off-Pump Transapical Aortic Valve Implantation. *Ann Thorac Surg*, Vol. 88, No. 6, (December 2009), pp. 2041, ISSN 0003-4975

Kong, W. K., Zhang, D. & Li, W. (2003). Palmprint Feature Extraction Using 2-D Gabor Filters. *Pattern Recognition*, Vol. 36, No. 10, (October 2003), pp. 2339-2347, ISSN 0031-3203

Li, M., Kapoor, A., Mazilu, D. & Horvath, K. A. (2011). Pneumatic Actuated Robotic Assistant System for Aortic Valve Replacement Under MRI Guidance. *Biomedical*

Engineering, IEEE Transactions on, Vol. 58, No. 2, (January 2011), pp. 443-451, ISSN 0018-9294

Li, M., Mazilu, D. & Horvath, K. (2008). Robotic System for Transapical Aortic Valve Replacement with MRI Guidance. *Medical Image Computing and Computer-Assisted Intervention.* Vol. 5242, (2008), pp. 476-484, DOI: 10.1007/978-3-540-85990-1_57

Nollert, G. & Wich, S. (2009). Planning A Cardiovascular Hybrid Operating Room: The Technical Point of View. *The heart surgery forum*, Vol.12, No. 3, (June 2009), pp. E125-130, ISSN 1098-3511

Pasic, M., Unbehaun, A., Dreysse, S., Drews, T., Buz, S., Kukucka, M., Mladenow, A., Gromann, T. & Hetzer, R. (2010). Transapical Aortic Valve Implantation in 175 Consecutive Patients: Excellent Outcome in Very High-Risk Patients. *Journal of the American College of Cardiology*, Vol. 56, No.10, (August 2010), pp. 813-20, ISSN 0735-1097

Siegel, R., Luo, H. & Biner, S. (2011). Transcatheter Valve Repair/Implantation. *The International Journal of Cardiovascular Imaging (formerly Cardiac Imaging)*, pp. 1-13, ISSN 1569-5794

Singh, I. M., Shishehbor, M. H., Christofferson, R. D., Tuzcu, E. M. & Kapadia, S. R. (2008). Percutaneous Treatment of Aortic Valve Stenosis. *Cleveland Clinic journal of medicine*, Vol.75, No.11, (November 2008), pp. 805-812, DOI 10.3949/ccjm.75.11.805

Thomas, M., Schymik, G., Walther, T., Himbert, D., Lefevre, T., Treede, H., Eggebrecht, H., Rubino, P., Michev, I., Lange, R., Anderson, W. N. & Wendler, O. (2010). Thirty-Day Results of the SAPIEN Aortic Bioprosthesis European Outcome (SOURCE) Registry: A European Registry of Transcatheter Aortic Valve Implantation Using the Edwards SAPIEN Valve. *Circulation*, Vol. 122, No.1, (July 2010), pp. 62-69, DOI 10.1161/circulationaha.109.907402

Valle-Fernández, R. d., Martinez, C. A. & Ruiz, C. E. (2010). Transcatheter Aortic Valve Implantation. *Cardiology Clinics*, Vol.28, No.1, (February 2010), pp. 155-168, ISSN 0733-8651

Van de Veire, N. (2010). Imaging to Guide Transcatheter Aortic Valve Implantation. *Journal of Echocardiography*, Vol. 8, No.1, (March 2010), pp. 1-6, ISSN 1349-0222

Walther, T., Dewey, T., Borger, M. A., Kempfert, J., Linke, A., Becht, R., Falk, V., Schuler, G., Mohr, F. W. & Mack, M. (2009). Transapical Aortic Valve Implantation: Step by Step. *Ann Thorac Surg*, Vol. 87, No. 1, pp. 276-83, ISSN 0003-4975

Walther, T., Schuler, G., Borger, M. A., Kempfert, J., Seeburger, J., Rückert, Y., Ender, J., Linke, A., Scholz, M., Falk, V. & Mohr, F. W. (2010). Transapical Aortic Valve Implantation in 100 Consecutive Patients: Comparison to Propensity-Matched Conventional Aortic Valve Replacement. *European Heart Journal*, Vol.31, No.11, (January 2009), pp. 1398-1403, DOI 10.1093/eurheartj/ehq060

Yan, T. D., Cao, C., Martens-Nielsen, J., Padang, R., Ng, M., Vallely, M. P. & Bannon, P. G. (2010). Transcatheter Aortic Valve Implantation for High-Risk Patients with Severe Aortic Stenosis: A Systematic Review. *The Journal of thoracic and cardiovascular surgery*, Vol.139, No.6, (Junary 2010)pp. 1519-28, ISSN 0022-5223

Zheng, Y., John, M., Liao, R., Boese, J., Kirschstein, U., Georgescu, B., Zhou, S. K., Kempfert, J., Walther, T., Brockmann, G. & Comaniciu, D. (2010). Automatic Aorta Segmentation and Valve Landmark Detection in C-arm CT: Application to Aortic Valve Implantation. *Med Image Comput Comput Assist Interv*, Vol. 13, No. Pt 1, pp. 476-83, DOI 10.1007/978-3-642-15705-9_46

Part 7

Congenital Anomalies of the Aortic Valve

14

Unicuspid Aortic Valve

Venkata Thota and Farouk Mookadam
Mayo Clinic College of Medicine, Scottsdale, AZ
USA

1. Introduction

Unicuspid aortic valve was first described more than half a century ago (Edwards, 1958). Although reported infrequently, the natural history of unicuspid aortic valve is poorly understood. Developmental abnormalities of aortic valve cusps in decreasing order of frequency include bicuspid (0.9%-1.3%), unicuspid (0.02%), quadricuspid (0.008%- 0.043%), and pentacupsid aortic valves (Cemri, 2000). Decreasing cusp number in the congenitally abnormal aortic valve has shown increasing male predilection, earlier valve failure and aggressive pathological changes compared to normal tricuspid aortic valve (Collins MJ, 2008).

2. Embryology

The normal aortic valve consists of three valve cusps, sinuses and coaptations (Angelini, 1989). During the embryological development, the bulbous cordis elongates and forms the proximal conus and distal truncus arteriosus. This initial single channel bifurcates into two separate trunks, namely, the aortic and pulmonary trunks by two spiral truncoconal ridges, derived from neural crest mesoderm. Simultaneous to this, cardiac mesoderm and cranial neural crest derivatives grow into the two separate lumens forming 3 leaflets for each trunk. These three leaflet structures will constitute the future aortic and pulmonary valves (Carlson, 1999). Abnormalities in the growth of this mesoderm into the lumen to form leaflets are believed to result congenital aortic valvular abnormalities. During the same time, out of the many buds which arise from the coronary sinuses of the aorta, generally only two buds establish a connection with the epicardial tree to form future coronary arteries. These developmental spatial associations can explain the frequent concurrence of abnormalities between the aortic valve and coronary arteries.

Two sub-types of UAV have been described. One is the pinhole shaped acommissural UAV and the second being the slit shaped unicommissural UAV. While the pinhole-shaped UAV presents early in infancy with severe aortic stenosis, the slit-shaped UAV presents relatively later in adults with a less aggressive course. Theoretically, if the leaflet mesoderm grows in circumferentially from annulus it results in pin-hole shaped UAV and if it grows in with two coaptation points, it results in the slit-shaped unicommisural UAV. (Fig. 1)

The association of UAV with various coronary artery anomalies, patent ductus arteriosus, aortic aneurysms and coarctation of aorta suggests a common abnormal embryological development. Temporal association of the aortic leaflet evolution with coronary artery development from sinuses of valsalva implies similar embryological derangements.

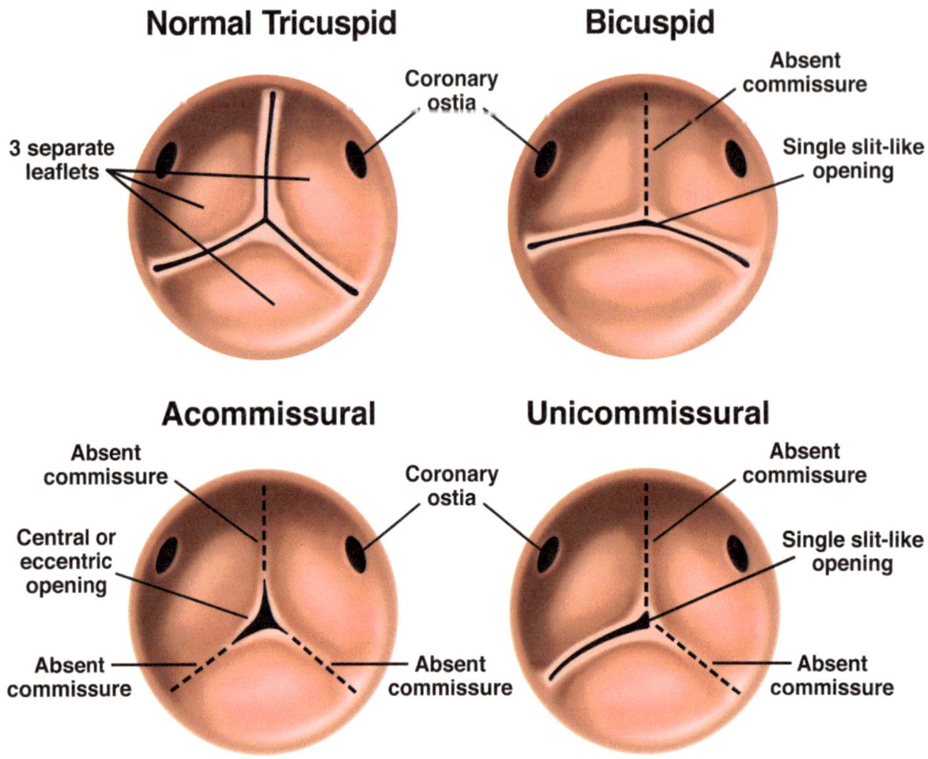

Fig. 1. Slit-shaped and pinhole shaped unicuspid aortic valves

Dilatation or aneurysm of aortic annulus/aortic root/ascending aorta
Patent ductus arteriosus
Coarctation of aorta
Aortic dissection
Anomalous coronary artery
Ventricular septal defect
Mycotic aneurysm of aorta

Table 1. Associated anomalies/complications of unicuspid aortic valve (Mookadam, 2010a and 2010b)

3. Epidemiology

While the more common bicuspid aortic valve has an incidence of 0.9-1.36% among the general population compared to unicuspid aortic valve which is about 50 fold less common with an incidence of 0.02% (Lewin, 2005; Mookadam, 2010a). Unicuspid aortic valve is more common in males with gender ratio of 4:1 in males:females (Mookadam, 2010a). It is relatively uncommon in adults when compared to neonates. Although an autosomal dominant pattern of inheritance with incomplete penetrance has been suggested for BAV, no familial cases of UAV have been reported in the literature to date.

4. Clinical presentation

The presenting features and associated anomalies/complications of UAV differ significantly in children as compared to adults.

	Pediatric Age<15yrs	Adult >15yrs
Mean age	14 months	42 years
Symptoms	Left heart failure, failure to thrive	Dyspnea,angina, syncope
Aortic stenosis	Common	Common
Aortic regurgitation	Uncommon	Fairly common
Aortic dilation	Very rare	Common
Coarctation of Aorta	Common	Rare
Ventricular septal defect	Common	Rare
Patent ductus arteriosus	Infrequent	Rare

Table 2. Clinical presentation of adult UAV and pediatric UAV

In the pediatric age group, the most common presentation included symptoms of left heart failure secondary to aortic stenosis. Pin hole shaped UAV is generally associated with a severe degree of stenosis compared to unicommissural UAV and tends to be symptomatic early in life. In the adults, reported symptoms in descending order of frequency include dyspnea, angina, dizziness and syncope. Most common aortic valve lesion included isolated aortic stenosis followed by combined AS with AR and isolated AR.

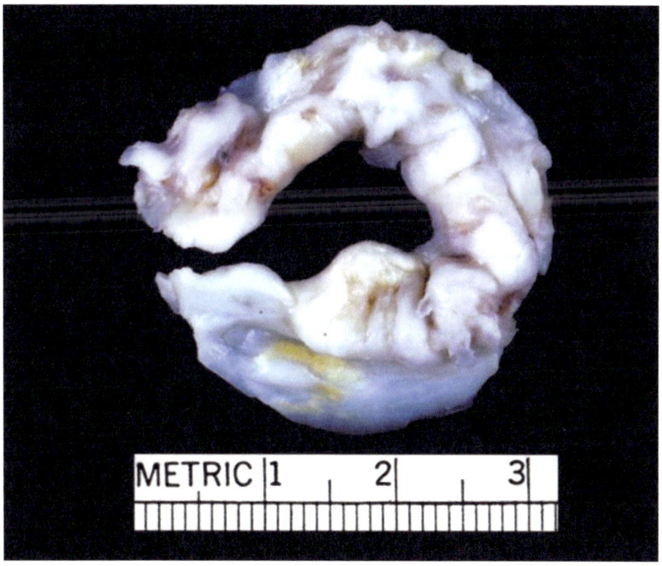

Fig. 2. Unicommissural AS-AI (1984, 2-630-422, Sawley 39F)

Associated anomalies in children included most commonly coarctation of aorta followed by ventricular septal defect and patent ductus arteriosus. However in adults, aortic aneurysm/dilatation was most common finding followed by aortic dissection, aortic mycotic aneurysm, coronary artery anomalies and ventricular septal defect.

UAV is more frequent among patients presenting to surgery with AS; approximately about 5% of patients presenting to surgery for pure AS will have UAV.
In adults, pathology of resected UAVs is characterized by heavy calcification implying early degeneration from hemodynamic stress. However, calcification is a very rare phenomenon in the pediatric age group. An important clinical implication of calcific UAV is the presence of calcification that extends into the interventricular septum, with possible damage to the conduction system during debridement at the time of surgery in preparation for replacement of the aortic valve.

5. UAV and aortopathy

Aortopathy is an important associated complication of UAV. Also a bimodal distribution of UAV has been described in the literature older UAV patients presenting without any pathological aortic dilatation and younger UAV patients with aggressive form of pathological aortic dilatation (Agnihotri, 2006). The UAV is also associated with pathological aortic dilatation over time which is thought to be secondary to hemodynamic stress and congenitally inherited weakness of aortic media. This congenitally inherited weakness in BAV is believed to be secondary to apoptosis of neural crest derivatives thereby predisposing to premature cystic medial necrosis. It is not known whether UAV shares similar pathological features of BAV. Aortic dissection also occurs at an increased rate in UAV patients compared to general population. And whenever it occurs, aortic dissection also presents at an earlier age in UAV patients compared to BAV and TAV.

6. Diagnosis

Clinically patients present with the usual and expected symptoms of syncope, chest pain, dyspnea and heart failure. As with any other etiology of aortic stensosi, however the age at presentation should alert the clinician as to the likely etiology as being unicuspid or bicuspid. Furhermore the aortopathy implies either unicupid or bicuspid abnormalities of the aortic valve. The presence of associated congenital heart abnormalities would suggest acommissural unicuspid aortic valve especially in the very young. Auscultation is significant for a third heart sound, systolic and diastolic murmurs depending on the predominant lesion. With at least moderate AS and concomitant moderate or higher degree of AR, the murmur may be confused for a coronocameral fistula, the machinery like murmur of PDA or mixed valve diseases. This difficulty can be reflected from the fact that approximately 60% of the adult UAV cases are diagnosed at autopsy/surgical resection, while only 20% are diagnosed by TTE and TEE. (Mookadam 2010a)
Transthoracic echocardiographic imaging remains the most common modality deployed for diagnosing UAVs preoperatively. Echocardiographic imaging allows satisfactory assessment of valve morphology, valve orifice, annular attachment zone and severity of aortic stenosis and regurgitation.
In addition the ascending aorta, left ventricular changes in response to the hemodynamic load, other valvualr structures and associated congenital anomalies (Table 2), can be identified. Other ancillary modalities including transesopahgeal echocardiography (TEE), real time 3-Dimensional echocardiographic imaging, cardiac computed tomography (CT) and magnetic resonance imaging (MRI) can also be used for better evaluation. All these ancillary imaging modalities have the capability to diagnose and identify preoperatively any associated anomalies.

Given the association, early progression and aggressive presentation between aortopathy and UAV, it is prudent to follow these patients regularly for timely intervention.

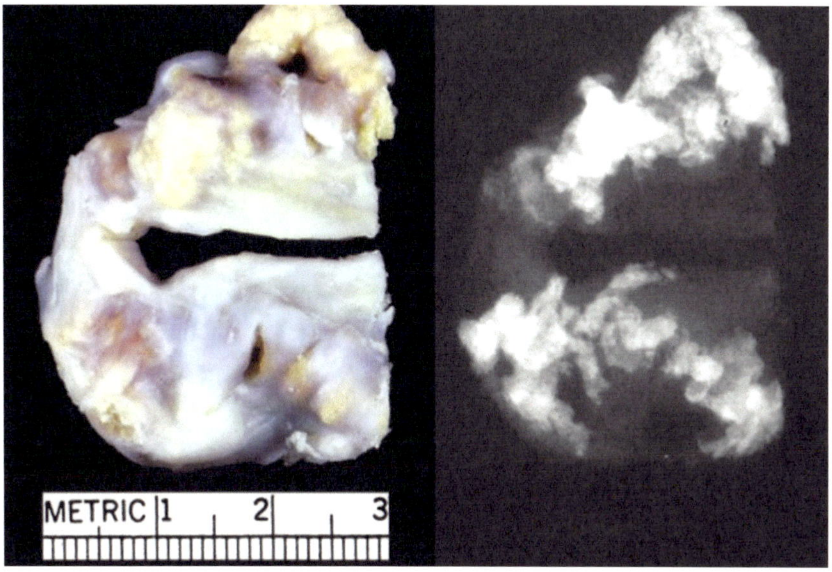

Fig. 3. Unicommissural AS (1983, 2-283-534, Eaton 42M), with x-ray

7. Management

The treatment approach differs significantly between adults and children. In children, treatment choices included aortic balloon valvoplasty, surgical valvotomy, and commissurotomy (Mookadam, 2010b). Repair of the aortic coarctation is also frequent among children, which was the most common associated anomaly. However, replacement of aortic root is uncommon in the pediatric age group.

In adults, most common treatment modality was aortic valve replacement associated with replacement of aortic annulus/aortic root/ascending aorta. Other treatment modalities included bicuspidization of UAV, Bentall's operation, aortic valvotomy and Ross procedure. Also in UAV, aortic valve replacement (AVR) was about 10-20 years earlier than BAV, and 20-30 years earlier than normal TAV. The current management approach of UAV is to follow valve sparing techniques in children and delaying AVR to allow aorta to grow to adult size.

8. References

Agnihotri AK, Desai SC, Lai YQ, et al. Two distinct clinical presentations in adult unicuspid aortic valve. *J Thorac Cardiovasc Surg* 2006; 131:1169-1170

Angelini A, Ho SY, Anderson RH, et al. The morphology of the normal aortic valve as compared with the aortic valve having two leaflets. *J Thorac Cardiovasc Surg* 1989; 98:362-367

Carlson BM. Human Embryology and Developmental Biology. 2nd edition. St. Louis, MO: Mosby, 1999; pp. 422-424. ISBN-10: 0815114583

Cemri M, Cengel A, Timurkaynak T. Pentacuspid aortic valve diagnosed by transoesophageal echocardiography. *Heart* 2000; 84:E9

Collins MJ, Butany J, Borger MA, Strauss BH, David TE. Implications of a congenitally abnormal valve: a study of 1025 consecutively excised aortic valves. *J Clin Pathol.* 2008 Apr; 61(4):530-6

Edwards JE. Pathologic aspects of cardiac valvular insufficiencies. *AMA Arch Surg* 1958; 77:634-649

Lewin MB, Otto CM. The bicuspid aortic valve: Adverse outcomes from infancy to old age. *Circulation* 2005; 111:832-834

Mookadam F, Thota VR, Garcia-Lopez AM, et al. Unicuspid aortic valve in adults: A systematic review. *J Heart Valve Dis* 2010; 19:79-85

Mookadam F, Thota VR, Garcia-Lopez AM, et al. Unicuspid aortic valve in children: A systematic review spanning four decades. *J Heart Valve Dis* 2010; 19:678-683.

15

Bicuspid Aortic Valve

Blerim Berisha, Xhevdet Krasniqi,
Dardan Kocinaj, Ejup Pllana and Masar Gashi
*Cardiology Department, Internal Clinic, University Clinical Centre of Kosovo
Republic of Kosovo*

1. Introduction

Bicuspid aortic valve (BAV) disease is the most common congenital cardiovascular malformation with prevalence of 1-2% in the human population (Hoffman, 1990; Hoffman & Kaplan, 2002). Current clinical and scientific studies reveal that bicuspid aortic disease is not a simple valve condition. It increasingly appears to be a genetically based connective tissue disorder. It has been reported that a molecular abnormality in the extracellular matrix may lead to abnormal cell differentiation during valvulogenesis; however, the exact mechanism remains unclear (Nataatmadja et al., 2003; Eisenberg et al., 1995; Fedak et al., 2002). An important problem is that the aorta of patients with BAV is not normal in strength or size. BAV is frequently associated with other cardiovascular malformations, including aortic root dilatation, aortic stenosis, coarctation of the aorta, and ventricular defects. Although symptoms often manifest in adulthood, there is a wide spectrum of presentations ranging from severe disease detected in utero to asymptomatic disease in old age. Complications can include aortic valve stenosis or incompetence, endocarditis, aortic aneurysm formation, and aortic dissection. Two large contemporary series have demonstrated that the life expectancy in adults with normally functioning BAV is not shortened when compared with that of the general population whereas age and severity of disease were associated with primary cardiac events (Michelena et al., 2008; Tzemos et al., 2008). The risk of aortic dilatation and aortic dissection is higher in patients with BAV than in the general population. In most of patients with BAV, symptoms and physical findings often are absent for many years, whereas the clinical consequences in patients with BAV are associated with regurgitation, endocarditis, and aortic aneurism and dissection. Endocarditis is an important complication for patients with BAV. It occurs particularly in patients with regurgitant or obstructive valves, although the risk of endocarditis may also be high also in hemodynamically stable patients. Prior studies reported significant mortality in patients with infected BAV. However, the last ACC/AHA guidelines recommend that antibiotic prophylaxis is not indicated in young patients and adolescents with BAV (Nishimura et al., 2008).

Patients with moderate valvular dysfunction and normal left ventricular dimensions should be systematically monitored using echocardiography. In adition hypertension should be carefully followed by a cardiologist or cardiac surgeon with specific interest in this valve pathology.

Adequate oral hygiene and antibiotic prophylaxis during dental procedures or when a poor cardiac condition is present are important for preventing endocarditis. Surgery is indicated for severe valvular dysfunction, symptomatic patients, and aortic dilatation.

This article addresses the embryology, genetic, pathophysiology, clinical presentation, diagnostic procedures, and therapeutic strategies for BAV. In this chapter we will present some cases with BAV with different prognoses from our clinic.

2. Embryology

The cardiac structure is evident from the second week of gestation, whereas separation of the heart into four chambers is completed during the sixth and seventh weeks of gestation, resulting in separated systemic and pulmonary circulation. The process of aortic valve morphogenesis begins from the cardiac cushions located in the ventricular outflow tract of the primary heart tube. The pathogenesis of BAV is still unclear. Studies in a Syrian hamster model with a high prevalence of BAV reported that fusion of the right and the left valve cushions is a key factor in the formation of BAV s (Sans-Coma et al., 2006). A previous study suggested that BAV is a consequence of the anomalous behavior of cells derived from the neural crest because BAV often is associated with congenital aortic arch malformations and other neural crest-derived systems (Kappetein et al., 1991). Other studies suggest that extracellular matrix proteins may affect the initiation of cell differentiation during valvulogenesis, while a molecular abnormality in this process may lead to the formation of abnormal cusps (Eisenberg et al., 1995; Fedak et al., 2002).
These abnormalities cause the fusion of two cusps and lead to one larger cusp; therefore, the BAV usually includes two unequally sized cusps, the presence of a central raphe, and smooth cusp margin (Figure 1). A previous clinicopathologic study of a large group surgically excised congenital BAVs showed that raphal position was between the right and left cusp in 86% of cases (Sabet et al., 1999). An anomalous origin of coronary arteries depends on the spatial orientation of the two cusps. When the orientation of the cusps is anteroposterior, the coronary arteries originate from the anterior sinus or if cusps later-lateral oriented the right coronary artery originate from the common trunk and right Valsava's sinus (Schang et al., 1975). An anomalous origin of coronary arteries may be associated with myocardial hypoperfusion and angina pectoris.

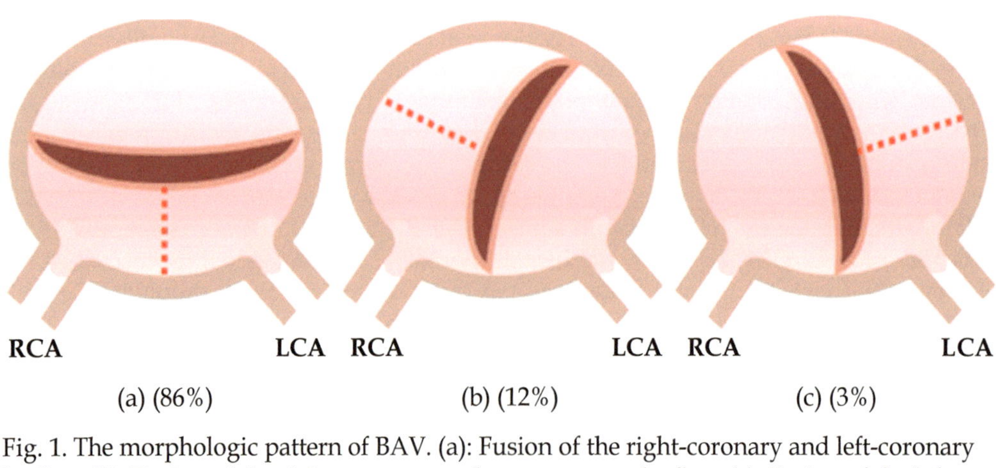

Fig. 1. The morphologic pattern of BAV. (a): Fusion of the right-coronary and left-coronary leaflets. (b): Fusion of the right-coronary and non-coronary leaflets. (c): Fusion of the left-coronary and non-coronary leaflet. RCA, right coronary artery. LCA, left coronary artery. The red dotted line indicate the raphal position

3. Genetics of the bicuspid aortic valve

BAV is a complex congenital disease; therefore, its etiology remains unclear, but genetic factors have been proposed. Most BAV s occur as an isolated congenital defect; however, a study on 41 families with a family member having surgically corrected BAV reported the prevalence of BAV to be at least 14.6% (Emanuel et al., 1978). A much more recent study in 50 probands with BAV concluded that the heritability (h) of BAV was 89%, and suggested that in this population, BAV is almost entirely genetic (Cripe et al., 2004). Two studies have identified genomic regions responsible for cardiovascular congenital disease associated with BAV. The first genetic cause of BAV is Anderson syndrome, which is reported to be a result of mutations in the KCNJ2 gene, whereas it clinically presents as ventricular arrhythmias, periodic paralysis, and scoliosis (Andelfinger et al., 2002). Another study in a large family with autosomal-dominant aortic valve disease diagnosed using genome-wide linkage analysis suggests that NOTCH1 gene mutations mapped to chromosome 9q-34 are responsible for the early developmental defect in the aortic valve (Garg et al., 2005). These studies are very important for understanding the complex etiology of congenital valvular disease, and they may help us to develop novel therapeutic strategies for preventing and treating BAV.

4. Congenital cardiovascular syndromes associated with bicuspid aortic valve

4.1 Coarctation of the aorta

It has been reported that BAV is presented in > 50 % of patients with coarctation of the aorta (COA) (Duran et al., 1995). Patients with COA and BAV are reported to have more severe disease associated with aortic stenosis, aortic regurgitation, and aortic aneurysm. The risk of dissection of the aorta and death is greater when COA and BAV are comorbid (Abbott, 1928). Microfibrilar proteins such us fibrillin -1 may be deficient during valvulogenesis, which could reduce the structural integrity both in the aortic valve and aorta. Aortic dysregulation is associated with increased activity of metalloproteinases, which may have impact on fibrillin-1 (McMillan ,et al., 1997).

4.2 Turner syndrome

Turner syndrome characterized by a defect in or the absence of one X chromosome. Except for gonadal dysgenesis, cardiovascular defects are commonly present in this group of patients. Clinical research on patients with Turner Syndrome reports that BAV is present in 30% of cases, that over 95% of BAV s result from fusion of the right and left coronary leaflets, and that aortic ascending diameters are significantly greater in this group of patients (Miller et al., 1983; Sachdev et al., 2008).

4.3 Patent ductus arteriosus

Patent ductus arteriosus is usually obliterated during the first month of life (Mitchell, 1957; Reller et al., 1988; Mandorla et al., 1990; Lim et al., 1992). Patent ductus arteriosus is usually present in pediatric patients with BAV and may be associated with hand anomalies (Gelb et al., 1999).

4.4 Williams syndrome

Williams Syndrome is arteriopathy characterized by supravalvular aortic stenosis which may be associated with COA, renal artery stenosis, and arterial hypertension. Williams syndrome has also been associated with complete atrioventricular septal defect (Nakamoto et al., 2003), and is reported to be commonly present in patients with BAV (Sugayama et al., 2003; Hallidie-Smith & Karas, 1988).

4.5 Ventricular septal defect

Ventricular architecture may be characterized by complex malformation during embryogenesis involving both septation and valve formation. Ventricular septal defects are often associated with BAV and other complex congenital malformations (Oppenheimer-Dekker et al., 1985) . BAV is reported to be present in up to 30 % of adult patients with small ventricular septal defects (Neumayer et al., 1988). However, BAV may also be associated with large ventricular septal defects and poor clinical outcome (Berisha et al., 2009).

5. Pathophysiology

Valve leaflet morphology and orientation are competent for pathophysiology of left heart. Adhesions of commissures and cusp calcifications predisposes to eventual stenosis, hemodynamically presented by different pressures between left ventricle (LV) and the ascending aorta during the systolic and diastolic period. Aortic stenosis is the most common complication of BAV, whereas aortic regurgitation is reported to be present in 13% of cases (Sabet et al., 1999). Turbulent flow along the abnormal structure of the BAV leads to fibrotic changes and stenotic progression. The pressure differences in stenotic patients with BAV are important because deviation from normal flow can cause important changes, in both the LV and the ascending aorta. High LV pressure in BAV increases wall stress, which results in the generation of concentric ventricle hypertrophy. Previous studies suggest that mechanical stimuli of myocytes can induce ventricular hypertrophy by specific gene expression, possibly via protein kinase C activation (Komuro et al., 1991, 1999). Progressively over time, the LV becomes more hypertrophic and less compliant, which contributes to a reduction of LV function. At this point, reduced stroke volume and cardiac output may lead to congestive heart failure. Post-stenotic dilatation may be a result of prolonged and severe aortic stenosis. Abnormal flow along the wall of the aorta can vibrate the vessel wall at different frequencies (Boughner & Roach, 1971), and may directly modulate elastin, whereas histopathological findings in congenital cardiac syndromes show medial degeneration and decreased fibrillin-1 in the aortic wall (Nataatmadja et al., 2003); however, the exact mechanism causing aortic dilatation in patients with BAV is unclear.

BAV may be associated with abnormal coronary arteries or the coronary ostium may be stenotic (Roberts, 1970), while angina pectoris is reported to be present in patients with severe aortic stenosis and without coronary disease (Julius et al., 1997) .Wall stress during systole and diastole, and impaired LV relaxation in severe aortic stenosis, reduces the coronary flow reserve and causes subendocardial underperfusion; however, the exact mechanisms of angina pectoris in BAV are not very clear.

Aortic regurgitation in patients with BAV is a result of cusp prolapse, fibrotic retraction, or dilatation of the sinotubular junction. BAV tends to become progressively more stenotic or regurgitant over time, and the valve becomes the site of infective endocarditis. Endocarditis is a result of turbulent flow, which induces chronic abrasion and abscess formation. Endocarditis can cause valve destruction and lead to severe aortic incompetence associated with a poor clinical outcome.

6. Clinical presentation

The clinical presentation of patients with BAV can vary from severe valve disease in infancy to asymptomatic valve disease in old age. Disease is more severe and has poor clinical outcomes in infants with BAV comorbid with aortic stenosis (Hastreiter et al., 1963; Moller et al., 1966).

Symptoms are a result of valvular stenosis, regurgitation, endocarditis, and aortic complications such as dilatation and dissection. Symptoms associated with aortic stenosis are angina pectoris, syncope, and congestive heart failure. Stenosis is more rapid if the aortic cusps are asymmetrical or anteroposteriorly oriented (Ward, 2008). Angina pectoris occurs in patients with severe aortic stenosis and in those who do not have coronary artery disease; it may be a result of ventricular hypertrophy.

Syncope is another common symptom in patients with BAV. Syncope reflects the cerebral hypoperfusion caused by the inability to increase stroke volume during physical activity.

The most common complication of aortic stenosis is congestive heart failure symptomatically presented with dyspnea, which is a result of combined diastolic and systolic dysfunction caused by elevated afterload and increased filling pressures.

Aortic regurgitation reported to be more common in young patients and caused by prolapse of the greater cusp, which may associated with aortic root dilatation. Although young patients with BAV often are asymptomatic, echocardiographic studies show that 47% of this group of patients have some degree of incompetence (Michelena et al., 2008). Aortic regurgitation in patients with BAV carries an increased risk of endocarditis. If a patient with BAV complians of fever, weakness, and chest pain, endocarditis may be present. Endocarditis occurs in 10-30% of patients with BAV and can lead to valve perforation or destruction (Ward, 2008).

Aortic dilatation and dissection can be echocardiographcally diagnosed in patients with minimal valvular dysfunction even when they are asymptomatic; therefore, the risk of aortic dissection in patients with BAV may be higher than clinical presentation. Aortic dilatation may be progressive and often requires surgical correction (Duran et al., 1990; Sabet et al., 1999).

The clinical presentation in patients with BAV and presence of other cardiac congenital defects depends from structural complexity of the heart. In patients with COA, the presence of hypertension increases the risk of aortic dissection, considering that congenital abnormalities of the aortic wall are also involved. Patient may complain of chest pain, hoarseness, and respiratory difficulties. In adult patients with interventricular septal defects, the clinical presentation depends on the size of the defect area and the grade of aortic stenosis. If the interventricular defect is small, the patient may be asymptomatic, but when the interventricular defect is large, cardiac output will decrease and Eisenmenger syndrome will develop. Eisenmenger syndrome clinically presents with central cyanosis and shortness of breath during physical activity. However, during that the BAV becomes thicker, more fibrotic, and more calcified, and if is not surgically corrected cardiac output will decrease dramatically and may lead to cardiac death.

Two large recent series reported that clinical course of unoperated patients with BAV depends on age, stenosis, and aortic incompetence (Michelena et al., 2008; Tzemos et al., 2008). The severe aortic stenosis, and severe aortic incompetence in older patients increases the risk of primary cardiac events including cardiac death. Both these studies suggest that intervention on the basis of early symptoms or incipient cardiac dysfunction may decreases the mortality of patients with BAV.

7. Diagnosis

7.1 Physical examination

A physical examination is very helpful for evaluating the complications of BAV. Munt et al. (1999) reported that the amplitude of the pulse in the carotid artery was a significant predictor of outcome in patients with valvular aortic stenosis. If stenosis is present, the arterial pulse is small or weak and rises slowly, described as "parvus et tardus". The cardiac pulse at the apex initially is normal; however, arterial pulse is delayed and reduced in amplitude if evaluated by palpation of the carotid artery. Auscultatory findings are best heard in the left second intercostal space. The S1 usually is normal but sometimes may be associated with ejection click. The S2 is soft, and when aortic stenosis is present, S2 occurs simultaneously with P2. In aortic stenosis, an ejection systolic murmur is heard in the left second intercostal space but may also be transmitted to the carotid arteries. If aortic incompetence is present, a diastolic murmur of aortic regurgitation may be heard.

7.2 ECG

The ECG changes are not specific in patients with BAV: left ventricular hypertrophy, atrial enlargement, and arrhythmias may be present.

7.3 Echocardiography

The most important diagnostic method for first detecting and evaluating complications in patients with BAV is echocardiography. A transthoracic echocardiogram (TTE) considered the method of choice for evaluating valvular structure, calcifications, vegetations, cardiac chamber structure, and ejection fraction. Doppler methods are the most common techniques used for evaluating valvular regurgitation. For BAV associated with stenosis, mean gradient and maximal flow velocity should be measured, but when regurgitation is present, the effective regurgitant area (ERO) and Doppler jet size should be evaluated (Quinones, et al., 2002; Zoghbi et al., 2003). Based on recommendations for evaluating the severity of native valvular regurgitation with two-dimensional and Doppler echocardiography, aortic regurgitation is classified as mild, moderate, and severe (Zoghbi et al., 2003). In 2006, ACC/AHA published guidelines for the management of patients with valvular disease in which aortic stenosis classified as mild, moderate, or severe (Table 1). For asymptomatic patients with aortic stenosis, echocardiography is recommended for evaluating disease progression. In asymptomatic patients, TTE recommended: every year for severe aortic stenosis, ever 1-2 years for moderate aortic stenosis and every 3-5 years for mild aortic stenosis (Bonow et al., 2006). Transesophageal echocardiography (TEE) is also very

Indicator	Mild	Moderate	Severe
Jet velocity (m per second)	< 3.0	3.0-4.0	> 4.0
Mean gradient (mmHg)	< 25	25-40	> 40
Valve area (cm^2)	< 1.5	1.0-1.5	< 1.0
Valve area index (cm per m^2)			< 0.6

Modified from Bonow et al.,(2006). ACC/AHA Practice Guidelines. *Circulation* 114, pp. e84-e231.

Table 1. Classification of the severity of aortic stenosis

important for evaluating the aortic valve and thoracic aorta, whereas the sensitivity and specifity of multiplane technique for assessing aortic valve morphology is high (Alegret et al., 2005; Espinal et al., 2000).

7.4 Other diagnostic procedures

In patients with poor acustic window, cardiac magnetic resonance (MR) and multidetector computed tomography (CT) are useful for measuring the aortic valve area and is an alternative method to echocardiography in selected cases (Shelton et al., 2003; Pouleur et al., 2007). MR imaging is an essential method for diagnosing COA and root aneurism.

8. Endocarditis prophylaxis

The most common bacteria that causes the formation of perivalvular abscess is Staphylococcus aureus. Indications for antibiotic prophylaxis in patients with BAV are before procedures expected to produce bacteremia; however, new ACC/AHA guidelines recommend that antibiotic prophylaxis is no longer indicated for preventing of infective endocarditis in adolescents and young adults with native heart valve disease (Nishimura et al., 2008). This committee concluded that infective endocarditis prophylaxis for dental procedures is reasonable only for patients with cardiac conditions associated with a high risk of adverse outcomes from infective endocarditis (Table 2).

Procedures	Antibiotics
Dental :	Amoxicillin, Ampicillin
Manipulation of gingival tissue	Penicillin allergic:
Manipulation of periapical region of teeth	Clindamycin, Cefalexin, Cefadroxil, Cefazolin
Perforation of oral mucosa	Azithromycin, Clarithromycin, Clindamycin

Prophylaxis is not recommended for patients who undergo a:
- Genitourinary procedure
- Gastrointestinal procedure

Nishimura et al., (2008). *J Am Coll Cardiol* 52,676-685.

Table 2. Recommendations for antibiotics for endocarditis prophylaxis before procedures

9. Treatment

When to surgically treat asymptomatic patients with BAV remains controversial. Sometimes aortic stenosis correlates poorly with clinical presentation; however, if it is combined with regurgitation, symtoms might be present. The risk of sudden death in asymptomatic adult patients with severe aortic stenosis is reported to be less than 1% per year (Pellika et al., 2005). Bonow et al., (2007) and Iung B et al. (2003) reported that valve replacement is not recommend for asymptomatic patients; however, current practice guidelines recommended aortic valve replacement in patients with reduced left ventricular systolic function (EF< 50%) without other explanation even when they are asymptomatic (Table 3).

Class I	Class II b
1. Indicated for symptomatic patients with severe aortic stenosis	1. Asymptomatic with severe aortic stenosis and abnormal response to exercise
2. Indicated for severe aortic stenosis and undergoing CABG	2. Asymptomatic Adults with severe aortic stenosis and rapid progression
3. Indicated for severe aortic stenosis and undergoing surgery on the aorta and other heart valves	3. Mild aortic stenosis, undergoing CABG, rapid progressions
4. Indicated for severe aortic stenosis and LV dysfunction EF less than 0.50	4. Asymptomatic with extremely severe aortic stenosis (when mortality ≤1%)
Class II a	**Class III**
1. Indicated for moderate aortic stenosis and undergoing CABG or surgery of the aorta and other heart valves	1. AVR is not recommended for preventing sudden cardiac death in patients who have non of the findings listed in IIa and IIb

CABG, coronary artery bypass graft. AVR, aortic valve replacement;
Bonow et al. (2006).

Table 3. Indications for aortic valve replacement in patients with aortic stenosis

Class I	Class IIa
Patients with bicuspid aortic valve and dilatation of the aortic root or ascending aorta (diameter > 4.0 cm) should undergo serial evaluation of aortic root/ascending aorta size and morphology by echocardiography, CMR or CT on a yearly basis.	It is reasonable to give b-adrenergic blocking agents to patients with BAV and dilated aortic roots (diameter >than 4.0 cm) who are not candidates for surgical correction and who do not have moderate to severe AR.
Surgery to repair the aortic root or replace the ascending aorta is indicated in patients with BAV if the diameter of aortic root or ascending aorta is greater than 5.0 cm or if the rate of increase in diameter is 0.5 cm per year or more.	CMR imaging or cardiac CT is reasonable in patients with BAV when aortic root dilatation is detected by echocardiography to further quantify severity of dilatation and involvement of the ascending aorta.
In patients with BAV undergoing AVR because of severe AS or AR, repair of the aortic root or replacement of the ascending is indicated if the diameter of the aortic root or ascending aorta is grater than 4.5 cm.	

CMR= cardiac magnetic resonance, CT= computed tomography. Bonow et al. (2006).

Table 4. Evaluation and Treatment of Dilated Ascending Aorta in patients with Bicuspid Aortic Valve ACC/AHA 2006 Guidelines for the management of patients with valvular heart disease

Risk factor	EuroSCORE Points
Age (years)	
< 60	0
60-64	1
65-69	2
70-74	3
75-79	4
80-84	5
85-89	6
90-94	7
>95	8
Sex	
Female	1
Chronic pulmonary disease	1
Extracardiac arteriopathy	2
Neurological dysfunction	2
Previous cardiac surgery	3
Serum creatinine > 200 μM/L	2
Active endocarditis	3
Critical preoperative state	3
Unstable angina	2
LV dysfunction :	
LVEF 30-50%	1
LVEF < 30%	3
Recent MI < 90 days	2
Pulmonary hypertension, PSAP>60mmHg	2
Emergency	2
Major cardiac procedure other than CABG	2
Surgery of thoracic aorta	3
Post- infarct septal rupture	4

LVEF=left ventricular ejection fraction, MI= myocardial infarction, CABG=coronary artery bypass grafting Roques et al. (1999).

Table 5. Score risk classification in the EuroScore

Elective surgery in patients with severe stenosis can prevent sudden cardiac death, and irreversible cardiac damage, and decrease operative risk. Coady et al., (1997) reported that the growth rate for the ascending segment of the aorta is 0.1 to 0.15 cm per year; therefore, older patients and those who have hypertension must be carefully followed-up and should be informed about the symptoms of aortic dissection. According to the ACC/AHA guidelines, patients with a dilated aortic root or an ascending aorta > 5.0 cm, or if the rate of increase in diameter > 0.5cm per year, should undergo simultaneous AVR and ascending aortic replacement (Table 4).
AVR carries a high risk for adverse events and poor clinical outcome when associated with LV dysfunction. In patients with functional class NYHA III-IV after aortic replacement, the one year mortality increased especially in patients with aortic stenosis (Rothenburger et al., 2003). Based on factors predicting operative mortality, which have been identified form large series of patients undergoing heart-valve surgery, The Task Force on the Management of Valvular Heart Disease of the European Society of Cardiology proposed risk classification scores for this group of patients (Vahanian et al., 2007) (Table 5).
For high-risk patients to undergo conventional novel methods including aortic balloon valvulotomy or transfemoral valve implantation may be helpful. This method reduced one-year mortality from 50.7% in the standard therapy group to 30.7% in transcatheter aortic-valve implantation group (Leon et al., 2010). A patient considered inoperable should be treated orally with angiotensin converting enzyme (ACE) inhibitors, diuretics, and digitalis. In patients with depressed LV associated with pulmonary congestion and atrial fibrillation, diuretics and digitalis may be used with the understanding that in some cases intensive hemodynamic monitoring is needed. Patients with aortic root dilatation > 4.0cm who are not candidate for surgical treatment should be given β-adrenergic blocking agents.

10. Case presentations

Case 1

History

- 42- year- old man referred for chest pain and shortness of breath.
- No previous cardiovascular disease
- CAD risk factors present: smoking, hypertension.

Physical examination

- BP: 140/80 mmHg, Hr: 64/min
- Arterial pulse is small and rises slowly, "parvus et tardus"
- Heart rhythm regular, fourth heart sound (S4), systolic murmur heard at the base of the heart Gr. 4/6

Other diagnostic procedures

- ECG: sinus rhythm, Hr: 64/min, biphasic T in D2, D3, AVF, ST segment depression for 0.5mm in V5 and V6 with biphasic T.
- TTE: cardiac chambers with normal dimensions, EF: 55%, aortic valve is bicuspid with vertical commissure, cusps are unequal, aortic valve area: 1.85cm^2, V mean: 131 cm/s, VTI: 41.9cm, Mean pressure gradient: 8 mmHg, aorta: 2.90 cm, (Figure 2 and 3).
- TEE: Bicuspid aortic valve with vertical commissure, cusps are unequal, aortal regurgitation (Figure 4).
- Coronary angiography: normal coronary arteries.

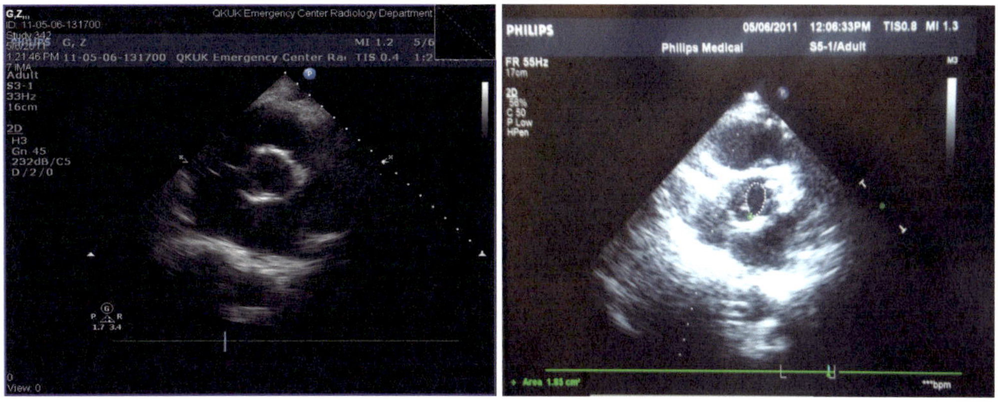

(a) (b)

Fig. 2. TTE: (a) Parasternal short axis view: BAV during systole, (b) Parasternal short axis view: aortic valve area

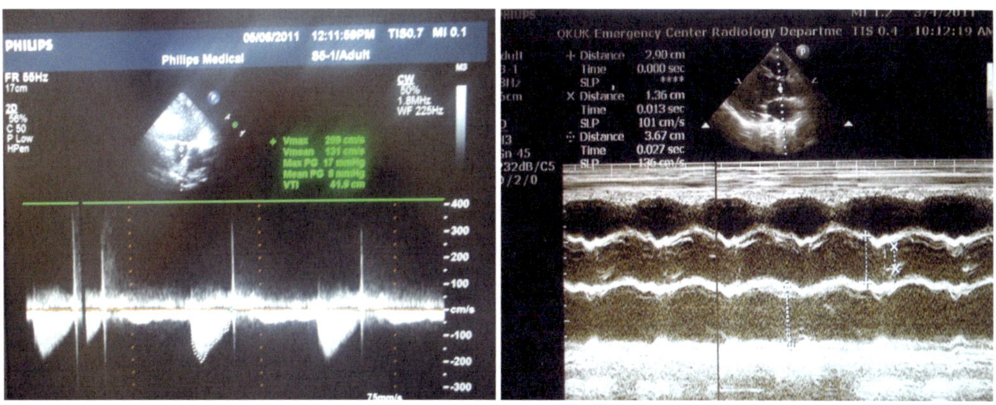

(a) (b)

Fig. 3. TTE: (a) Normal haemodinamic parameters , (b) Parasternal long axis view: Aortic diameter

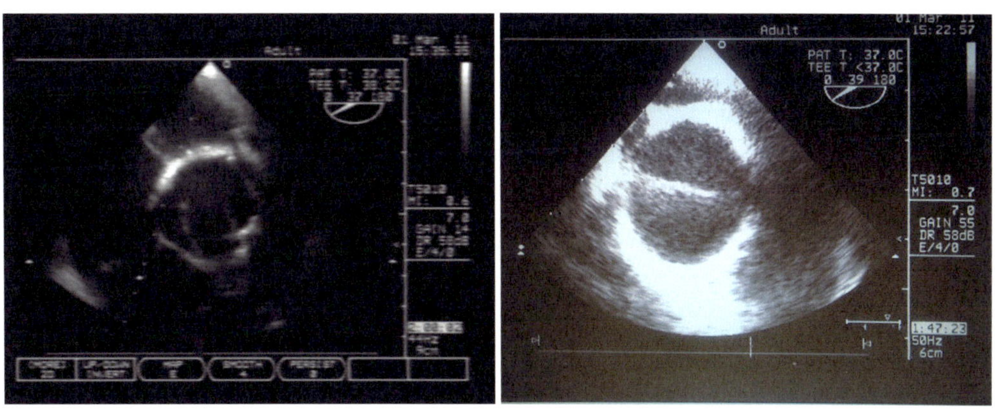

(a) (b)

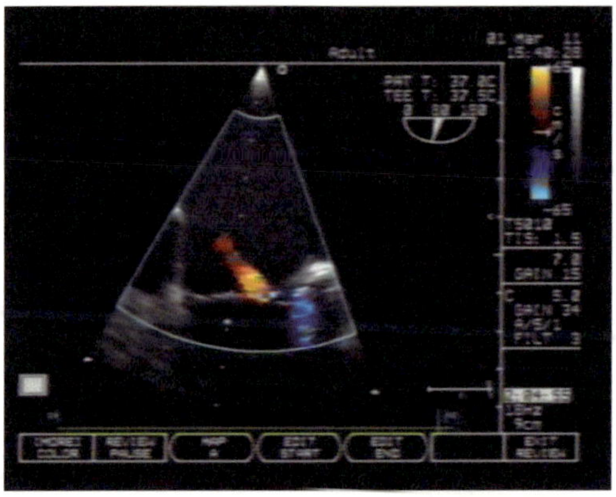

(c)

Fig. 4. TEE: (a) Short axis view: BAV during systole, (b) Short axis: BAV during diastole, (c) Aortic regurgitation

Comments

- Aortic valve replacement was not indicated in this patient because has no more symptoms, valve area is 1.85cm^2, aortic dimensions are normal, and LV systolic function is normal at rest (EF> 50)

Treatment

- Prescribed ACE inhibitor, endocarditis prophylaxis therapy, recommended serial evaluation using echocardiograpy.

Case 2

History

- 57- year- old man referred for chest pain, shortness of breath and syncope.
- No previous cardiovascular disease.
- No CAD risk factors present.

Physical examination

- BP: 120/80 mmHg, Hr: 85/min.
- Arterial pulse in apex is normal while in carotid artery is small.
- Heart rhythm iregular, soft systolic murmur heard at the base of the heart and radiated at the apex.

Other diagnostic procedures

- ECG: atrial fibrillation, Hr: 85/min, ST segment depression for 0.5mm in DI, AVL, V2 -V6.
- TTE: Left cardiac chambers enlarged especially LA,

EF: 45%, aortic valve is artificial, Vel: 1.82m/s, PG: 13.2mmHg, incipient dilatation of aorta (Figure 5).

Treatment

- Before surgical treatment: prescribed β-adrenergic blocking agents, anti-angina drugs, endocarditis prophylaxis therapy and recommended surgical correction of BAV.
- After surgical treatment: β-adrenergic blocking agents, anticoagulation therapy, recommended serial evaluation using echocardiography.

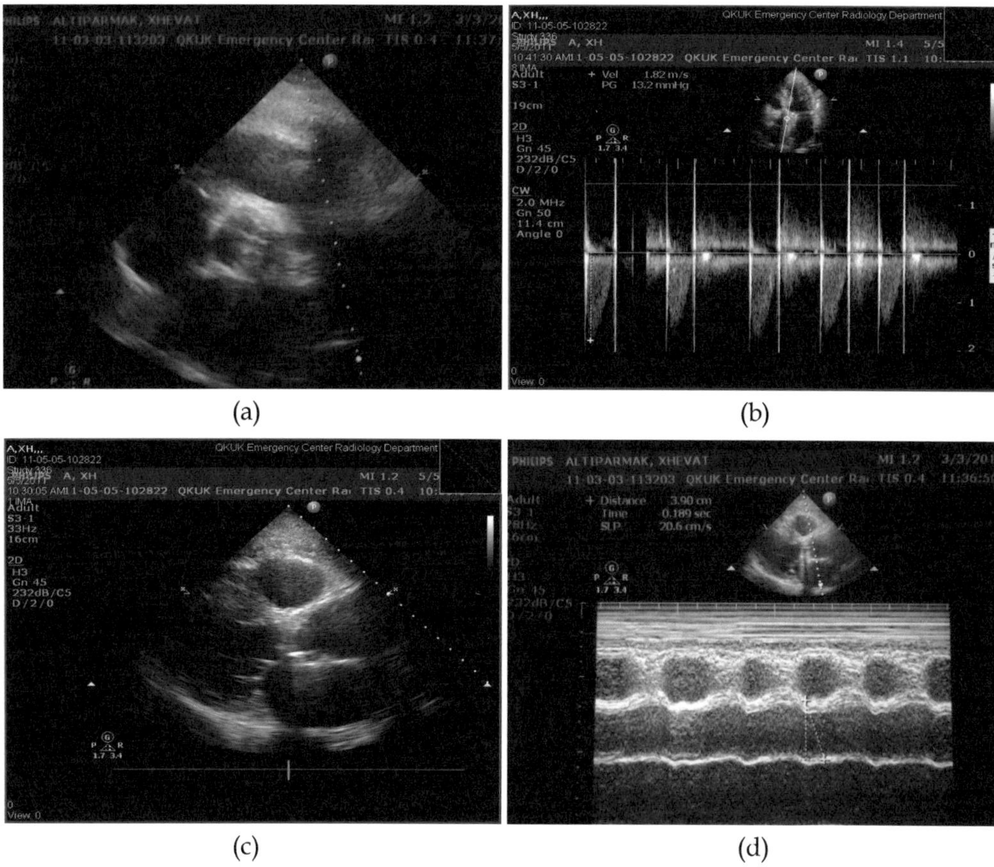

Fig. 5. TTE: (a) Artificial aortic valve (parasternal short axis view), (b) Apical five chamber view, (c) and (d) Parasternal long axis view: incipient aortic dilatatation and LA enlargement

Comments

- In this patient we recommended aortic valve replacement because he was symptomatic for several months, he had aortic regurgitation, incipient aortic dilatation, decreased systolic function at rest (EF> 45%).
- After surgical treatment, patient remained stable and without any postoperative complication.

11. References

Abbott, M. (1928) Coarctation of the aorta of adult type; II. A statistical study and historical retrospect of 200 recorded cases with autopsy, of stenosis or obliteration ofdescending arch in subjects above age of two years. *Am Heart J*, 3:574-618.

Alegret, J., Palazon, O., Duran, I. & Vernis, J. (2005) Aortic valve morphology definition with transthoracic combined with transesophageal echocardiography in a population with high prevalence of bicuspid aortic valve. *Int J Cardiovasc Imaging* 21, 213–217.

Andelfinger, G., Tapper AR., Welch, RC.,Vanoye, CG., George, AL. & Benson, W. (2002) KCNJ2 mutation results in Andersen syndrome with sex-specific cardiac and skeletal muscle phenotypes. *Am J Hum Genet* 71,663–668.

Berisha, B., Krasniqi, X., Thaqi, A., Gashi, M & Kocinaj, D. (2009) Single ventricle, bicuspid aorta and interatrial wall aneurysm as a rare adult congenital heart disease: a case report. *Cases Journal*, 2:109.

Bonow, RO., Carabello, BA., Kanu, C., et al. (2006) ACC/AHA 2006 guidelines for the management of patients with valvular heart disease: a report of the American College of Cardiology/American Heart Association. *Circulation* 114,e84-e231

Boughner, DR & Roach, MR. (1971) Effect of low frequency vibration on the arterial wall. *Circ Res*, 29:136.

Caruthers, SD., Lin, SJ., Brown, P., Watkins, MP., Williams, TA., Katherine, A. Lehr & Samuel A. Wickline, SA. (2003) Practical Value of Cardiac Magnetic Resonance Imaging for Clinical Quantification of Aortic Valve Stenosis: Comparison With Echocardiography. *Circulation* 108, 2236-2243.

Coady, MA., Rizzo, JA., Hammond, GL., et al. (1997) What is the appropriate size criterionfor resection of thoracic aortic aneurysms? J Thorac Cardiovasc 113,476-91.

Cripe, L., Andelfinger, G., Martin, LJ., Shoner, K& Benson W. (2004) Bicuspid aortic valve is heritable. J Am Coll Cardiol 44,138-43.

Duran, A.C., Frescura, C., Sans-Coma, V., Angelini, A., Baso, C. & Thiene, G. (1995) Bicuspid aortic valves in hearts with other congenital heart disease. *J Heart Valve Dis* 4, 581-90.

Eisenberg, LM& Markwald, RR. (1995) Molecular regulation of atrioventricular valvuloseptal morphogenesis. Circ Res 77,1-6.

Emmanuel, R., Withers, R., O'Brien, K., Ross, P and Feizi, O.,. (1978) Congenitally bicuspid aortic valves, clinicogenetic study of 41 families. Br Heart J 40,1402-7.

Espinal, M., Fuisz, AR., Nanda NC., Aaluri SR., Mukhtar, O & Sekar PC. (2000) Sensitivity and specificity of transesophageal echocardiography for determination of aortic valve morphology. Am Heart J 139,1071-6.

Fedak PW, Verma S, David TE., Leask Rl, Weisel, RD & Butany J. (2002) Clinical and pathophysiological implications of a bicuspid aortic valve. Circulation 106,900-4.

Garg, V., Muth, AN., Ransom, JF., Schluterman, MK., Barnes, R., King, IN., Grossfeld, PD & Srivatava D. (2005) Mutations in NOTCH1 cause aortic valve sdisease. Nature, 437:270–274.

Gelb, BD., Zhang, J., Sommer, RJ., Wasserman, JM., Reitman, MJ & Willner, JP.(1999) Familial patent ductus arteriosus and bicuspid aortic valve with hand anomalies: a novel heart-hand syndrome. *Am J Med Genet* 19,87:175-9.

Hallidie-Smith, KA. & Karas S.(1988) Cardiac anomalies in Williams-Beuren syndrome. *Arch Dis Child.* 63, 809-13.

Hastreiter, AR., Oshima, M., Miller, RA., Lev, M. & Paul, MH. (1963) Congenital aortic stenosis syndrome in infancy. Circulation 28,1084 –95.

Hoffman, JI. (1990). Congenital heart disease: incidence and inheritance. Pediatr Clin North Am 37:25–43.

Hoffman, JI. & Kaplan, S. (2002) The incidence of congenital heart disease. J Am Coll Cardiol 39:1890–1900

Iung, B., Gohlke- Barwold, C., Tornos, P., Tribouilloy, C., Hall, R., Butchart, E & Vahanaian, A . (2003) Recommendations on the management of the asymptomatic patient with valvular heart disease. Eur Heart J 23,1252-1266.

Julius, BK., Spillmann, M., Vassalli, G., Villari, B., Eberli, FR and Hess OM. Angina pectoris in patients with aortic stenosis and normal coronary arteries: mechanisms & pathophysiological concepts. (1997) *Circulation* 95,892-898.

Kappetein A.P., Gittenberger-de Groot A.C., Zwinderman A.H., Rohmer, J., Poelmann, RE. & Huysmans HA. (1991) The neural crest as a possible pathogenetic factor in coartation of the aorta and bicuspid aortic valve . *J Thorac Cardiovasc Surg* 102,830-836.

Komuro, I., Kaida, T., Shibazaki, Y., Kurabayashi, M., Katoh, Y., Hoh, E., Takaku, F & Yzaki Y.(1990) Stretching cardiac myocytes stimulates protooncogene expression. *J Biol Chem*, 265:3595.

Komuro, I., Katoh, Y., Kaida, T., Shibazaki, Y., Kurabayashi, M., Hoh, E., Takaku, F. & Yzaki, Y. (1991) Mechanical loading stimulates cell hypertrophy and specific gene expression in cultured rat cardiac myocytes: possible role of protein kinase C activation. *J Biol Chem* 266,1265–1268.

Leon, MB., Smith, CR., Mack, M., Miller, DC., Moses, JW., Svensson, LG., et al. (2010) PARTNER Trial Investigators. Transcatheter aortic-valve implantation for aortic stenosis in patients who cannot undergo surgery. N Engl J Med 363, 1597–607.

Lim, MK., Hanretty, K., Houston, AB., Lilley, S., & Murtagh, EP. (1992) Intermittent ductal patency in healthy newborn infants: demonstration by colour Doppler flow mapping. *Arch Dis Child.* 67,1217–1218.

Mandorla, S. (1990) The ductus arteriosus in healthy newborn infants studied by continuous Doppler guided by two-dimensional Doppler color echocardiography. *G Ital Cardiol.* 20,705–712.

Miller, MJ., Geffner, ME., Lippe, BM., Itami, RM., Kaplan, SA., Disesa, TG., Isabel-Jones, JB & Friedman, WF. (1983) Echocardiography reveals a highincidence of bicuspid aortic valve in Turner syndrome. J Pediatr 102,47-50.

Michelena, HI., Desjardins, VA., Avierinos, JF., Ruso, A., Nkomo, VT., Sundt, TM., Pellikka, PA., Tajik, J & Enriques-Sarano, M . (2008) Natural history of asymptomatic patients with normally functioning or minimally dysfunctional bicuspid aortic valve in the community. Circulation 117,2776–84.

Mitchell, SC. (1957) The ductus arteriosus in the neonatal period. *J Pediatr.* 51,12–17.

McMillan, WD., Tamarina, NA., Cipollone, M., Johnson, DA., Parker, MA., Perace, WH. (1997) Size matters: the relationship between MMP-9 expression and aortic diameter. *Circulation* 96,2228–32

Moller, JH., Nakib, A., Eliot, RS & Edwards JE. (1966) Symptomatic congenital aortic stenosis in the first year of life. J Pediatr 69,728 –34.

Munt, B, Legget, ME, Kraft, CD, Miyake-Hull, CY., Fujioka, M & Otto, CM . (1999) Physical examination in valvular aortic stenosis: Correlation with stenosis severity and prediction of clinical outcome. Am Heart J , 137:298.

Nakamoto, S., Saga, T., & Shinohara, T. (2003) Williams syndrome associated with complete atrioventricular septal defect. *Heart*, 89:e15.

Nataatmadja, M., West, M., West, J., Summers, K., Walker, P., Nagata, M & Watanabe, T. (2003) Abnormal extracellular matrix protein transport associated with increased apoptosis of vascular smooth muscle cells in Marfan syndrome and bicuspid aortic valve thoracic aortic aneurysm. *Circulation* 108, II329–II334.

Neumayer, U., Stone, S. & Somerville, J. (1998) Small ventricular septal defects in the adult. Eur Heart J 9, 1573-82.

Nishimura, RA., ta al. (2008) ACC/AHA 2008 Guideline Update on Valvular Heart Disease: Focused Update on Infective Endocarditis. J Am Coll Cardiol 52,676-685.

Oppenheimer- Dekker, A., Gittenberger -de Groot, AC., Bartelings, MM., Wenink, AC., Moene, RJ., & van der Haerte, JJ. (1985) Abnormal architecture of the ventricles in hearts with an overriding aortic valve and a perimembranous ventricular septal defect ("Eisenmenger VSD"). Int J Cardiol. 9,341-55.

Pellika, PA., Sarano, ME., Nishimura, RA., Malouf, JF., Bailey, KR., Scott, CG., Barnes, ME & Tajik, J. (2005) Outcome of 622 adults with asymptomatic, hemodinamically significant aortic stenosis during prolonged follow-up. Circulation 111,3290-3295.

Pouleur, A., Waroux, JB., Pasquet, A., Vanoverschelde, J. & Gerber, B. (2007) Aortic valve area assessment: multidetector CT compared with cine MR imaging and transthoracic and transesophageal echocardiography. *Radiology* 244,745–754.

Quinones, MA., Otto, CM., Stoddard, M., Waggoner, A., & Zoghbi, WA. (2002) Doppler Quantification Task Force of the Nomenclature Standards Committee of the American Society of Echocardiography.Recommendations for quantification of Doppler echocardiography: a report from the Doppler Quantification Task Force of the Nomenclature and Standards Committee of the American Society of Echocardiography. *J Am Soc Echocardiogr* 15,167–184.

Reller, MD., Ziegler, ML., Rice, MJ., Solin, RC and McDonald, RW. (1988) Duration of ductal shunting in healthy preterm infants: an echocardiographic color flow Doppler study. *J Pediatr.*112,441–446

Roberts WC. (1970) The congenitally bicuspid aortic valve. A study of 85 autopsy cases. *Am J Cardiol* 26,72-83.

Roques F, Nashef SA, Michel P, Gauducheau E, de Vincentiis C, Baudet E, Cortina J, David M, Faichney A, Gabrielle F, Gams E, Harjula A, Jones MT, Pintor PP, Salomon R, Thulin L. (1999) Risk factors and outcome in European cardiac surgery: analysis of the EuroSCORE muntinational database of 19030 patients. Eur J Cardiothorac Surg 15, 816-822;discussion 822-823

Rothenburger, M., Dreber, K., Tjan, T., Schmidt, C., Schmid, C., Wichter, T., Scheld, HH. & Dewick, M. (2003) Aortic valve replacement for aortic regurgitation and stenosis, in patients with severe left ventricular dysfunction . Eur J of Cardiothorac Surgery 23,703–709.

Sabet, HY., Edwards, WD., Tazelaar, HD & Daly, RC.(1999) Congenitally bicuspid aortic valves: a surgical pathology study of 542 cases (1991 through 1996) and a literature review of 2,715 additional cases. *Mayo Clin Proc* Jan 74,14-26.

Sachdev, V., Matura, LA., Sidenko, S., Ho, VB., Arai, AE., Rosing, DR. & Bondy, CA. (2008) Aortic valve disease in Turner syndrome. *J Am Coll Cardiol* 51,1904-9.

Sans-Coma, V., Fernandez, B., Duran, AC., Thiene, G., Arque, JM., Munoz, CR., & Cardo, M. (1996) Fusion of valve cushions as a keyfactor in the formation of congenital bicuspid aortic valves in Syrian hamsters. Anat Rec 244,490–498.

Schang, SJ., Pepine, CJ. & Bemiller, CR. (1975) Anomalous coronary artery origin and bicuspid aortic valve. *Vasc Surg*, 9, 67–72.

Sugayama, SM., Moises, RL., Wagenfur, J, Ikari, NM., Abe, KT, Leone, C., Silva, CA., Chauffaille, M& Kim, CA . (2003) Williams-Beuren syndrome:cardiovascular abnormalities in 20 patients diagnosed with fluorescent in situ hybridization. Arq Bras Cardiol 81,462-73.

Tzemos, N., Therrien, J., Yip, J., Thanassoulis, G., Tremblau, S., Jamorski, MT., Webb, GD & Siu, SC. (2008) Outcomes in adults with bicuspid aortic valves. JAMA 300,1317-25.

Vahanian A, Baumgartner H, Bax J et al. (2007) Guidelines on the management of valvular heart disease. The Task Force on the Management of Valvular Heart Disease of the European Society of Cardiology . European Heart Journal 28, 230–268

Ward, C. (2000) Clinical significance of the bicuspid aortic valve. *Heart* 83,81–85

Zoghbi, WA., Enriquez-Sarano, M., Foster, E., et al. (2003) Recommendations for evaluation of the severity of native valvular regurgitation with two-dimensional and Doppler echocardiography. *J Am Soc Echocardiogr* 16, 777-802.

16

A Case-Control Investigation of the Relationship Between Bicuspid Aortic Valve Disease and Coronary Heart Disease

Mehmet Necdet Akkus
Mersin University
Turkey

1. Introduction

Bicuspid aortic valve disease is the most common congenital heart defect, affecting 1% to 2% of the general population, with a higher prevalence in males (Hoffman & Kaplan, 2002; Movahed et al., 2006). Quite often, the diagnosis of bicuspid aortic valve disease is an incidental finding during an echocardiogram. However, the disease may be associated with significant valvular dysfunction and lead to aortic stenosis (Subramanian et al., 1984; Roberts & Ko, 2005) or aortic regurgitation (Roberts et al., 1981; Olson et al., 1984) and is a risk for infective endocarditis (Lamas & Eykyn, 2000; Fenoglio et al., 1977). Aortic regurgitation is probably more common in younger patients, and aortic stenosis becomes more frequent with age (Movahed et al., 2006). In this paper we reviewed the current literature on bicuspid aortic valve disease, particularly its etiopathogenesis, and report a case-control investigation of the relationship between this disease and coronary heart disease.

1.1 History

The earliest description of a bicuspid aortic valve has been attributed to Leonardo da Vinci, who over 400 years ago sketched the bicuspid variant of the aortic valve (Mills et al., 1978, as cited in Braverman et al., 2005). In 1844, Paget brought attention to the propensity of the bicuspid aortic valve to develop disease, and in 1858, Peacock reported the tendency of these valves to develop obstructive lesions initially, with subsequent incompetence (Roberts, 1970, as cited in Braverman et al., 2005). The clinical significance of the bicuspid aortic valve was also emphasized by Osler in 1886 when he described 18 cases of bicuspid aortic valve with the predilection of these valves to develop infective endocarditis (Wauchope, 1928, as cited in Braverman et al., 2005). In the 1950s, investigators observed that the propensity to develop isolated calcific aortic stenosis occurring in the setting of bicuspid aortic valve was the result of an intrinsic property of the bicuspid aortic valve rather than the result of rheumatic disease (Campbell et al., 1953, Smith & Matthews, 1955, and Bacon & Matthews, 1959, as cited in Braverman et al., 2005). Wauchhope's autopsy studies established that the bicuspid aortic valve is the commonest congenital anomaly of the heart (Mills et al., 1978 and Wauchope, 1928, as cited in Braverman et al., 2005). Furthermore, the association of bicuspid aortic valve with diseases of aorta was first commented on by Abbott in 1927 with the description of an association between congenital bicuspid aortic valve with aortic dissection (Acierno, 1994, as cited in Braverman et al., 2005).

1.2 Morphogenesis of bicuspid aortic valve

Bicuspid aortic valve likely results from a complex developmental process, not simply the fusion of two normal cusps (Sans-Coma et al., 1996). However, the exact mechanism remains unclear. Some researchers have implicated the anomalous behaviour of cells derived from the neural crest as a possible etiology (Kappetein et al., 1991; Fernández et al., 1998; Mancuso et al., 2002). The proponents of this theory note that bicuspid aortic valve is associated with congenital malformations of the aortic arch and other neural crest derived systems (Duran et al., 1995; Kappetein et al., 1991). In particular, some researchers suggest that a molecular abnormality in the extracellular matrix may lead to abnormal valvulogenesis, becouse matrix proteins help direct cell differentiation and cusp formation during valvulogenesis (Hinton et al., 2006; Eisenberg & Markwald, 1995; Fedak et al., 2002). This could also explain why bicuspid aortic valve is often linked to other cardiovascular anomalies, which will be mentioned below (Duran et al., 1995). In an another study Lee et al. (2000) reported that mice lacking endothelial nitric oxide synthase had a predisposition to forming bicuspid aortic valve, which suggests that abnormalities in this protein may lead to the disruption of intricate cell signals required for proper valvulogenesis in the mammalian heart. In human development, organogenesis is completed during the first trimester of pregnancy, after which further maturation and growth predominate. The first organ to form is the heart, with the earliest recognizable cardiac structure evident on day 15 of gestation, when the cardiac progenitor cells have been specified and are organized in a crescent shape. At three weeks of gestation, these bilaterally symmetric heart primordial cells migrate to the midline and fuse to form a single linear heart tube with an inner endothelial lining surrounded by an outer myocardial cell layer, which are separated by extracellular matrix. During the sixth and seventh weeks of gestation, the heart divides into four distinct chambers and an aorta and pulmonary artery, respectively, resulting in separated pulmonary and systemic circulations (Rabkin-Aikawa al., 2004; van den Hoff et al., 1999). The process of valvular morphogenesis begins from the time at which the heart is a simple tube. The initial endocardial cushions, which will contribute to all four cardiac valves, are formed by the thickening of the extracellular matrix in the region of the atrioventricular and outflow tract. Within the next day, there is a complex interplay of myocardial and endocardial signaling, which is necessary for proper endothelial-to-mesenchymal transformation. This process is initiated by the secretion of extracellular matrix proteins such as fibronectin and transferrin across the cardiac jelly to the adjacent endocardium. The endocardium then secretes transforming growth factor beta family members, which act synergistically with bone morphogenetic protein-2 secreted by the myocardium, to increase mesenchyme formation and proliferation, which results in the growth of the endothelial cushions. The myocardial cells then invade the margins of the cellular endothelial cushions. In the outflow tract, the truncal cushion swellings contribute to form three leaflet valves of the aorta and pulmonary artery. When this process is distrupted in the aorta, the primordial leaflets do not separate or remain fused, which results in bicuspid aortic valve (reviewed in De Mozzi et al., 2008).

1.3 Genetics

Although most cases of bicuspid aortic valve disease are sporadic, familial clusters have been identified (Emmanuel et al., 1978; Glick & Roberts, 1994; Hungtington et al., 1997). The earliest studies suggesting that bicuspid aortic valve disease was the consequence of an underlying genetic abnormality were case reports describing familial clustering of bicuspid aortic valve disease and reports of bicuspid aortic valve disease in monozygotic twins (McKusick, 1972; Gale et al., 1977; Godden et al., 1987; McDonald & Maureer, 1989; Brown et al., 2003). Subsequently, other authors sought to evaluate the relatives of patients with bicuspid aortic valve disease to investigate the prevalence of bicuspid aortic valve disease in the family members of affected patients. Emmanuel et al. (1978) studied 41 families with a member having surgically proven bicuspid aortic valve disease. Six of the families had more than one affected member. Of note, the diagnosis of bicuspid aortic valve disease in this study was based largely on the findings of the clinical examination, chest radiograph, and electrocardiogram; only a limited number were examined using M-mode echocardiography (Emmanuel et al., 1978). In contrast, Glick and Roberts (1994) studied the genetics of six families in whom greater than one member had aortic valve disease; 11 members had bicuspid aortic valve disease confirmed during surgery. They noted that of the 71 family members investigated, 17 (24%) had evidence of aortic valve disease likely secondary to a bicuspid aortic valve. In a prospective study, Hungtington et al (1997) assessed the frequency of familial clustering of congenital bicuspid aortic valve using two-dimensional echocardiography. They identified 39 consecutive patients with bicuspid aortic valve disease in their database and attempted to enroll 210 first-degree relatives. They were able to obtain echocardiographic evaluations in 89% of the first-degree relatives and reported that 9% of the relatives had a definitive diagnosis of bicuspid aortic valve. This was a significantly higher prevalence than the 1% prevalence that has generally been described in the literature for the general population. However, given the asymmetric clustering of a number of cases in some of the families, the inheritance pattern in those families was felt to be more compatible with an autosomal-dominant inheritance pattern with reduced penetrance (Hungtington et al., 1997).

Other studies have suggested multiple complex modes of inheritance for bicuspid aortic valve disease. Statistical genetic models have been tested to demonstrate that the regions of the genome are responsible for the phenotype of bicuspid aortic valve. However, to date, only a few studies have identified responsible genomic regions. Interestingly, some of the genes identified appear to account for inheritance in only a small proportion of the familial cases of bicuspid aortic valve disease reported. One of these genes identified is *NOTCH1*. Analyses of mouse and zebrafish Notch mutants revealed an essential role for NOTCH1 in promoting the epithelial-to-mesenchymal transition process (Timmerman et al., 2004). During the development of aortic valve in mice, *NOTCH1*, is highly expressed and represses the activity of a central transcriptional regulator of osteoblast cell fate (reviewed in Artavanis-Tsakonas et al., 1999). In 2005, Garg et al. (2005) identified a five-generation European-American family showing linkage for bicuspid aortic valve to a single locus on chromosome 9q34-35. Direct sequencing of all coding exons of the *NOTCH1* gene revealed a heterozygous C-to-T transition of nucleotide 3322 leading to a premature stop codon at position 1108 (p.R1108X). Additionally, in a second and smaller Hispanic family, a second mutation (p.H1505del) in *NOTCH1* co-segregated with the disease in three affected family members. None of these mutations could be found in the 1138 controls. The authors suggested that mutations of the *NOTCH1* gene may have caused an early developmental defect in the aortic valve and later led to a de-repression of calcium deposition and an aortic valve disease.

Other genes identified in bicuspid aortic valve disease are the potassium channel gene *KCNJ2* (chromosome 17q24.3) (Andelfinger et al., 2002) and the ubiquitin fusion degradation 1-like gene *UFD1L* (chromosome 22q11.2) (Mohamed et al., 2005). The *UFD1L* gene encodes a component of a multi-enzyme complex involved in the degradation of ubiquitin fusion proteins, and is highly expressed during embryogenesis in certain tissues. It seems to play a key role in the development of ectoderm-derived structures, including neural crest cells. Downregulation of the *UFD1L* gene, hypothetically resulting from an anomalous behavior of neural crest cells, may lead to reduced degradation activities, and may finally lead to fusion of valve cushions, a key factor in the development of congenital bicuspid aortic valve (Yamagishi et al., 2003). The presence of multiple genomic regions associated with bicuspid aortic valve disease demonstrates genetic heterogeneity and further supports complex inheritance. Given that a large proportion of bicuspid aortic valve disease familial cases are of unknown etiology, it is expected that other regions of the genome also predispose individuals to develop bicuspid aortic valve or associated cardiovascular malformations. Martin et al. (2007) have recently identified some regions of the human genome that harbor genes influencing the inheritance of bicuspid aortic valve disease or associated cardiovascular malformations. In particular, three novel loci for bicuspid aortic valve and associated cardiovascular malformations were identified on chromosomes 18, 5, and 13.

1.4 Bicuspid aortic valve anatomy, variants, and pathologic features

An intraoperative appearance of bicuspid aortic valve is shown in Figure 1. The anatomy of the bicuspid aortic valve usually includes unequal cusp size (due to fusion of two cusps leading to one larger cusp), the presence of a central raphe (usually in the center of the larger of the two cusps), and smooth cusp margins. The leaflets are usually oriented right to left, with the true commissures oriented anterior and posterior. Three morphologies are identified: type 1, fusion of right coronary cusp and left coronary cusp; type 2, fusion of

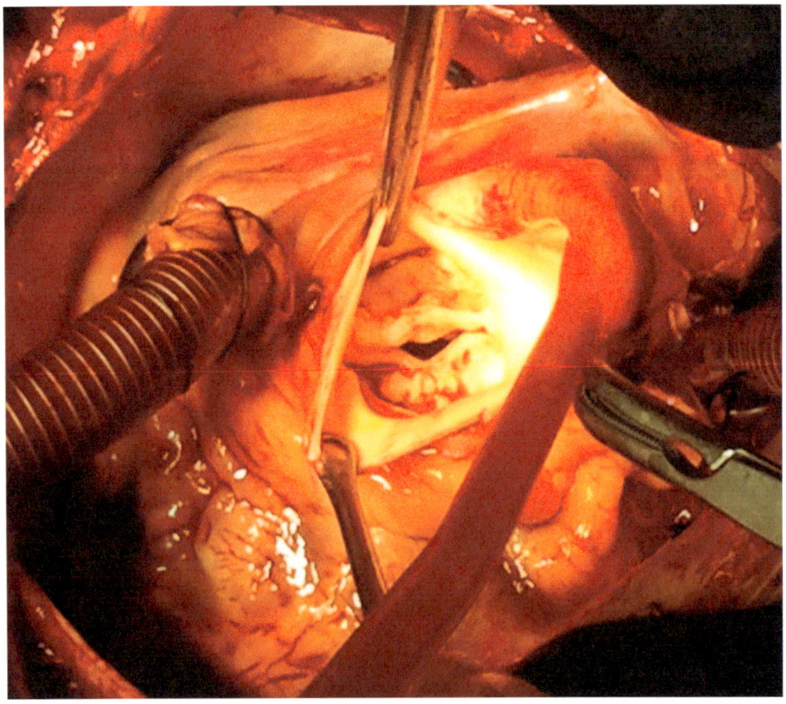

Fig. 1. An intraoperative appearance of bicuspid aortic valve

right coronary cusp and noncoronary cusp; and type 3, fusion of left coronary cusp and noncoronary cusp (Schaefer, 2008; Sievers & Schmidtke, 2007). The most common is type 1 (70% to 86%), followed by type 2 (12% to 28%) and type 3 (1% to 3%) (Fernandes et al., 2004; Sabet et al., 1999). The raphe or fibrous ridge is the site of congenital fusion of the two components of the conjoined cusps and is identifiable in most bicuspid aortic valve patients (Sabet et al., 1999). Of interest, pathologic examination of the raphe has shown that it does not contain valve tissue (Pomerance, 1972). Sometimes it shows a deep indentation, which gives a false image of a tricuspid valve on two-dimensional echocardiography. Valvular incompetence is usually caused by the redundancy of one cusp, since the two cusps usually have different dimensions (reviewed in De Mozzi et al., 2008). Few cases of congenital bicuspid aortic valve are accompanied by an abnormal fibrous band stretched from the center of the conjoined cusp to the aortic wall, and they appear to be associated with valve insufficiency (Nakamura et al., 1999).

1.5 The bicuspid aortic valve and associated congenital or acquired cardiovascular lesions

Despite its importance, our understanding of bicuspid aortic valve disease is incomplete, and questions remain unanswered about this common condition. Although much of the original focus centered on the abnormal bileaflet valve, the disease is significantly more complex. Bicuspid aortic valve disease is not only a disorder of valvulogenesis, but also represents the coexistent aspect of a genetic disorder of aorta or cardiac development. Accordingly, associated congenital cardiovascular anomalies have been reported in as many as 25% of patients. Patent ductus arteriosus and ventricular septal defect are the most frequent heart defects associated with bicuspid aortic valve disease (Deshpande & Kinare, 1991; Suzuki et al., 1994). Hypoplastic left heart syndrome, complete atrioventricular canal defect, Ebstein's anomaly, and partial or total anomalous pulmonary venous return. Tetralogy of Fallot, double-outlet right ventricle (Fernandes, et al., 2004), Williams syndrome (Lopez-Rangel et al., 1992), and Down syndrome (Weinhouse et al., 1995) are occasionally associated with bicuspid aortic valve disease. Shone's complex, which is defined by four cardiovascular defects (supravalvular mitral membrane, valvular mitral stenosis with a parachute mitral valve, subaortic stenosis, and aortic coarctation), is rare and forms another association in bicuspid aortic valve disease cases (Popescu et al., 2008).
Moreover, many vascular abnormalities, such as aortic dilatation (Sabet et al., 1999; Ward, 2000; Fedak et al., 2002; Bauer et al., 2002; Alegret et al., 2003), aortic aneurysm (Sabet et al., 1999; Ward, 2000; Fedak et al., 2002; Bauer et al., 2002; Alegret et al., 2003), aortic dissection (Larson & Edwards, 1984; Ward, 2000; Fedak et al., 2002), coarctation of the aorta (Ward, 2000; Lindsay, 1988; Warnes, 2003), interrupted aortic arch (Roberts et al., 1962), cervicocephalic arterial dissection (Schievink & Mokri, 1995), ductus diverticulum aneurysm (Sagic et al., 1997), and annuloaortic ectasia (Oyonarte et al., 1992) have been described in association with bicuspid aortic valve disease. Aortic dilatation, with an estimated prevalence of approximately 50%, is the most common abnormality among these vascular abnormalities that have been reported in association with bicuspid aortic valve disease (Pachulski et al., 1991 Hahn et al., 1992; Fedak et al., 2002; Alegret et al., 2003).

1.6 The bicuspid aortic valve and associated disorders in coronary arteries

Besides these abnormalities involving different arteries, some reports have also suggested the involvement of coronary arteries, including congenital coronary artery anomalies

(Rashid et al., 2005; Palomo et al., 1985; Doty, 2001), coronary artery fistulas (Oomman & Mao, 2000), spontaneous coronary artery dissection (Labombarda et al., 2009), reversal of coronary dominance (Hutchins et al., 1978; Higgins & Wexler, 1975), and immediate bifurcation and a shorter length of the left main coronary artery (Hutchins et al., 1978; Higgins & Wexler, 1975; Yuan et al., 2010).

There have also been some case reports describing patients with bicuspid aortic valve disease associated with coronary heart disease (Shimuzu et al., 1984; Bensaid et al., 1978; Yokoyama et al., 2002; Theleman et al., 2006) and even with acute myocardial infarction (Demir, 2009). There are also some studies in which the prevalence rate of angiographic coronary heart disease among the patients with bicuspid aortic valve disease has been given (Yuan et al., 2010; Goland et al., 2007). However, to the best of our knowledge, there is only one study in the current literature comparing the prevalence rate of angiographic coronary heart disease between patients with and without bicuspid aortic valve disease (Yuan et al., 2010). However, that study was retrospective in nature and was not designed primarily to compare the prevalence rate of angiographic coronary heart disease in bicuspid aortic valve disease patients with the rate in an age- and gender-matched control group.

On the other hand, it has been suggested that from 15% to 50% of patients with coronary heart disease lack any of the four conventional risk factors for this disease (i.e., hypercholesterolemia, hypertension, diabetes mellitus, and cigarette smoking) (Hennekens, 1998; Futterman & Lemberg, 1998; Khot et al., 2003; Greenland et al., 2003). Atherosclerosis is a complex disease process resulting from the interaction of a number of environmental and genetic factors. Evidence from epidemiologic studies has consistently demonstrated that there is a substantial heritable component to atherosclerosis susceptibility (Hunt et al., 2002; Fox et al., 2003).

1.7 Aim of the study

Based on the above-mentioned knowledge, in the present study, we aimed to determine whether or not there is a relationship between the presence of bicuspid aortic valve disease and the occurrence, severity, and extent of angiographic coronary heart disease. We also sought to determine whether the relationship, if any, between bicuspid aortic valve disease and coronary heart disease is due to the changes in flow dynamics secondary to stenosis or regurgitation in the aortic valve. We also sought to determine any possible relationship between the type of bicuspid aortic valve and occurrence of coronary heart disease.

2. Material and methods

2.1 Study design

Over a 9-year period, 11,702 consecutive patients who underwent coronary angiography at our institution for the first time for suspected coronary heart disease (mainly for the evaluation of typical, atypical, or non-anginal chest pain or electrocardiogram findings suggesting the disease) were subjected to routine transthoracic Doppler echocardiography to detect bicuspid aortic valve disease. Based on echocardiographic examinations, a diagnosis of bicuspid aortic valve disease was made in 115 (0.98%) of the patients (bicuspid aortic valve disease group). From the same population and during the same period, for each case patient, we randomly selected a control from the patients who had no bicuspid aortic valve disease, age- (within 1 year) and gender-matched to the case patient (control group, n = 115). For the purposes of the study, from the coronary angiograms, we determined the prevalence rate of coronary heart disease and the scores derived using three different scoring systems, which reflect severity and extent of the disease, in the bicuspid aortic valve disease group and control group, and we compared these variables between these two groups.

The median number of diseased vessels, the distribution of the coronary arteries disease, and conventional risk factors for coronary heart disease (hypercholesterolemia, hypertension, diabetes mellitus, cigarette smoking, and family history for premature coronary heart disease), the frequency of patients with an associated congenital coronary artery anomaly and with a comorbid condition, median of length of the left main coronary artery, and the frequency of coronary artery dominance patterns were also determined and compared between the groups.

To determine whether bicuspid aortic valve disease is an independent risk factor for coronary heart disease, we also conducted a multivariate logistic regression analysis with coronary heart disease as the dependent variable, and with age, gender, hypercholesterolemia, diabetes, smoking, family history for premature coronary heart disease, and bicuspid aortic valve disease as independent variables. We also compared the prevalence rates of the four conventional risk factors for coronary heart disease and the prevalence rate of the patients without any of these risk factors between patient groups, which consisted of patients in the total study population with and without angiographic coronary heart disease.

Furthermore, to determine whether the association, if any, between bicuspid aortic valve disease and coronary heart disease was due to functional alterations in the aortic valve, we first determined the presence and severity of aortic stenosis and aortic regurgitation and the presence of aortic dilatation in the bicuspid aortic valve disease group, and then compared the frequency of patients with moderate or severe aortic stenosis, moderate or severe aortic regurgitation, moderate or severe aortic stenosis or regurgitation, and aortic dilatation between coronary heart disease-present and coronary heart disease-absent subgroups of this group.

Finally, to determine whether there is a relationship between the type of the bicuspid aortic valve and occurrence of coronary heart disease, we compared the prevalence rates of coronary heart disease within each of the three subgroups, which were divided according to the type of the bicuspid aortic valve in the bicuspid aortic valve disease group.

2.2 Angiographic measurements

All patients underwent coronary angiography, using standard techniques. Angiograms were assessed independently by two experienced interventional cardiologists (M.N.A., A.C.) who were blinded to the patients' clinical parameters. Coronary heart disease was defined as the presence of angiographic coronary stenosis greater than or equal to 50% of the luminal diameter in at least one of the three major epicardial arteries or in a major branch on quantitative coronary analysis. The patients with no irregularities or with minor irregularities of the coronary vasculature, or with a moderate diameter reduction less than 50%, were classified as without coronary heart disease.

All coronary angiographies classified as coronary heart disease were assessed using the modified Gensini index as previously described (Gensini, 1983; Ringqvist et al., 1983). Briefly, location, degree of stenosis (severity), and number of occluded segments (extent) were evaluated. Coronary vasculature was divided into 27 coronary segments, and each involved segment was weighted by a value from 0.5 (least important) to 5.0 (critical location), reflecting the location of coronary artery lesions. The severity (percentage of stenosis) was weighted as follows: < 25%, 2; 26-50%, 4; 51-75%, 8; 76-90%, 16; 91-99%, 32; 100%, 64. Extent was determined by the number of occluded segments (from 1 to 27) and constitutes score III. Score II is the sum of the weighted severity for all involved segments. The product of the weights for location and severity is the total weight for each arterial segment, and the sum of all segments involved constitutes score I (the modified Gensini index), reflecting location, severity and extent (Ringqvist et al., 1983). The length of the left main coronary artery was measured on the right anterior oblique view of the archived coronary angiography images.

2.3 Echocardiographic measurements

Comprehensive two-dimensional and Doppler echocardiographic examinations were performed in a systemic manner by experienced cardiologists who were blinded to the study. In addition to the other routine examinations, aortic valve morphology and function, as well as aortic arterial dimensions were determined. Aortic valve morphology was assessed in the parasternal long- as well as short-axis views. The diagnosis of bicuspid aortic valve was based on previously defined criteria (Brandenburg et al., 1983) as the presence of only two cusps was clearly identified in systole and diastole in the short-axis view. Patients with fusion of the commissures attributable to rheumatic disease (Rose, 1986; Passik et al., 1987) were not included as having bicuspid aortic valve. An example for the echocardiograms of our patients with bicuspid aortic valve is shown in Figure 2. In this transthoracic two-dimensional echocardiogram in parasternal short-axis view at the aortic valve level, a clear systolic "fish-mouth" appearance of the aortic valve in mid-systole (arrow) is seen. The type of bicuspid aortic valve was determined from the short-axis view of transthoracic echocardiograms as previously described (Schaefer et al., 2008). Three morphologies, namely, type 1 (fusion of right and left coronary cusps), type 2 (fusion of right and noncoronary cusps), and type 3 (fusion of left and noncoronary cusps), were identified based on orientation of the valve cusps.

Aortic regurgitation was evaluated by color Doppler in the parasternal long-axis and short-axis views, and in the apical long-axis and five-chamber views. The severity of aortic regurgitation was assessed by the ratio of proximal jet area to left ventricular outflow tract area in combination with the ratio of jet height to left ventricular outflow tract height. In addition, the rate of deceleration of the velocity signal of aortic regurgitation and the presence of retrograde flow in the abdominal aorta on continuous-wave Doppler echocardiography were also considered in our assessment. These combined indices were analyzed to grade aortic regurgitation as mild, moderate, or severe, according to the American Society of Echocardiography criteria (Zoghbi et al., 2003).

Aortic stenosis was evaluated by both pulsed-wave and continuous-wave Doppler. Aortic stenosis was defined as present when the aortic peak velocity obtained by continuous-wave Doppler was > 2.5 m/s, and was classified as mild (valve area > 1.5 cm^2; mean pressure gradient < 25 mmHg), moderate (valve area, 1.0-1.5 cm^2; mean pressure gradient = 25-40 mmHg), or severe (valve area < 1.0 cm^2; mean pressure gradient > 40 mmHg) (Bonow et al., 2006). Figure 3 shows an example of the continuous wave Doppler images of severe aortic stenosis and mild aortic regurgitation in a patient with bicuspid aortic valve disease.

Thoracic aortic diameter measurements were taken in the parasternal long-axis view at the end of diastole at the level of the aortic annulus, sinus of Valsalva, sinotubular junction, and proximal ascending aorta (measured 1 cm from the sinotubular junction), as previously described (Roman et al., 1989). Measurements were made perpendicular to the long axis of the aorta using the leading-edge-to-edge method in views showing the largest aortic dimensions. The average of two measurements taken at every level was recorded. A dilated aorta was defined as an ascending aorta with a diameter greater than 37 mm, which is near the 95th percentile for this region for gender and body surface area (Roman et al., 1989; Vasan et al., 1995).

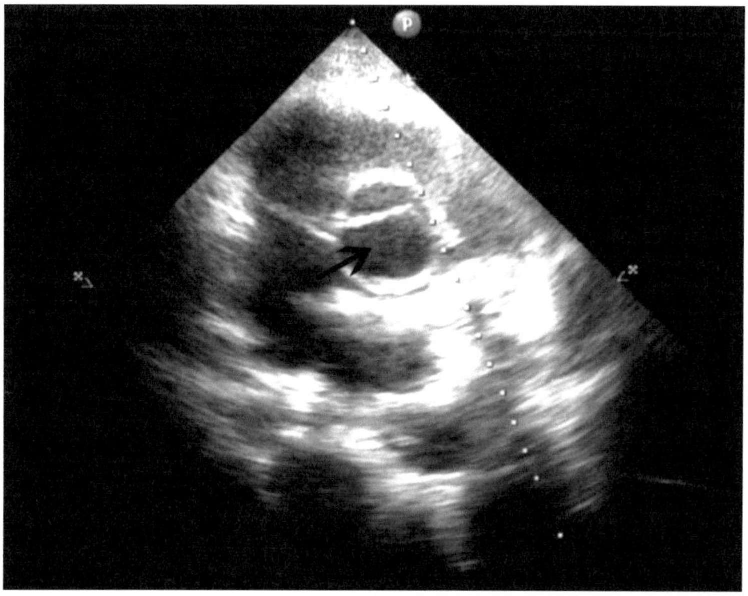

Fig. 2. Transthoracic two-dimensional echocardiogram in parasternal short-axis view of the aortic valve in mid-systole showing a clear systolic "fish-mouth" appearance of the bicuspid aortic valve orifice (arrow)

2.4 Other definitions

The five conventional risk factors for coronary heart disease were defined as follows: hypercholesterolemia: having a serum total cholesterol level of greater than or equal to 200 mg/dL, or an LDL-cholesterol level of greater than or equal to 130 mg/dL, or current treatment with lipid-lowering agents; hypertension: having an average blood pressure of greater than or equal to 140 mmHg systolic or 90 mmHg diastolic on three different occasions, or using antihypertensive medication; diabetes mellitus: having a fasting serum glucose of greater than or equal to 126 mg/dL (if confirmed on a subsequent day) or a 2-hour post load glucose of greater than or equal to 200 mg/dL, or using antidiabetic medication; family history of premature coronary heart disease: having a history of coronary heart disease in a first-degree male relative less than 55 years old or in a female first-degree relative less than 65 years old; and cigarette smoking: smoking more than or equal to 5 cigarettes per day for at least one year.

2.5 Exclusion criteria

Patients with a history or evidence of current or previous acute coronary syndrome, or with a history of percutaneous coronary intervention or coronary artery bypass grafting were excluded from the study.

The study protocol was approved by the Institutional Ethics Committee, and written informed consent was obtained from all study participants.

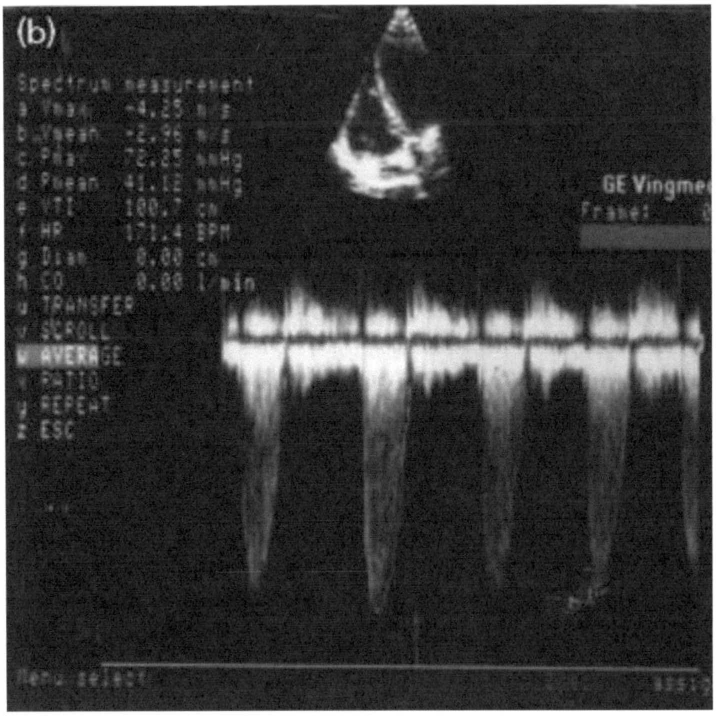

Fig. 3. Continuous wave Doppler recording of a bicuspid aortic valve (from apical five-chamber approach) showing severe stenosis across the valve and mild regurgitation

2.6 Statistical analyses

Statistical calculations were done using SPSS 17 (SPSS Inc., Chicago, IL, USA). Before the comparisons between the groups, the continuous variables were tested for normality using the Kolmogorov-Smirnov test. Data are expressed as mean ± standard deviation for normally distributed continuous variables, as median (25th, 75th percentile) for non-normally distributed continuous variables, and as numbers and percentages [n (%)] for categorical variables. All tests were two-sided, and alpha was set at = 0.05. For comparisons, Student's *t*-test was used for normally distributed data, and the Mann–Whitney U-test was used for data that was non-normally distributed. A $\chi 2$ test with Yates's correction or Fisher's exact test was used for categorical data.

3. Results

3.1 Study population

As seen in Table 1, the bicuspid aortic valve disease group and control group were not significantly different in age, gender, the frequency of the indications for coronary angiography (i.e., presence or absence of typical, atypical, or non-anginal chest pain), conventional risk factors for coronary heart disease, the presence of an associated congenital cardiovascular anomaly, or comorbidity status.

	Bicuspid Aortic Valve Disease Group (n = 115)	Control Group (n = 115)	p
Age (years)	56.4 ± 13.8	56.4 ± 13.6	N.S.
Gender (male)	96 (83.5)	96 (83.5)	N.S.
Indications for angiography			
Typical chest pain	71 (61.7)	67 (58.3)	N.S.
Atypical or non-anginal chest pain	34 (29.6)	36 (31.3)	N.S.
No chest pain	10 (8.7)	12 (10.4)	N.S.
Conventional risk factors for coronary heart disease			
Hypertension	25 (21.7)	20 (17.4)	N.S.
Diabetes	7 (6.1)	8 (7.0)	N.S.
Ever smoker	27 (23.5)	30 (26.3)	N.S.
Hypercholesterolemia	20 (17.4)	15 (13.0)	N.S.
Family history of premature coronary heart disease	6 (5.2)	7 (6.1)	N.S.
Associated congenital cardiovascular anomaly present	3[1] (2.6)	0 (0.0)	N.S.
Comorbidity			
Atrial fibrillation	5 (3.8)	2 (1.7)	N.S.
Renal failure	2 (1.7)	1 (0.9)	N.S.
Hypothyroidism	1 (0.9)	1 (0.9)	N.S.
Hyperthyroidism	0 (0.0)	1 (0.0)	N.S.
Marfan's syndrome	1 (0.9)	0 (0.0)	N.S.
Iron deficiency anaemia	1 (0.9)	1 (0.9)	N.S.

[1]Coarctation of the aorta in 1, secundum type atrial septal defect in 1, and operated patent ductus arteriosus in 1 case.

Table 1. Baseline characteristics of the groups. N.S.: Not significant

	Number and percentage of patients
a) Functional alterations of the aortic valve	
Aortic regurgitation	**38 (33.0)**
Severe	10 (8.7)
Moderate	15 (13.0)
Mild	13 (11.3)
Aortic stenosis	**32 (27.8)**
Severe	9 (7.8)
Moderate	13 (11.3)
Mild	10 (8.7)
Combined aortic stenosis and regurgitation	**28 (24.4)**
Severe or moderate stenosis	10 (8.7)
Severe or moderate regurgitation	10 (8.7)
Severe or moderate stenosis and regurgitation	4 (3.5)
Mild stenosis and regurgitation	4 (3.5)
No functional abnormalities	17 (14.8)
b) Aortic dilatation	**47 (40.9)**

Table 2. Functional alterations of the aortic valve and prevalence of aortic dilatation in 115 patients with bicuspid aortic valve disease

In the bicuspid aortic valve disease group, data on the type of the bicuspid aortic valve were not available in 25 (21.7%) patients. Among the remaining 90 patients, the most common morphology of the bicuspid aortic valve was type 1 (n = 70 [77.8%]), followed by type 2 (n = 18 [%20.0]) and type 3 (2 [2.2%]). Among the 115 patients with bicuspid aortic valve disease, the bicuspid aortic valve was regurgitant in 38 (33.0%) patients, stenotic in 32 (27.8%) patients, combined regurgitant and stenotic in 28 (24.4%) patients, and functionally normal in 17 (14.8%) patients, and aortic dilatation was present in 47 (40.9%) patients (Table 2).

3.2 Angiographic results

Coronary angiography revealed a significantly higher incidence of coronary heart disease in the bicuspid aortic valve disease group than in the control group (73.9% vs. 60.0%; p = 0.035). The median (25th; 75th percentile) number of diseased vessels (2.0 [2.0; 2.0] vs. 2.0 [1.0; 2.0]; p = 0.021) and indices of severity (score II, 99.0 [77.0; 122.0] vs. 88 [77.0; 111.0]; p = 0.029) and extent (score III, 10.9 [7.8; 12.55] vs. 8.9 [6.7; 11.65]; p = 0.026), and the modified Gensini index (score I, 106.0 [84.0; 129.0] vs. 95.0 [84.0; 118.0]; p = 0.016), which reflects location, severity, and extent, were also significantly higher in the bicuspid aortic valve disease group than in the control group (Table 3). Additionally, the median (25th; 75th percentile) length of

	Bicuspid Aortic Valve Disease Group (n = 115)	Control Group (n = 115)	p
Coronary heart disease on angiogram	85 (73.9)	69 (60.0)	0.035
No of diseased vessels	2.0 (2.0; 2.0)	2.0 (1.0; 2.0)	0.021
Indexes of severity and extent of coronary heart disease			
Score I (location/severity/extent)	106.0 (84.0;129.0)	95.0 (84.0;118.0)	0.016
Score II (severity)	99.0 (77.0;122.0)	88.0 (77.0;111.0)	0.029
Score III (extent)	10.9 (7.8;12.55)	8.9 (6.7;11.65)	0.026
1-vessel disease	11 (12.9)	18 (26.1)	0.062
Multi-vessels disease	74 (87.1)	51 (73.9)	0.062
Left main coronary artery	3 (1.7)	1 (0.8)	0.641
Left anterior descending artery	81 (46.8)	61 (48.4)	0.877
Circumflex artery	31 (17.9)	32 (25.4)	0.155
Right coronary artery	58 (33.5)	32 (25.4)	0.166
Length of the left main coronary artery, mm	7.7 (6.0;9.0)	8.9 (4.7;9.7)	0.019
Coronary artery anomaly	2[1]2.4)	1[2] (1.5)	1.000
Coronary dominance patterns			
Dominant right coronary artery	90 (78.3)	103 (89,6)	0.031
Dominant circumflex artery	22 (19.1)	10 (8.7)	0.036
Co-dominant arteries (right coronary artery, circumflex artery)	3 (2.6)	2 (1.7)	0.645

[1]Split right coronary artery in one patient and a fistula from the right coronary artery to the right ventricle in the other one patient.

[2]Circumflex artery arising from the proximal right coronary artery.

Table 3. Coronary angiographic findings in the groups

the left main coronary artery was significantly shorter (7.7 [6.0; 9.0] vs. 8.9 [4.7; 9.7]; p = 0.019) and the prevalence of left dominance (19.1% vs. 8.7%, p = 0.036) was significantly higher in the bicuspid aortic valve disease group than in the control group than in the control group (Table 3). Furthermore, although the difference was not significant, the test showed a higher frequency of multi-vessel disease in the bicuspid aortic valve disease group than in the control group (87.1% vs. 73.9%; p = 0.062). There were no significant differences between the two groups with regard to the distribution of the diseased coronary arteries (Table 3).

3.3 Results of the logistic regression analysis

The results of the logistic regression analysis are presented in Table 4. This analysis revealed that together with age (Odds ratio: 1.03; 95% confidence interval: 1.002-.048; p = 0.031), the presence of bicuspid aortic valve disease (Odds ratio: 1.90; 95% confidence interval: 1.070-3.357; p = 0.028) was an independent risk factor for coronary heart disease. In this analysis, none of the other independent variables, namely, gender, hypercholesterolemia, diabetes, smoking, and family history for premature coronary heart disease, was significant.

	Odds ratio	95% Confidence intervals	p
Age	1.03	1.00-1.05	0.019
Male gender	0.81	0.37-1.75	N.S.
Hypercholesterolemia	1.24	0.54-2.83	N.S.
Hypertension	1.42	0.63-3.18	N.S.
Diabetes	1.94	0.57-6.59	N.S.
Smoking	1.02	0.508-2.029	N.S.
Family history for premature coronary heart disease	0.92	0.27-3.09	N.S.
Bicuspid aortic valve disease	1.90	1.07-3.37	0.028

Table 4. Results of the multivariable logistic regression for the presence of angiographically proven coronary heart disease. N.S.: Not significant

3.4 Comparison of the demographic data and the frequency of patients with a risk factor for coronary heart disease and those without any of these factors between the coronary heart disease-present and -absent groups in the total study population

The mean age was significantly higher and the prevalence of patients without any of the four risk factors for coronary heart disease were significantly lower the coronary heart disease-present group than in the coronary heart disease-absent group. However, none of the four risk factors for coronary heart disease were significantly different between the groups, although there was a trend toward a higher prevalence of hypertension, diabetes, and hypercholesterolemia in the coronary heart disease-present group (Table 5).

3.5 Relationship between the functional alterations in aortic valve and aortic dilatation and the presence of coronary heart disease in the bicuspid aortic valve disease group

No significant changes were detected between the coronary heart disease-present and coronary heart disease-absent subgroups of the bicuspid aortic valve disease group with respect to the frequency of patients with moderate or severe aortic stenosis, moderate or severe aortic regurgitation, moderate or severe aortic stenosis or aortic regurgitation, and aortic dilatation, although all of these variables tended to be higher in the former than the latter subgroup (Table 6).

	Coronary Heart Disease		
	Present (n = 154)	Absent (n = 76)	p
Age	57.9 ± 13.7	53.2 ± 13.2	0.014
Gender (male)	128 (83.1)	64 (84.2)	0.983
Hypertension	34 (22.1)	11 (14.5)	0.234
Diabetes	11 (7.1)	4 (5.3)	0.795
Ever smoker	38 (24.7)	19 (25.0)	1.000
Hypercholesterolemia	25 (16.2)	10 (13.2)	0.678
Family history for premature coronary heart disease	8 (5.2)	5 (6.6)	0.901
Absence of these risk factors	50 (32.5)	37 (48.7)	0.025

Table 5. Comparison of the demographic data and the prevalence of the coronary heart disease risk factors and of absence of any of these risk factors between the coronary heart disease-present and -absent groups in the total study population

	Coronary Heart Disease Present (n = 85)	Coronary Heart Disease Absent (n = 30)	p
Moderate or severe aortic stenosis	26 (30.6)	6 (17.0)	0.381
Moderate or severe aortic regurgitation	28 (32.9)	7 (23.3)	0.452
Moderate or severe aortic stenosis or regurgitation	57 (67.1)	14 (46.7)	0.079
Aortic dilatation	37 (43.5)	10 (33.3)	0.447

Table 6. Comparison of coronary heart disease-present and -absent subgroups of the bicuspid aortic valve disease group by the presence of moderate or severe aortic stenosis, moderate or severe aortic regurgitation, moderate or severe aortic stenosis or aortic regurgitation, and aortic dilatation

3.6 Comparison of the prevalence rates of coronary heart disease within subgroups which were divided according to the type of bicuspid aortic valve

None of the comparisons of the prevalence rates of coronary heart disease within subgroups which were divided according to the type of bicuspid aortic valve among 90 bicuspid aortic valve disease patients showed a significant difference (Table 7).

	Coronary Heart Disease-Present (n = 66)	Coronary Heart Disease-Absent (n = 24)	p
Type 1	54 (81.8)	16 (66.7)	N.S.
Type 2	12 (18.2)	6 (25.0)	N.S.
Type 3	0 (0.0)	2 (8.3)	N.S.

Table 7. Comparison of the prevalence rates of coronary heart disease within subgroups which were divided according to the type of bicuspid aortic valve. N.S.: Not significant

4. Discussion

In the present study, in a specific population consisting of patients who underwent coronary angiography for suspected coronary heart disease (i.e., a population in which the incidence of coronary heart disease is expected to be high), we found a significantly higher prevalence of coronary heart disease in those patients with bicuspid aortic valve disease than in their age- and gender-matched counterparts without bicuspid aortic valve disease (73.9% vs. 60.0%). The indices of angiographic severity and extent of coronary heart disease were also significantly higher in the bicuspid aortic valve disease group than in the control group.

As mentioned earlier, there have been some case reports describing patients with bicuspid aortic valve disease associated with coronary atherosclerosis (Shimuzu et al., 1984; Bensaid et al., 1978; Yokoyama et al., 2002; Theleman et al., 2006) and even with acute myocardial infarction (Demir, 2009). However, to the best of our knowledge, there are only two studies in which the frequency of angiographic coronary heart disease has been given for patients with bicuspid aortic valve disease (Yuan et al., 2010; Goland et al., 2007). In one of these studies (Goland et al., 2007), which included 252 bicuspid aortic valve disease patients (mean age: 61 ± 15, 66.3% male) undergoing aortic valve replacement, the prevalence of coronary heart disease was 40.5%. In the other study (Yuan et al., 2010), the prevalence of angiographic coronary heart disease was not significantly different between the group consisting of the patients with bicuspid aortic valve disease who underwent cardiac surgery (n = 241), and the control group consisting 225 patients without bicuspid aortic valve disease who underwent an operation for an isolated aortic dilation, a combined aortic dilation and aortic valve abnormality, coarctation of the aorta, Marfan's syndrome, aortic dissection, infective endocarditis, or aortic valve disorders (22.82% vs. 28.9%; p = not significant). However, that study was not designed primarily to compare the frequency of coronary heart disease in bicuspid aortic valve disease patients with that in an age- and gender-matched control group. Accordingly, there were significant differences between these two groups, mainly with regard to mean age (56.1 ± 15.1 vs. 62.8 ± 14.7; $p < 0.0001$) and gender distribution (male/female: 3.38/1 vs. 1.78/1). To our knowledge, the present study is unique in prospectively examining the relationship between the presence of bicuspid aortic valve disease and the occurrence, severity, and extent of angiographic coronary heart disease. According to our knowledge, neither the above-mentioned two studies (Yuan et al., 2010; Goland et al., 2007) nor the five case reports (Shimuzu et al., 1984; Bensaid et al., 1978; Yokoyama et al., 2002; Theleman et al., 2006; Demir, 2009) nor any other publication in the literature have suggested any explanation for a possible association between bicuspid aortic valve disease and coronary heart disease.

First, it must be emphasized that since both of these diseases have high prevalences, there is a great possibility that their coexistence is not uncommon. Moreover, in some of the above-mentioned reported cases, in addition to bicuspid aortic valve disease and coronary heart disease, a third disorder, which may be relevant to coronary heart disease, namely rheumatoid arthritis in one case (Shimuzu et al., 1984) and mitral annular calcification in an another case (Theleman et al., 2006), was also present.

On the other hand, two possible explanations for the coexistence of the aforementioned congenital vascular abnormalities with bicuspid aortic valve disease or for long-term complications of bicuspid aortic valve disease have been proposed: (1) they may be secondary to flow dynamics (e.g., post-stenotic dilatation), and (2) there may be a common underlying developmental defect involving the aortic valve and the arterial wall (Niwa et al., 2001; Bonderman et al., 1999; Hahn et al., 1992; Pachulski et al., 1991). In favor of the latter mechanism, the ascending aorta above a bicuspid aortic valve was reported to be dilated, irrespective of the presence or absence of aortic stenosis or regurgitation (Hahn et al., 1992; Pachulski et al., 1991). Moreover, the study by Niwa et al. (2001) reported that light and electron microscopic abnormalities in the tunica media of the ascending aorta above a bicuspid aortic valve were also identical irrespective of the functional state of the valve. The authors concluded that this observation was in favor of the view that there is an inherent fault in the ascending aortic media. Accordingly, we believe that similar mechanisms may also have been involved in our finding that the presence of bicuspid aortic valve disease is associated with the occurrence, severity, and extent of coronary heart disease. In favor of the former of the above two mechanisms, we observed trends toward an increased frequency of patients with moderate or severe aortic stenosis, aortic regurgitation, aortic stenosis or aortic regurgitation, and aortic dilatation in the coronary heart disease-present subgroup of the bicuspid aortic valve disease group. However, none of these differences were significant, perhaps because of the limited size of the study population.

Of interest is that in some earlier papers it was suggested that more than 50% of patients with coronary heart disease lacked any of the aforementioned four conventional risk factors for atherosclerosis (Futterman & Lemberg, 1998; Hennekens, 1998). However, in some more recent studies, this percentage was reported to be between 15 and 20 (Khot et al., 2003; Greenland et al., 2003). In the present study, the percentage of patients without any of these risk factors was 27.1% in the coronary heart disease-present subgroup of the bicuspid aortic valve disease group and 39.1% in the coronary heart disease-present subgroup of control group (data not shown). Atherosclerosis, the major underlying cause of coronary heart disease, is present in all humans at an advanced age, and it progresses over a lifetime, but its extent and progression is dependent on its risk factors (Berenson et al., 1998). In addition, genetic factors are important. Twin studies indicate that the heritability of coronary heart disease, defined as the proportion of the interindividual differences resulting from genetic factors, is 30% to 60% (Marenberg et al., 1994). Existing research into the genetic basis of coronary heart disease falls into two categories. Firstly, earlier studies investigated candidate genes on which suspicion fell as result of evidence that the gene influenced one of the mechanisms by which coronary heart disease arose, such as lipoprotein metabolism or inflammation. More recently, genome-wide association studies have investigated many variants across the genome, without any underlying hypotheses. With the availability of high-density genome-wide association studies, and as studies become larger and more numerous, significant positive findings are emerging. These studies have resulted in the identification of 17 loci associated with coronary heart disease (reviewed in Sivapalaratnam et al., 2011). Still, only part of the heritability of coronary heart disease is currently explained. Accordingly, it can be also stated that there is a possibility for a common genetic basis for the association between bicuspid aortic valve disease and coronary heart disease.

It is interesting that degenerative-calcific aortic stenosis, which predominantly affects older people, is a presentation of atherosclerosis (Faggiano et al., 2011; Otto et al., 1999; Branch et al., 2002). However, according to our knowledge, there are no studies in the literature reporting such an association for aortic stenosis of rheumatic origin or due to bicuspid valves and for aortic regurgitation or aortic dilatation of any origin.

Among the findings of this study was the lack of independent predictiveness of the five conventional risk factors for coronary heart disease, namely hypercholesterolemia, hypertension, diabetes mellitus, cigarette smoking, and a family history of premature coronary heart disease. Accordingly, none of these five risk factors was significantly different between the coronary heart disease-present and -absent groups in the total study population, although a trend toward a higher prevalence of hypertension, diabetes, and hypercholesterolemia in the former group was observed. We believe that these findings may probably be partly due to the relatively high prevalence of patients who were using medications against these risk factors (i.e., antihypertensive, antidiabetic, and lipid-lowering drugs).

Finally, it should be also stated that, our findings that the increased prevalence of left dominance (Hutchins et al., 1975; Higgins & Wexler, 1975) and significantly shorter left main coronary artery length (Hutchins et al., 1975; Higgins & Wexler, 1975; Yuan et al., 2010) in patients with bicuspid aortic valve disease are in general in accord with the studies in the literature.

5. Limitations of the study

Because it is unethical to do coronary angiography on every patient with bicuspid aortic valve disease, the study was done on patients who underwent coronary angiography for suspected coronary heart disease (i.e., on patients in whom the probability of coronary heart disease was high). It is clear that this is not an ideal design to investigate a probable relationship between bicuspid aortic valve disease and coronary heart disease.

6. Conclusion

In conclusion, there may be an association between bicuspid aortic valve disease and coronary heart disease. It is both possible that this association is due to structural changes in the walls of the coronary arteries secondary to flow dynamics in bicuspid aortic valve disease or to a common underlying congenital cause involving both the aortic valve and coronary arteries. It is also possible that both of these factors may make the coronary arteries prone to atherosclerosis. More studies are needed to confirm our findings and to study the potential mechanisms of this association.

7. Acknowledgements

I thank everyone who worked with me in all phases of the study for their effort and commitment. I especially thank Caner Bozali, MD, for providing Figure 1.

8. References

Alegret, JM., Duran, I., Palazon, O., Vernis, JM., Ameijide, A., Rabassa, A. & Masana, L. (2003). Prevalence of and predictors of bicuspid aortic valves in patients with dilated aortic roots. *The American Journal of Cardiology*, Vol. 91, No. 5, (March 2003), pp. (619-622).

Andelfinger, G., Tapper, AR., Welch, RC., Vanoye, CG., George, AL. Jr. & Benson, DW. (2002). KCNJ2 mutation results in Andersen syndrome with sex-specific cardiac and skeletal muscle phenotypes. *American Journal of Human Genetics*, Vol. 71, No. 3, (July, 2002), pp. (663-668).

Artavanis-Tsakonas, S., Rand, MD. & Lake, RJ. (1999). Notch signaling: cell fate control and signal integration in development. *Science,* Vol. 284, No. 5415, (April, 1999), pp. (770-776).

Bauer, M., Pasic, M., Schaffarzyk, R., Siniawski, H., Knollmann, F., Meyer, R. & Hetzer, R. (2002). Reduction aortoplasty for dilatation of the ascending aorta in patients with bicuspid aortic valve. *The Annals of Thoracic Surgery,* Vol. 73, No. 3, (March 2002), pp. (720-724).

Bensaid, J., Christides, C., Renaudin, D., Virot, P., Aldigier, JC., Blanc, P., Gandjbakhch, I. & Cabrol, C. (1978). Association of an aortic bicuspid calcification with an obstructive myocardiopathy and a stenosing coronary atherosclerosis, Triple surgical correction. *Annales de Cardiologie et d'Angéiologie,* Vol. 27, No. 4, (July-September 1978), pp. (303-309).

Berenson, GS., Srinivasan, SR., Bao, W., Newman, WP., 3rd., Tracy, RE. & Wattigney WA. (1998). Association between multiple cardiovascular risk factors and atherosclerosis in children and young adults. The Bogalusa Heart Study. *The New England Journal of Medicine,* Vol. 338, No. 23, (June, 1998), pp. (1650-1656).

Bonderman, D., Gharehbaghi-Schnell, E., Wollenek, G., Maurer G., Baumgartner, H., & Lang, IM. (1999). Mechanisms underlying aortic dilatation in congenital aortic valve malformation. *Circulation,* Vol. 99, No. 16, (April 1999), pp. (2138–2143).

Bonow, RO., Carabello, BA., Kanu, C., de Leon, AC Jr., Faxon, DP., Freed, MD., Gaasch, WH., Lytle, BW., Nishimura, RA., O'Gara, PT., O'Rourke, RA., Otto, CM., Shah, PM., Shanewise, JS., Smith, SC Jr., Jacobs, AK., Adams, CD., Anderson, JL., Antman, EM., Faxon, DP., Fuster, V., Halperin, JL., Hiratzka, LF., Hunt, SA., Lytle, BW., Nishimura, R., Page, RL. & Riegel, B. (2006) ACC / AHA 2006 guidelines for the management of patients with valvular heart disease: a report of the American College of Cardiology/American Heart Association Task Force on Practice Guidelines (writing committee to revise the 1998 Guidelines for the Management of Patients With Valvular Heart Disease): developed in collaboration with the Society of Cardiovascular Anesthesiologists: endorsed by the Society for Cardiovascular Angiography and Interventions and the Society of Thoracic Surgeons. *Circulation,* Vol. 11, No. 5, (August 2006), pp. (e84-231).

Branch, K., O'Brien, KD. & Otto, CM. (2002). Aortic valve sclerosis as a marker of active atherosclerosis. *Current Cardiology Reports,* Vol. 4, No. 2, (March 2002), pp. (111-117).

Brandenburg, RO. Jr., Tajik, AJ., Edwards, WD., Reeder, GS., Shub, C. & Seward, JB. (1983). Accuracy of 2-dimensional echocardiographic diagnosis of congenitally bicuspid aortic valve: echocardiographic-anatomic correlation in 115 patients. *The American Journal of Cardiology,* Vol. 51, No. 9, (May 1983), pp. (1469-1473).

Braverman, AC., Guven, H., Beardslee, MA., Makan, M., Kates, AM., & Moon MR. (2005). The bicuspid aortic valve. *Current Problems in Cardiology,* Vol. 30, No. 9, (September 2005), pp. (470-522).

Brown, C., Sane, DC. & Kitzman, DW. (2003). Bicuspid aortic valves in monozygotic twins. *Echocardiography,* Vol. 20, No. 2, (February, 2003), pp. (183-184).

Chang, CP., Neilson, JR., Bayle, JH., Gestwicki, JE., Kuo, A., Stankunas, K., Graef, IA & Crabtree, GR. (2004). A field of myocardial-endocardial NFAT signaling underlies heart valve morphogenesis. *Cell,* Vol. 118, No. 5, (September, 2004), pp. (649-663).

Demir, M. Acute myocardial infarction in a young patient with bicuspid aortic valve. *Turk Kardiyoloji Dernegi Arsivi,* Vol. 37, No. 7, (October 2009), pp. (490-492).

De Mozzi, P., Longo, UG., Galanti, G. & Maffulli, N. (2008). Bicuspid aortic valve: a literature review and its impact on sport activity. *British Medical Bulletin*, Vol. 85, (February 2008), pp. (63-85).
Deshpande, J. & Kinare, SG. (1991). The bicuspid aortic valve - an autopsy study. *Indian Journal of Pathology & Microbiology*, Vol. 34, No. 2, (April 1991), pp. (112-118).
Doty, DB. (2001). Anomalous origin of the left circumflex coronary artery associated with bicuspid aortic valve. *The Journal of Thoracic and Cardiovascular Surgery*, Vol. 122, No. 4, (October 2001), pp. (842-843).
Duran, AC., Frescura, C., Sans-Coma, V., Angelini, A., Basso, C. & Thiene, G. (1995). Bicuspid aortic valves in hearts with other congenital heart disease. *The Journal of heart valve disease*, Vol. 4, No. 6, (November, 1995), pp. (581-590).
Eisenberg, LM. & Markwald, RR. (1995). Molecular regulation of atrioventricular valvuloseptal morphogenesis. *Circulation Research*, Vol. 77, No. 1, (July 1995), pp. (1-6).
Emanuel, R., Withers, R., O'Brien, K., Ross, P., & Feizi, O. (1978). Congenitally bicuspid aortic valves. Clinicogenetic study of 41 families. *British Heart Journal*, Vol. 40, No. 12, (December 1978), pp. (1402-1407).
Faggiano, P., Frattini, S., Zilioli, V., Rossi, A., Nistri, S., Dini, FL., Lorusso, R., Tomasi, C., & Cas, LD. (2011). Prevalence of comorbidities and associated cardiac diseases in patients with valve aortic stenosis. Potential implications for the decision-making process. *International Journal of Cardiology*, (2011 March). [Epub ahead of print].
Fedak, PW., Verma, S., David, TE., Leask, RL., Weisel, RD. & Butany, J. (2002). Clinical and pathophysiological implications of a bicuspid aortic valve. *Circulation*, Vol. 106, No. 8, (August 2002), pp. (900-904).
Fenoglio, JJ., Jr., McAllister, HA., Jr., DeCastro, CM., Davia, JE. & Cheitlin, MD. (1977). Congenital bicuspid aortic valve after age 20. *The American Journal of Cardiology*, Vol. 39, No. 2, (February 1977), pp. (164-169).
Fernandes, SM., Sanders, SP., Khairy, P., Jenkins, KJ., Gauvreau, K., Lang, P., Simonds, H. & Colan, SD. (2004). Morphology of bicuspid aortic valve in children and adolescent. *Journal of the American College of Cardiology*, Vol. 44, No. 8, (October 2004), pp. 1648-1651.
Fernández, B., Fernández, MC., Durán, AC., López, D., Martire, A. & Sans-Coma, V. (1998). Anatomy and formation of congenital bicuspid and quadricuspid pulmonary valves in Syrian hamsters. *The Anatomical record*, Vol. 250, No. 1, (January 1998), pp. (70-79).
Fox, CS., Polak, JF., Chazaro, I., Cupples, A., Wolf, PA., D'Agostino, RA. & O'Donnel,l CJ. (2003). Genetic and environmental contributions to atherosclerosis phenotypes in men and women: heritability of carotid intima-media thickness in the Framingham Heart Study. *Stroke*, Vol. 34, No. 2, (February 2003), pp. (397-401).
Futterman, LG. & Lemberg, L. (1998). Fifty percent of patients with coronary artery disease do not have any of the conventional risk factors. *American Journal of Critical Care*, Vol. 7, No. 3, (May 1998), pp. (240-244).
Gale, AN., McKusick, VA., Hutchins, GM. & Gott, VL. (1977). Familial congenital bicuspid aortic valve: secondary calcific aortic stenosis and aortic aneurysm. *Chest*, Vol. 72, No. 5, (November, 1977), pp. (668-670).
Garg, V., Muth, AN., Ransom, JF., Schluterman, MK., Barnes, R., King, IN., Grossfeld, PD. &, Srivastava D. (2005). Mutations in NOTCH1 cause aortic valve disease. *Nature*, Vol. 437, No. 7056, (July, 2005), pp. (270-274).

Gensini, GG. (1983). A more meaningful scoring system for determining the severity of coronary heart disease. *The American Journal of Cardiology*, Vol. 51, No. 3, (February 1983), pp. (606).

Glick, BN. & Roberts, WC. (1994). Congenitally bicuspid aortic valve in multiple family members. *The American Journal of Cardiolog*, Vol. 73, No. 5, (February 1994), pp. (400-404).

Godden DJ, Sandhu PS, & Kerr, F. (1987). Stenosed bicuspid aortic valves in twins. *European Heart Journal*, Vol. 8, No. 3, (Martch, 1987), pp. (316-318).

Goland, S., Czer, LS., De Robertis, MA., Mirocha, J., Kass, RM., Fontana, GP., Chang, W. & Trento, A. (2007). Risk factors associated with reoperation and mortality in 252 patients after aortic valve replacement for congenitally bicuspid aortic valve disease. *The Annals of Thoracic Surgery*, Vol. 83, No. 3, (March 2007), pp. (931-937).

Greenland, P., Knoll, MD., Stamler, J., Neaton, JD., Dyer, AR., Garside, DB., & Wilson, PW. (2003). Major risk factors as antecedents of fatal and nonfatal coronary heart disease events. *The Journal of the American Medical Association*, Vol. 290, No. 7, (August 2003), pp. (891-897).

Hahn, RT., Roman, MJ., Mogtader, AH., & Devereux, RB. (1992). Association of aortic dilation with regurgitant, stenotic and functionally normal bicuspid aortic valves. *Journal of the American College of Cardiology*, Vol. 19, No. 2, (February 1992), pp. (283-288).

Hennekens, CH. (1998). Increasing burden of cardiovascular disease: current knowledge and future directions for research on risk factors. *Circulation*, Vol. 97, No. 11, (March 1998), pp. (1095-1102).

Higgins, CB. & Wexler, L. (1975). Reversal of dominance of the coronary arterial system in isolated stenosis and bicuspid aortic valve. *Circulation*, Vol. 52, No. 2, (August 1975), pp. (292-296).

Hinton, RB., Jr., Lincoln, J., Deutsch, GH., Osinska, H., Manning, PB., Benson, DW. & Yutzey, KE. (2006). Extracellular matrix remodeling and organization in developing and diseased aortic valves. *Circulation Research*, Vol. 98, No. 11, (AprilJune, 2006), pp. (1431-1438).

Hoffman, JI. & Kaplan, S. (2002). The incidence of congenital heart disease. *Journal of the American College of Cardiology*, Vol. 39, No. 12, (June 2002), pp. (1890-1900).

Hunt, KJ., Duggirala, R., Goring, HH., Williams, JT., Almasy, L., Blangero, J., O'Leary, DH. & Stern, MP. (2002). Genetic basis of variation in carotid artery plaque in the San Antonio family heart study. *Stroke*, Vol. 33, No. 12, (December 2002), pp. (2775-2780).

Huntington, K., Hunter, AG. & Chan, KL. (1997). A prospective study to assess the frequency of familial clustering of congenital bicuspid aortic valve. *Journal of the American College of Cardiology*, Vol. 30, No. 7, (December, 1997), pp. (1809-1812).

Hurlstone, AF., Haramis, AP., Wienholds, E., Begthel, H., Korving, J., Van Eeden, F., Cuppen, E., Zivkovic, D., Plasterk, RH. & Clevers, H. (2003). The Wnt/beta-catenin pathway regulates cardiac vaive formation. *Nature*, Vol. 425, No. 6958, (October, 2003), pp. (633-637).

Hutchins, GM., Nazarian, IH. & Bulkley, BH. (1978). Association of left dominant coronary arterial system with congenital bicuspid aorta. *The American Journal of* Cardiology, Vol. 42, No. 1, (July 1978), pp. (57-59).

Kappetein, AP., Gittenberger-de Groot, AC., Zwinderman, AH., Rohmer, J., Poelmann, RE. & Huysmans, HA. (1991). The neural crest as a possible pathogenetic factor in coarctation of the aorta and bicuspid aortic valve. *The Journal of Thoracic and Cardiovascular Surgery*, Vol. 102, No. 6, (December 1991), pp. (830-836).

Khot, UN., Khot, MB., Bajzer, CT., Sapp, SK., Ohman, EM., Brener, SJ., Ellis, SG., Lincoff, AM. & Topol, EJ. (2003). Prevalence of conventional risk factors in patients with coronary heart disease. *The Journal of the American Medical Association*, Vol. 290, No. 7, (August 2003), pp. (898-904).

Labombarda, F., Legallois, D., & Sabatier, R. (2009). Spontaneous coronary artery dissection and bicuspid aortic valve. *Archives of Cardiovascular Disease*, Vol. 102, No. 12, (December 2009) pp. (857-858).

Lamas, CC. & Eykyn SJ. (2000). Bicuspid aortic valve--A silent danger: analysis of 50 cases of infective endocarditis. *Clinical Infectious Diseases*, Vol. 30, No. 2, (February 2000), pp. (336-341).

Larson, EW. & Edwards, WD. (1984). Risk factors for aortic dissection: a necropsy study of 161 cases. *The American Journal of Cardiology*, Vol. 53, No. 6, (March 1984), pp. (849-855).

Lee, TC., Zhao, YD., Courtman, DW. & Stewart, DJ. (2000). Abnormal aortic valve development in mice lacking endothelial nitric oxide synthase. *Circulation*, Vol. 101, No. 20, (May, 2000), pp. (2345-2348).

Lindsay, J., Jr. (1988). Coarctation of the aorta, bicuspid aortic valve and abnormal ascending aortic wall. *The American Journal of Cardiology*, Vol. 61, No. 1, (January 1988), pp. (182–184).

Lopez-Rangel, E., Maurice, M., McGillivray, B. & Friedman, JM. (1992). Williams syndrome in adults. *American Journal of Medical Genetics*, Vol. 44, No. 6, (December 1992), pp. (720-729).

Mancuso, D., Basso, C., Cardaioli, P. & Thiene, G. (2002). Clefted bicuspid aortic valve. *Cardiovascular Pathology*, Vol. 11, No. 4, (July-August, 2002), pp. (217-220).

Marenberg, ME., Risch, N., Berkman, LF., Floderus, B. & de Faire, U. (1994). Genetic susceptibility to death from coronary heart disease in a study of twins. *The New England Journal of Medicine*, Vol. 330, No. 15, (April, 1994), pp. (1041-1046).

Martin, LJ., Ramachandran, V., Cripe, LH., Hinton, RB., Andelfinger, G., Tabangin, M., Shooner, K., Keddache, M. & Benson, DW. (2007). Evidence in favor of linkage to human chromosomal regions 18q, 5q and 13q for bicuspid aortic valve and associated cardiovascular malformations. *Human Genetics*, Vol. 121, No. 2, (January 2007), pp. (275-284). McDonald, K. & Mauree, BJ. (1989). Familial aortic valve disease: evidence for a genetic influence? *European Heart Journal*, Vol. 10, No. 7, (July, 1989), pp. (676-677).

McKusick, VA. (1972). Association of congenital bicuspid aortic valve and erdheim's cystic medial necrosis. *Lancet*, Vol. 1, No. 7758, (May, 1972), pp. (1026-1027).

Mohamed, SA., Hanke, T., Schlueter, C., Bullerdiek, J. & Sievers, HH. (2005). Ubiquitin fusion degradation 1-like gene dysregulation in bicuspid aortic valve. *The Journal of thoracic and cardiovascular* surgery, Vol. 130, No. 6, (December, 2005), pp. (1531-1536).

Movahed, MD., Hepner, AD. & Ahmadi-Kashani, M. (2006). Echocardiographic prevalence of bicuspid aortic valve in the population. *Heart, Lung & Circulation*, Vol. 15, No. 5, (October 2006), pp. (297-299).

Nakamura, K., Onitsuka, T., Nakamura, E., Yano, M., Matsuzaki, Y. & Nabeshima, K. (1999) Rare cases of congenital bicuspid aortic valve with an abnormal fibrous band.

Annals of Thoracic and Cardiovascular Surgery, Vol. 5, No. 5, (October 1999), pp. 343-346.

Niwa, K., Perloff, JK., Bhuta, SM., Laks, H., Drinkwater, DC., Child, JS. & Miner, PD. (2001). Structural abnormalities of great arterial walls in congenital heart disease: light and electron microscopic analyses. *Circulation*, Vol. 103, No. 3, (January 2001), pp. (393–400).

Olson, LJ., Subramanian, R. & Edwards, WD. (1984). Surgical pathology of pure aortic insufficiency: a study of 225 cases. *Mayo Clinic Proceedings*, Vol. 59, No. 12, (December 1984), pp. (835-841).

Oomman, A. & Mao, R. (2000). Coronary artery fistula from both coronaries to pulmonary artery in association with congenital bicuspid aortic stenosis. *Indian Heart Journal*, Vol. 52, No. 2, (March-April 2000), pp. (201-202).

Otto, CM., Lind, BK., Kitzman, DW., Gersh, BJ., & Siscovik, DS. (1999) Cardiovascular Health Study Association of aortic valve stenosis with cardiovascular morbidity and mortality in the elderly. *The New England Journal of Medicine*, Vol. 341, No. 3, (July 1999), pp. (142-147).

Oyonarte, M., Moyano, C., Terra, E. & Barrientos, C. (1992). Fatal infectious endocarditis in a patient with annulo-aortic ectasia and predominant bicuspid valve aortic stenosis. Anatomoclinical case. *Revista médica de Chile*, Vol. 120, No. 1, (January, 1992), pp. (62-68).

Pachulski, RT., Weinberg, AL. & Chan, KL. (1991). Aortic aneurysm in patients with functionally normal or minimally stenotic bicuspid aortic valve. *The American Journal of* Cardiology, Vol. 67, No. 8, (April 1991), pp. (781-782).

Palomo, AR., Schrager, BR. & Chahine, RA. (1985). Anomalous origin of the right coronary artery from the ascending aorta high above the left posterior sinus of Valsalva of a bicuspid aortic valve. *American Heart Journal*, Vol. 109, No. 4, (April 1985), pp. (902-904).

Passik, CS., Ackermann, DM., Pluth, JR., & Edwards, WD. (1987). Temporal changes in the causes of aortic stenosis: a surgical pathologic study of 646 cases. *Mayo Clinic Proceedings*, Vol. 62, No. 2, (Feb 1987), pp. (119–123).

Pomerance, A. (1972). Pathogenesis of aortic stenosis and its relation to age. *British Heart Journal*, Vol. 34, No. 6, (June 1972), pp. (569-574).

Popescu, BA., Jurcut, R., Serban, M., Parascan, L. & Ginghina, C. (2008). Shone's syndrome diagnosed with echocardiography and confirmed at pathology. *European Journal of Echocardiography*, Vol. 9, No. 6, (July 2008), pp. (865-867).

Rabkin-Aikawa, E., Farber, M., Aikawa, M. &,Schoen, FJ. (2004). Dynamic and reversible changes of interstitial cell phenotype during remodeling of cardiac valves. *The Journal of heart valve disease*, Vol. 13, No. 5, (September, 2004), pp. (841-847).

Rashid, A., Saucedo, JF. & Hennebry, TA. (2005). Association of single coronary artery and congenital bicuspid aortic valve with review of literature. *Journal of Interventional Cardiology*, Vol. 18, No. 5, (October 2005), pp. (389-391).

Ringqvist, I., Fisher, LD., Mock, M., Davis, KB., Wedel, H., Chaitman, BR., Passamani, E., Russell, RO Jr,. Alderman, EL., Kouchoukas, NT., Kaiser, GC., Ryan, TJ., Killip, T. & Fray, D. (1983). Prognostic value of angiographic indices of coronary artery disease from the Coronary Artery Surgery Study (CASS). *The Journal of Clinical Investigation*, Vol. 71, No. 6, (June 1983), pp. (1854-1866).

Roberts, WC., Morrow, AG. & Braunwald, E. (1962). Complete interruption of the aortic arch. *Circulation*, Vol. 26. (July 1962), pp. (39–59).

Roberts, WC. & Ko, JM. (2005). Frequency by decades of unicuspid, bicuspid, and tricuspid aortic valves in adults having isolated aortic valve replacement for aortic stenosis, with or without associated aortic regurgitation. *Circulation*, Vol. 111, No. 7, (February 2005), pp. (920-925).

Roberts WC, Morrow, AG., McIntosh, CL., Jones, M. & Epstein, SE. (1981). Congenitally bicuspid aortic valve causing severe, pure aortic regurgitation without superimposed infective endocarditis. Analysis of 13 patients requiring aortic valve replacement. *The American Journal of Cardiology*, Vol. 47, No. 2, (February 1981), pp. (206-209).

Roman, MJ., Devereux, RB., Kramer-Fox. R., & O'Loughlin J. (1989) Two-dimensional echocardiographic aortic root dimensions in normal children and adults. *The American Journal of Cardiology*, Vol. 64, No. 8, (September 1989), pp. (507-512).

Rose, AG. (1986). Etiology of acquired valvular heart disease in adults: a survey of 18,132 autopsies and 100 consecutive valve-replacement operations. *Archives of Pathology & Laboratory Medicine*, Vol. 110, No. 5, (May 1986), pp. (385-388).

Sabet, HY., Edwards, WD., Tazelaar,. HD. & Daly, RC. (1999). Congenitally bicuspid aortic valves: a surgical pathology study of 542 cases (1991 through 1996) and a literature review of 2715 additional cases. *Mayo Clinic Proceedings*, Vol. 74, No. 1, (January 1999), pp. (14–26).

Sagic, D., Miric, M., Popovic, Z., Grujicic, S., & Bojic, M. (1997). Ductus diverticulum aneurysm associated with bicuspid aortic valve and dilatation of ascending aorta. *The Journal of Cardiovascular Surgery (Torino)*, Vol. 38, No. 2, (April 1997), pp. (137-140).

Sans-Coma, V., Fernández, B., Durán, AC., Thiene, G., Arqué, JM., Muñoz-Chápuli, R. & Cardo, M. (1996). Fusion of valve cushions as a key factor in the formation of congenital bicuspid aortic valves in Syrian hamsters. *The Anatomical Record*, Vol. 244, No. 4, (April 1996), pp. (490-498).

Schaefer, BM., Lewin, MB., Stout, KK,, Gill, E., Prueitt, A., Byers, PH. & Otto, CM. (2008). The bicuspid aortic valve: an integrated phenotypic classification of leaflet morphology and aortic root shape. *Heart*, Vol. 94, No. 12, (February, 2008) pp. (1634-1638).

Schievink, WI. & Mokri, B. (1995). Familial aorto-cervicocephalic arterial dissections and congenitally bicuspid aortic valve. *Stroke*, Vol. 26, No. 10, (October 1995), pp. (1935–1940)

Shimuzu, M., Chang, N., Kawai, S., Okada, R. & Fukoda, Y. (1984). An autopsy case of rheumatoid arthritis with aortic steno-insufficiency, angina pectoris and severe heart failure. *Japanese circulation journal*, Vol. 48, No. 9, (Septeber 1984), pp. (1045-1049).

Sievers, HH. & Schmidtke, C. (2007). A classification system for the bicuspid aortic valve from 304 surgical specimens. *The Journal of Thoracic and Cardiovascular Surgery*, Vol. 133, No. 5, (May 2007), pp. (1226-1233).

Subramanian, R., Olson, LJ. & Edwards, WD. (1984). Surgical pathology of pure aortic stenosis: a study of 374 cases. *Mayo Clinic Proceedings*, Vol. 59, No. 10, (October 1984), pp. (683-690).

Sivapalaratnam, S., Motazacker, MM., Maiwald, S., Hovingh, GK., Kastelein, JJ., Levi M., Trip, MD. & Dallinga-Thie GM. (2011). Genome-wide association studies in atherosclerosis. *Current Atherosclerosis Reports*, Vol. 13, No. 3, (June, 2011), pp. (225-232).

Suzuki, T., Nagai, R., Kurihara, H, Yamazaki, T., Ho, E., Maemura, K., Shiojima, I., Yamaoki, K., Furuse, A., & Yazaki, Y. (1994). Stenotic bicuspid aortic valve associated with a ventricular septal defect in an adult presenting with congestive heart failure: a rare observation. *European Heart Journal*, Vol. 15, No. 3, (March 1994), pp. (402-403).

Theleman, KP., Grayburn, PA. & Roberts WC. (2006). Mitral "annular" calcium forming a complete circle "O" causing mitral stenosis in association with a stenotic congenitally bicuspid aortic valve and severe coronary artery disease. *American Journal Geriatric Cardioly*, Vol. 15, No. 1, (January-February 2006), pp. (58-61).

Timmerman, LA., Grego-Bessa, J., Raya, A., Bertrán, E., Pérez-Pomares, JM., Díez, J., Aranda, S., Palomo, S., McCormick, F., Izpisúa-Belmonte, JC. & de la Pompa, JL. (2004). Notch promotes epithelial-mesenchymal transition during cardiac development and oncogenic transformation. *Genes & Development*, Vol. 18, No. 1, (December, 2004), pp. (99-115).

van den Hoff, MJ., Moorman, AF., Ruijter, JM., Lamers, WH., Bennington, RW., Markwald, RR. & Wessels. (1999). A. Myocardialization of the cardiac outflow tract. *Developmental biology*, Vol. 212, No. 2, (August, 1999), pp. (477-490).

Vasan, RS., Larson, MG., Benjamin, EJ. & Levy, D. (1995). Echocardiographic reference values for aortic root size: the Framingham Heart Study. *Journal of the American Society of Echocardiography*, Vol. 8, No. 6, (November-December 1995), pp. (793-800).

Ward, C. (2000). Clinical significance of the bicuspid aortic valve. *Heart*, Vol 83, No. 1, (January 2006), pp. (81-85). Warnes, CA. (2003). Bicuspid aortic valve and coarctation: two villains part of a diffuse problem. *Heart*, Vol. 89, No. 9, (September 2003), pp. (965–966).

Weinhouse, E., Riggs, T. W. & Aughton, D. J. (1995). Isolated bicuspid aortic valve in a newborn with Down syndrome. *Clinical Pediatrics (Phila)*, Vol. 34, No. 2, (February 1995), pp. (116-117).

Yamagishi, C., Hierck, BP., Gittenberger-De Groot, AC., Yamagishi, H. & Srivastava D. (2003). Functional attenuation of UFD1l, a 22q11.2 deletion syndrome candidate gene, leads to cardiac outflow septation defects in chicken embryos. *Pediatric Research*, Vol. 53, No. 4, (February, 2003), pp. (546-553).

Yokoyama, S., Ashida, T., Sugiyama, T., Ebihara, A., Fujii, J., Chida, K., Ezaki, Y., & Ohkawa, S. (2002). An autopsied case with a bicuspid aortic valve who had progressive angina pectoris and heart failure during follow-up of 27 years. *Nippon Ronen Igakkai Zasshi*, Vol. 39, No. 4, (July 2002), pp. (444-447).

Yuan, SM., Jing, H. & Lavee, J. (2010). The bicuspid aortic valve and its relation to aortic dilation. *Clinics (Sao Paulo)*, Vol. 65, No. 5, (May 2010), pp. (497-505).

Yutzey, KE., Colbert, M. & Robbins, J. (2005). Ras-related signaling pathways in valve development: ebb and flow. *Physiology (Bethesda)*, Vol. 20, (December, 2005), pp. (390-397).

Zoghbi, WA., Enriquez-Sarano, M., Foster, E., Grayburn, PA., Kraft, CD., Levine, RA., Nihoyannopoulos, P., Otto, CM., Quinones, MA., Rakowsk,i H., Stewart, WJ., Waggoner, A. & Weissman, NJ., American Society of Echocardiography. (2003). Recommendations for evaluation of the severity of native valvular regurgitation with two-dimensional and Doppler echocardiography. *Journal of the American Society of Echocardiography*, Vol. 16, No. 7, (July 2003), pp. (777-802).

17

Novel Phenotypes in Bicuspid Aortic Valve Disease

Evaldas Girdauskas[1], Michael A. Borger[2] and Thomas Kuntze[1]
[1]*Zentralklinik Bad Berka*
[2]*Heart Centre Leipzig, University Leipzig*
Germany

1. Introduction

Bicuspid aortic valve (BAV) is the most common congenital abnormality of the human heart, affecting approximately 1-2% of the general population (Williams, 2006). It is widely accepted that BAV is a very heterogeneous disease and that the different phenotypes of BAV disease may be caused by unique pathogenetic mechanisms. Because the heterogeneous nature of BAV disease has been recognized by many researchers, attempts have been made to stratify the most common anatomic-clinical forms.

The clinically observed linkage between specific BAV morphology and the associated lesions of the proximal aorta has recently led to several phenotypic classifications which incorporate both valve and proximal aortic anatomy. These different BAV phenotypes may be caused by unique pathogenetic mechanisms and may require different therapeutic approaches. The clarification of this phenomenon will undoubtedly affect the individual treatment strategy of BAV disease.

In the face of these novel findings, this chapter deals with recent controversies in BAV disease.

2. Phenotypes in BAV disease

The recently identified BAV phenotypes incorporate specific aortic valve anatomy (or a predominant type of aortic valve dysfunction) and concomitant lesions of the proximal aorta. To begin with, these empirical observations were based on the surgical and echocardiographic findings of an association between specific BAV disease and concomitant lesions of aortic root, ascending aorta, or both. Configuration of the proximal aorta is undoubtedly different in patients with BAV stenosis versus BAV insufficiency. Moreover, there are apparently distinct forms of proximal aortic lesions in patients with fusion of right coronary and left coronary cusps versus fusion of right coronary and non-coronary cusps in BAV disease.

These specific associations of BAV anatomy and proximal aortic disease have been analyzed by a large number of *in vitro*, rheological and biomolecular investigations. These novel BAV phenotypes and the corresponding fundamental research articles will be addressed in detail in the following paragraphs.

2.1 BAV stenosis versus BAV insufficiency

The strong correlation between specific aortic dilatation patterns and the functional status of BAV (i.e., BAV stenosis versus insufficiency) has been demonstrated by some investigators based on the empirical analysis of clinical data. In particular, the presence of BAV stenosis is typically associated with asymmetrical dilatation of the mid-ascending aorta and a nearly normal aortic root diameter (Cotrufo & Della Corte, 2009). In contrast, aortic root dilatation is more often associated with a concomitant or consequent BAV insufficiency (i.e., root dilatation phenotype).

Different pathogenetic mechanisms have been proposed for those two apparently different BAV phenotypes (Cotrufo & Della Corte, 2009). Importantly, significant differences in the expression and spatial distribution of extracellular matrix (ECM) proteins have been found between these two subgroups of BAV disease (i.e., aortic valve stenosis versus insufficiency). Both BAV phenotypes have been linked to the specific patient's characteristics and will be discussed in detail.

2.1.1 BAV stenosis with an asymmetric mid-ascending aortic dilatation

This most common anatomical-clinical BAV phenotype includes stenosis of the BAV, an unaffected or only mildly dilated aortic root, and an asymmetric dilation of the mid-ascending aorta, starting from the sinotubular junction and involving mostly the convexity (i.e., the greater curvature) of the vessel (Fig. 1). The association between BAV stenosis and asymmetric mid-ascending aortic dilatation has been proposed to be pathogenetic (Della Corte *et al.*, 2007).

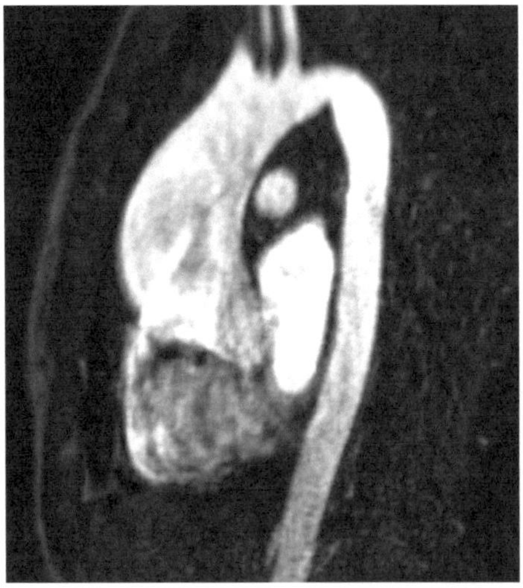

Fig. 1. Magnetic resonance imaging demonstrating an asymmetric mid-ascending aortic aneurysm in a patient with BAV stenosis

It has been proved that stenosis of the BAV, which is geometrically asymmetrical, produces an eccentric turbulent transvalvular blood flow that results in asymmetrical wall stress distribution in the ascending aorta (Fig. 2) (Robicsek *et al.*, 2004). It has been hypothesized that this uneven wall stress distribution may be important in promoting early localized aortic wall changes, which may lead subsequently to an asymmetric ascending aortic dilatation. These flow-dependant changes in the microstructure of the vessel wall are known as a *flow-induced vascular remodeling* (Lehoux *et al.*, 2002).

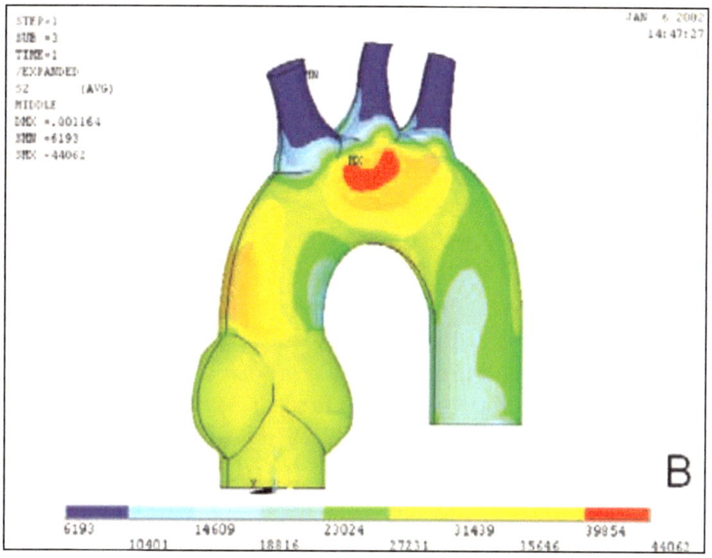

Fig. 2. Stress patterns in the proximal aorta in the setting of an eccentric BAV. The red and yellowish brown segments of the proximal aorta are the most stressed by the eccentric transvalvular blood flow; the blue segments are the least stressed (published in *Annals of Thoracic Surgery* 2004; 77:177-185)

According to these data, this pathogenetically linked anatomical-clinical BAV phenotype (i.e., BAV stenosis with an asymmetric mid-ascending aortic dilatation) may represent the predominantly hemodynamically triggered form of BAV aortopathy. In compliance with these findings, some most recent *in vitro* and *in vivo* studies provide further evidence of the hemodynamic nature of this BAV phenotype.

2.1.1.1 Correlation between BAV stenosis and the extent of mid-ascending aortic dilatation

Given the marked heterogeneity of BAV disease and the co-existence of different clinical-anatomical phenotypes, the data on the correlation between the type of BAV dysfunction and the extent of proximal aortic dilation are very controversial. However, when the analysis has been focused on the mid-ascending aortic dilatation form alone, a strong correlation has been found between the degree of BAV stenosis and the extent of ascending aortic dilatation at maximum diameter (Della Corte *et al.*, 2007).
Similar findings have been recently reported by some other investigators (Davies *et al.*, 2007). These authors were able to clearly demonstrate a strong association between the presence of aortic valve stenosis and all adverse aortic events in the BAV subgroup. Moreover, a significant correlation has been demonstrated most recently between the degree of eccentricity of the systolic transvalvular flow through the BAV and the severity of the proximal aortic dilatation in the pediatric BAV subpopulation (i.e., the larger the angle of misdirected blood flow with the aortic axis, the larger the proximal aortic diameter) (den

Reijer *et al.*, 2010). These correlations were most significant at the more distal level of the ascending aorta, where aortic wall stress is expectedly highest.

These results favour the hemodynamic hypothesis of BAV-associated aortopathy (i.e. abnormal blood flow patterns induced by BAV stenosis are directly involved in the development of ascending aortic dilatation).

2.1.1.2 Functioning of the "clinically normal" BAV

There is emerging evidence that the "clinically normal" BAV (i.e., one without a quantitatively detectable transvalvular pressure gradient by continuous-wave Doppler methods of grading) is morphologically stenotic and is associated with an abnormal eccentric systolic transvalvular flow, which results in asymmetrical wall stress distribution in the ascending aorta (Robicsek *et al.*, 2004).

This has been recently demonstrated in a sophisticated mathematical analysis, using a dynamic three-dimensional (3D) finite element model of the bicuspid aortic root (Conti *et al.*, 2010). These investigators were able to convincingly demonstrate that the mere fusion of the two aortic valve cusps restricts the opening motion of the conjoined cusp, which causes subclinical BAV stenosis. Moreover, the longitudinal stress at the convexity of the ascending aorta has been found to be increased by 36% in BAV versus the tricuspid aortic valve (TAV) aortic root finite element model.

The *in vitro* data have been supported most recently by an *in vivo* analysis of systolic transvalvular flow in BAV patients using sophisticated four-dimensional magnetic resonance imaging (MRI) (Hope *et al.*, 2010). The authors of this study demonstrated convincingly a nested helical systolic flow pattern in the proximal aorta in patients with BAV, including those without ascending aortic dilatation or significant BAV stenosis (Fig. 3). These abnormal systolic transvalvular flow patterns were shown to be different and unique for the two most common cusp fusion types in patients with BAV.

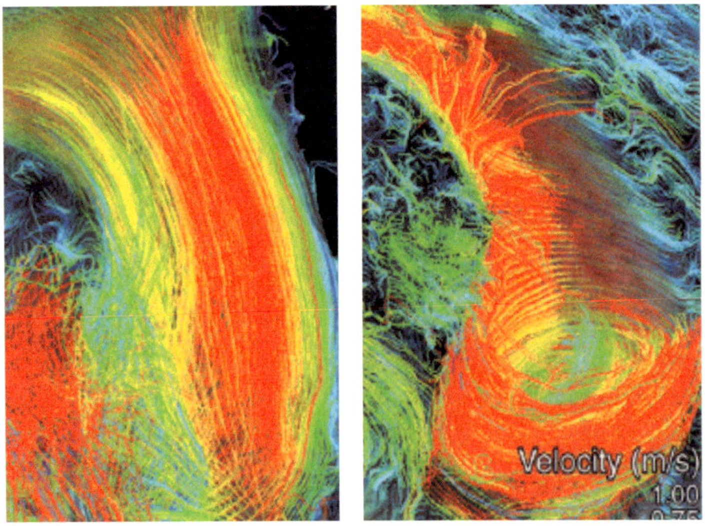

(a) (b)

Fig. 3. Systolic transvalvular flow patterns in the proximal aorta in a patient with TAV (a) and BAV (b) (published in *Radiology* 2010; 77:177-185)

All above-mentioned studies clearly indicate that the eccentric opening of "clinically normal" BAV is enough to generate significant flow disturbances downstream (e.g., turbulence, vortices, nested helical flow patterns, asymmetrically arranged flow), which may induce permanent mechanical stimuli to the ascending aortic wall, and, subsequently, asymmetric aortic dilation.

2.1.1.3 Asymmetric pattern of aortopathy in BAV disease

The concept of asymmetry in ascending aortic disease was first introduced by Cotrufo *et al.* (2001). This was based on the empirical macroscopic surgical observations of asymmetric ascending aortic aneurysms propagating from the right anterolateral aortic wall (i.e., convexity or a greater curvature).

The enlargement of the tubular mid-ascending aorta in patients with BAV disease has a typical asymmetric configuration at the convexity of the vessel, as shown in the retrospective analysis of aortic angiograms (Bauer *et al.*, 2006). Moreover, the distance between the aortic valve level and the level of the maximal ascending aortic diameter was found to be greater in BAV patients versus TAV patients.

The asymmetric pattern of the ascending aortic wall alterations has been confirmed by a series of consecutive histological and biomolecular investigations by Cotrufo *et al.* (2005). Consecutive studies have shown an asymmetric spatial pattern of extracellular matrix (ECM) protein expression and smooth muscle cell (SMC) changes in the convexity versus the concavity of the dilated ascending aorta in BAV patients (Cotrufo *et al.*, 2005; Della Corte *et al.*, 2006, 2008). Moreover, this asymmetric pattern of microstructural aortic wall changes has been found in non-dilated aortas in the setting of BAV stenosis.

This proven asymmetry of BAV aortopathy, which may be interpreted as a result of aortic wall stress-induced vascular remodeling, lends more credence to the hemodynamic nature of BAV stenosis-associated aortopathy.

In conclusion, the identified predominant anatomical-clinical BAV phenotype of BAV stenosis with an asymmetric mid-ascending aortic dilatation may include those patients in whom the hemodynamic factors play a determinant role.

2.1.2 BAV insufficiency with a dilatation of aortic root (root dilatation phenotype)

There is a relatively small subset of BAV patients (10-15%), who present with the predominant aortic root dilatation at the level of aortic annulus and the sinuses of Valsalva. This form of proximal aortic dilatation is commonly associated with a varying degree of concomitant or consequent aortic valve insufficiency. This relatively rare clinical-anatomical form of BAV disease has been described in the literature as a "root dilatation phenotype" (Della Corte *et al.*, 2007) (Fig. 4).

The prevalence of the root phenotype does not increase with age (it occurs primarily in the young BAV population) and shows a strong predilection for the male gender. It has been hypothesized, that this phenotype may be subtended by a less flow-dependent mechanism of aortic wall failure than is asymmetric mid-ascending aortic dilatation, and that it may coexist with every possible degree of aortic valve dysfunction. It has also been proposed that the root dilatation phenotype may be a purely genetic form of BAV disease and a completely different disease from BAV stenosis and asymmetric mid-ascending aortic dilatation (Cotrufo & Della Corte, 2009).

A subgroup of young male BAV patients with the predominant aortic dilatation at the level of the aortic root that occurred independently of age, body size, and aortic valve function has been also prospectively identified in a echocardiographic study (Nistri *et al.*, 1999). The authors of this report hypothesized that there may be a subgroup of BAV patients who are affected by the congenital weakness of the aortic wall structure that causes premature aortic root dilatation, independent of any hemodynamic perturbations.

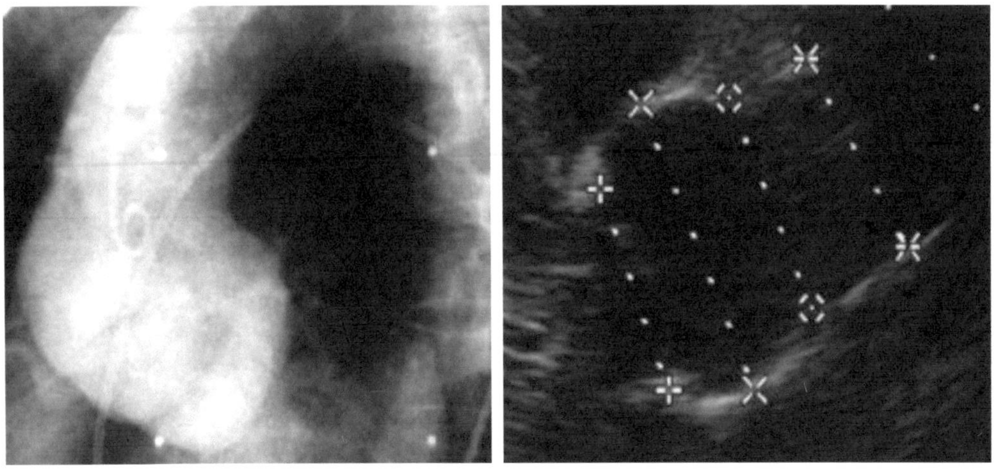

(a) (b)

Fig. 4. Images of aortic angiography (a) and transthoracic echocardiography (b) in BAV patient with a "root phenotype"

Although the genetic nature of the root dilatation phenotype has been postulated by all the above-mentioned studies, no specific gene defect responsible for this type of BAV disease has been ever identified. Moreover, there is a notable paucity of clinical and biomolecular data on the BAV subgroup with a "root phenotype".
Nonetheless, some important indices of the genetic origin of this clinical-anatomical form of BAV disease may be identified in the recent literature and will be discussed in detail as follows.

2.1.2.1 Evidence of the genetic nature of the root dilatation phenotype

A recent study by Loscalzo *et al.* (2007) analyzed a small number of selected families with a high prevalence of BAV disease and familial thoracic aortic aneurysms (TAA). Based on the genetic analysis of thirteen affected families, the authors concluded that BAV and familial thoracic aortic aneurysms are variably penetrant independent manifestations of a single gene defect which may be associated with a wide spectrum of left outflow tract disorders.
However, only fifteen family members of the analyzed probands (13%) had BAV in this study and only ten of them (9%) had a concomitant thoracic aortic aneurysm (i.e., the study included only a small subgroup of patients with a combined BAV/TAA phenotype). Moreover, three patients in the BAV/TAA subgroup had a significant aortic valve dysfunction (i.e., moderate or greater valve insufficiency or stenosis). Therefore, conclusions should be only cautiously drawn from such a limited number of affected patients.

The recently published echocardiographic study by Biner *et al.* (2009) focused on aortopathy in first-degree relatives of BAV patients. Unfortunately, this study included only a small proportion of first-degree relatives of BAV patients (i.e., 48 relatives of 54 BAV patients) and compared them with a highly selective control group (i.e., 45 healthy individuals without structural heart disease, who were included during a study period of 4 years). Irrespective of those methodological flaws, this study has demonstrated a high prevalence of mild aortic root dilatation, which was associated with abnormal elastic properties of proximal aorta in the first-degree relatives of BAV patients. Notably, this series included predominantly BAV patients with aortic dilatation at the level of aortic annulus and sinuses of Valsalva (i.e., the root dilatation phenotype of BAV disease).

We reported most recently on a patient with familial BAV disease and the root dilatation phenotype, who was operated on for proximal aortic aneurysm (Girdauskas *et al.*, 2011a). The surgery was complicated by intraoperative aortic dissection. Multi-generational genetic analysis was performed thereafter and revealed a mutation in the transforming growth factor-beta receptor type II (TGFBR2) gene in our patient and her father.

Some specific features were indicative of a genetic origin of the BAV-associated aortopathy in this patient. The strong family history of BAV disease associated with the root dilatation phenotype, the marked fragility of the aortic wall (which led to the intraoperative aortic dissection), and the histological pattern of symmetric medial degeneration (i.e., cystic medial necrosis) were indices of a Marfan-syndrome-like connective tissue disorder.

BAV has been previously described to be an associated feature of an uncommon connective tissue disorder known as Loeys-Dietz syndrome, which is characterized by progressive aortic dilatation and the triad of hypertelorism, cleft palate or bifid uvula, and craniosynostosis. However, no predictive clinical signs of this syndrome were found in the affected family in our case.

Mutations in the TGFBR1 and TGFBR2 genes have been recently demonstrated to result in a wide spectrum of Marfan syndrome-related genetic disorders (e.g., Loeys-Dietz syndrome, and familial thoracic aortic aneurysms and dissections). However, thus far, mutations in the TGFBR1 and TGFBR2 genes have not been found in patients with BAV disease (Arrington *et al.*, 2008; Loscalzo *et al.*, 2007). The possible explanation for this finding may be the heterogeneous nature of BAV disease (i.e., genetic analysis in these studies was not focused on BAV patients with the root dilatation phenotype).

Because there are no targeted genetic studies or detailed surgical reports that have focused on the root dilatation phenotype of BAV disease, the true incidence of TGFBR mutations in BAV disease is not known.

In conclusion, the above discussed data suggest that the proximal aortic dilatation associated with BAV stenosis versus that associated with BAV insufficiency should be considered as different diseases that are possibly amenable to different therapeutic approaches. The heterogeneous nature of BAV disease and the above-discussed pathogenetic insights should be considered when advocating novel surgical treatment guidelines for BAV-associated aortopathy (Guntheroth, 2008).

The widespread belief that BAV disease is a congenital disorder of vascular connective tissue has led to more aggressive treatment recommendations of the proximal aorta in BAV patients, approaching the aortic management recommendations for patients with Marfan syndrome. However, given the heterogeneity of the complex and multifaceted BAV disease,

there is an urgent need for diagnostic tools to reliably distinguish the more from the less "malignant" phenotypes of BAV disease (Girdauskas *et al.*, 2011b).
In the view of above-presented data, it would seem unjustified to extend the surgical procedure to the sinuses of Valsalva in BAV patients with aortic valve stenosis and asymmetric mid-ascending aortic dilatation. In contrast, the relatively small proportion of young male BAV patients with the root dilatation phenotype may benefit from the more radical and aggressive surgical treatment strategy.

2.2 Different cusps fusion patterns in BAV disease

There are two most common patterns of cusp fusion in BAV disease (Fig. 5): the most commonly seen fusion of the left and right coronary cusps, occurs in 70-85% of cases, and union of the right and non-coronary cusps, occurs in the remaining 15-30% of BAV cases. A more detailed classification system of all BAV morphologic variants has been presented by Sievers & Schmidtke (2007).

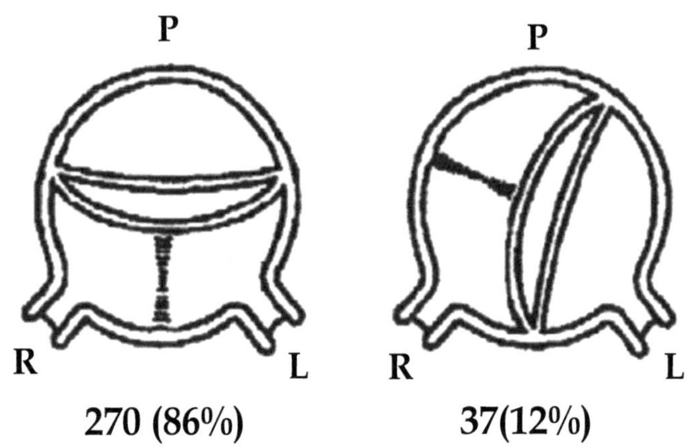

Fig. 5. Schema of morphologic BAV classification (published in *Mayo Clinic Proceedings* 1999; 74:14-26)

There is emerging evidence from the recent literature that the different cusp fusion patterns in BAV disease are associated with specific lesions of the proximal aorta. The histopathological grading of the of aortic wall changes in patients who underwent surgery for BAV disease demonstrated a more severe degree of wall degeneration in the ascending aorta in patients with fusion of the left coronary and right coronary cusps versus fusion of the right coronary and non-coronary cusps (Russo *et al.*, 2007). The prevalence of fibrosis, cystic medial necrosis, elastic fragmentation, and inflammation has been shown to be significantly higher in patients with fusion of the left coronary and right coronary cusps.
Moreover, BAV patients with fusion of the left coronary and right coronary cusps were significantly younger at the time of surgery and had a significantly larger aortic root diameter versus BAV patients with fusion of the right coronary and non-coronary cusps.
The investigators of this study concluded that the presence of more severe histopathological changes at a younger age, and a significantly larger aortic root diameter in BAV patients with fusion of the left coronary and right coronary cusps, may be predictive of a more accelerated and "malignant" BAV phenotype (Russo *et al.*, 2007).

A comparative echocardiographic evaluation of BAV patients with different aortic valve cusp fusion patterns brought comparable findings: fusion of the left coronary and right coronary cusps was associated with a larger aortic root diameter and a smaller aortic arch, than was fusion of the right coronary and non-coronary cusps (Schaefer *et al.*, 2007). Moreover, fusion of the left coronary and right coronary cusps correlated with a higher aortic stiffness index and lower distensibility at the level of the aortic root.
The authors hypothesized that the differences in the spatial propagation of blood flow through the BAVs with fusion of the left coronary and right coronary cusps versus fusion of the right coronary and non-coronary cusps may lead to an inhomogeneous distribution of shear stress and, consequently, to differential alterations of the proximal aortic wall.
The same authors advocated, in their subsequent retrospective analysis (Schaefer *et al.*, 2008), an integrated phenotypic classification of BAV disease that includes both the cusp fusion pattern and the proximal aortic shape. Three different proximal aortic shapes in BAV disease were identified (Fig. 6).

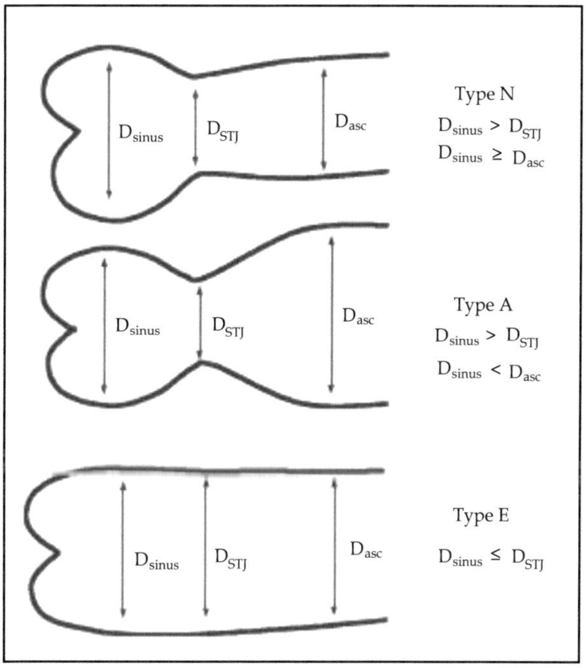

Fig. 6. Proximal aortic shapes in BAV disease (published in *Heart* 2008; 94:1634-1638)

Schaefer *et al.* arrived at very similar findings: fusion of the left coronary and right coronary cusps was associated with normal aortic shape (Type N) but a larger diameter of the aortic annulus and sinuses of Valsalva. In contrast, fusion of the right coronary and non-coronary cusps resulted in ascending aortic dilatation (Type A) and larger aortic arch dimensions. This phenotypic classification has been proposed as a clinical and a research tool in order to precisely define BAV subgroups based on the combination of cusp morphology and proximal aortic shape.
Another retrospective echocardiographic study demonstrated, analogously with Schaefer *et al.* (2007, 2008), that fusion of the right coronary and non-coronary cusps correlated with the

more rapid growth of ascending aortic diameter in the pediatric population (Holmes *et al.*, 2007).

The pathogenetic background for clinical observation of the specific aortic shapes in BAV patients with different morphologic cusp fusion patterns has been elucidated in detailed *in vivo* rheological studies using sophisticated 4D magnetic resonance imaging (Hope *et al.*, 2010). Hope *et al.* analyzed most recently the transvalvular systolic flow patterns in BAVs and demonstrated a markedly abnormal helical flow in patients with BAV, including those without ascending aortic dilatation or aortic valve stenosis. This suggests that the abnormal systolic flow pattern is not secondary to a dilated aorta or to aortic valve stenosis, but that it may be implicated in the pathogenesis of BAV-associated aortopathy.

Interestingly, Hope *et al.*, (2010) were able to convincingly demonstrate in their study two different nested helical flow patterns that are unique for the two most common cusp fusion types in patients with BAV (i.e., fusion of the left coronary and right coronary cusps versus fusion of the right coronary and non-coronary cusps).

The most common fusion pattern of the left coronary and right coronary cusps was associated with a right-anteriorly directed eccentric systolic flow jet, with a resulting marked peripheral skewing towards the convexity of the proximal aorta (Fig. 7a). A left-handed nested systolic helical flow, which was observed specifically in patients with fusion of the right coronary and non-coronary cusps, was associated with a left-posteriorly directed eccentric flow jet (Fig. 7b).

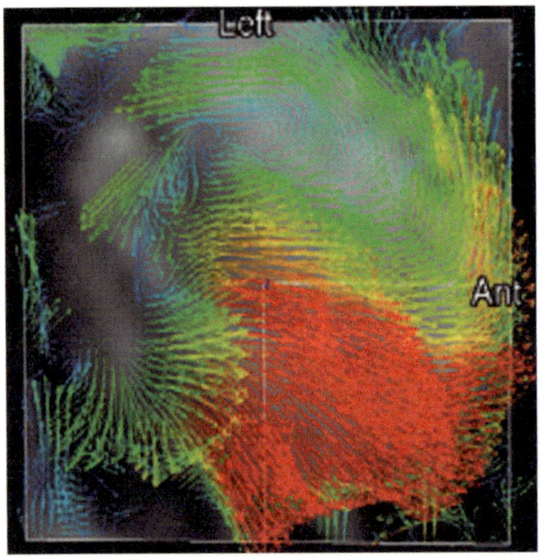

(a)

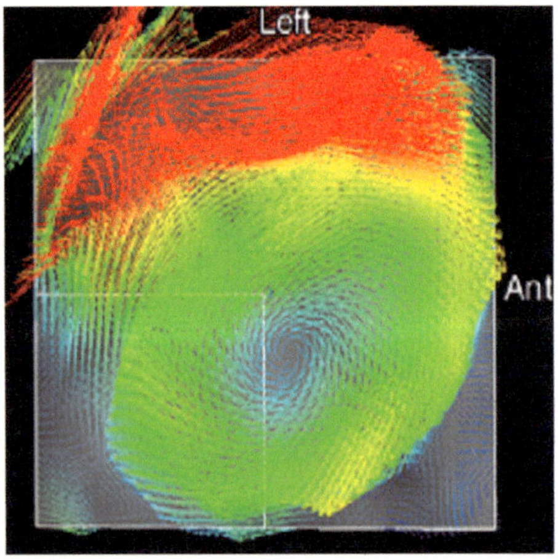

(b)

Fig. 7. Different eccentric transvalvular flow patterns in the proximal aorta in a patient with BAV and fusion of the left coronary and right coronary cusps (a) and in a patient with BAV and fusion of the right coronary and non-coronary cusps (b) (published in *Radiology* 2010; 77:177-185)

Most importantly, Hope *et al.* (2010) convincingly showed that different morphologic patterns of aortic valve cusp fusion in patients with BAV result in the specific orientation of systolic flow jets in the proximal aorta. As a logical consequence of this, it may be assumed that the direction of eccentric systolic flow would be crucial in determining the specific pattern of segmental aortic aneurysm formation in patients with a BAV. Specifically, fusion of the left coronary and right coronary cusps, which generates a right-anterior eccentric flow jet, may be linked to asymmetric dilatation of the mid-ascending tubular aorta. Fusion of the right coronary and non-coronary cusps, which produces a left-posteriorly directed eccentric flow jet, might explain the increased aortic arch dimensions in this subgroup of BAV patients.

Nonetheless, the above-mentioned rheological studies are not able to sufficiently answer all relevant questions concerning the pathogenesis of BAV aortopathy. The paucity of data on the "root dilatation phenotype" precludes any reasonable explanation for the larger aortic root dimensions in BAV patients with fusion of the left coronary and right coronary cusps. Asymmetric involvement of the aortic root (i.e., sinuses of Valsalva) in BAV patients has not been systematically addressed and, accordingly, there are no specific data on aortic root morphology in BAV patients with the "root dilatation phenotype". Additional in-depth studies are required, especially those that correlate the data of rheological studies with the results of detailed histological/ biomolecular analyses from the proximal aorta in BAV patients.

In summary, those detailed rheological data provide a unique hemodynamic insight into the different clinically observed phenotypes of BAV disease. This pathogenetic background should be considered when advocating treatment guidelines for BAV-associated aortopathy.

2.3 Clustering of patients with BAV aortopathy

Some efforts have been made to cluster BAV patients according to the anatomical pattern of proximal aortic dilatation and to propose "individualized" degrees of aortic replacement for these subgroups (Fazel *et al.*, 2008). Hierarchic cluster analysis was proposed by Fazel *et al.* to stratify BAV patients into four distinct patterns of proximal aortic involvement.

Based on four identified dilatation patterns of the proximal aorta, Itoh *et al.* (2010) argue that a custom-tailored approach to aortic resection is reasonable in patients with BAV and should involve the aortic arch in the majority of cases (i.e., in 73% BAV patients undergoing surgery) (Itoh *et al.*, 2010). All these surgical considerations are limited by the theoretical assumption that all patients with BAV have an underlying connective tissue disorder and that aneurismal aortic dilation is not a consequence of the co-existent hemodynamic abnormalities.

There are some major limitations of the study by Fazel *et al.* (2008), which should be stressed when considering such aggressive treatment guidelines for the dilated proximal aorta in the setting of a BAV. As discussed in the previous subparagraphs, there is a growing amount of evidence supporting the notion that hemodynamic factors are involved in the genesis of aortopathy in patients with BAV disease. Therefore, BAV morphology (i.e., different aortic valve cusps fusion patterns) and BAV function (i.e., BAV stenosis versus BAV insufficiency) should undoubtedly be considered when trying to better discriminate between specific subgroups of BAV disease (Della Corte & Cotrufo, 2008).

Interestingly, Fazel *et al.* (2008) found the highest prevalence of right coronary and non-coronary cusp fusion and the highest mean grade of aortic valve insufficiency in the cluster of BAV patients with dilatation of the tubular ascending aorta and aortic arch. These findings correlate appropriately with the data from the rheological and echocardiographic studies by Hope *et al.*, (2010), and Schaefer *et al.*, (2008). Moreover, the retrospective study by Fazel et al., (2008) included only a selected (i.e., non-consecutive) cohort of BAV patients, for whom thoracic aortic imaging data were available for analysis.

Fazel *et al.*, (2008) acknowledged in the discussion of their manuscript that there are no follow-up data to support the hypothesis that such an aggressive aortic replacement strategy results in decreased postoperative morbidity and mortality over the long term. The progression rate of aortic arch aneurysms over years after surgery is currently unknown and the 1.9 mm/year growth rate that Fazel *et al.* (2008) cited refers to the mid-ascending aortic tract.

Moreover, the aforementioned study lacks an accurate comparison of the study population with a matched TAV group, as already stressed in the invited commentary by Della Corte & Cotrufo (2008). Therefore, it is unclear whether the observed proximal aortic dilation patterns are unique to the BAV setting.

In summary, the presented novel treatment recommendations for the identified BAV clusters may not be drawn from purely observational studies, which include only a limited number of selective BAV patients and do not respect the hemodynamic background of different BAV phenotypes.

3. Conclusion

The clinically observed linkage between specific BAV morphology and the associated lesions of the proximal aorta has recently led to several phenotypic classifications which incorporate both aortic valve and proximal aortic anatomy. These novel BAV phenotypes and the fundamental research contributions have been addressed in detail in this chapter.

The predominant anatomical-clinical BAV phenotype of BAV stenosis with an asymmetric mid-ascending aortic dilatation may include those patients in whom the hemodynamic factors play the determinant role. The root dilatation phenotype may be subtended by a less flow-dependent mechanism of aortic wall failure and may be a purely genetic form of BAV disease. This is clearly a completely different disease from BAV stenosis and asymmetric mid-ascending aortic dilatation.

The evidence suggests that the proximal aortic dilatation associated with BAV stenosis versus that with BAV insufficiency should be considered as different diseases that may be amenable to specific therapeutic approaches. According to discussed in this chapter, it seems not justified to extend the surgical procedure to the sinuses of Valsalva in BAV patients with aortic valve stenosis and asymmetric mid-ascending aortic dilatation. In contrast, a relatively small proportion of young male BAV patients with the root dilatation phenotype should probably be treated more radically.

There is emerging evidence from the recent literature that different cusp fusion patterns in BAV disease are associated with specific lesions of the proximal aorta. The presence of more severe aortic histopathological changes at a younger age, and a significantly larger aortic root diameter in BAV patients with fusion of the left coronary and right coronary cusps may be predictive of a more accelerated and "malignant" BAV phenotype.

It has been convincingly demonstrated that fusion of the left coronary and right coronary cusps generates a right-anterior eccentric flow jet, which may hemodynamically explain the resulting asymmetric dilatation of the mid-ascending tubular aorta. Fusion of the right coronary and non-coronary cusps, which produces a left-posteriorly directed eccentric flow jet, might explain the increased aortic arch dimensions in this subgroup of BAV patients. However, the paucity of data on the "root dilatation phenotype" precludes any reasonable hemodynamic explanation for the larger aortic root dimensions in BAV patients with fusion of the left coronary and right coronary cusps. The aortic root (i.e., sinuses of Valsalva) has not been systematically addressed in BAV patients and, accordingly, there are no specific data on aortic root morphology in BAV patients with the "root dilatation phenotype". Additional in-depth studies are required, especially those that correlate the data of rheological studies with the results of detailed histological/ biomolecular analyses from the proximal aorta in BAV patients.

The pathogenetic background of different BAV phenotypes should be considered when advocating treatment guidelines for BAV-associated aortopathy. Data from recent studies requires a reevaluation of the overwhelming support of the genetic nature of BAV aortopathy, and they oblige us to acknowledge that hemodynamic factors are significantly involved in the development of this disease process. Given the described heterogeneity of BAV disease, additional studies are under way to more precisely describe which hypothesis is the "correct" one for explaining the apparently different phenotypes of BAV disease.

From a clinical standpoint, there is an urgent need for diagnostic tools to reliably distinguish the more from the less "malignant" phenotypes of BAV disease. The combination of protein assays (i.e., metalloproteinase 2 plasma levels) and magnetic resonance imaging tests (i.e., quantitative measurement of the angle of the misdirected blood flow) has been most recently proposed as a future diagnostic tool for clinical risk stratification of different BAV phenotypes (den Reijer *et al.*, 2010). Prospective multicenter studies will be needed to prove the predictive value of this novel concept. The identification of a BAV phenotype representing the more "malignant" form of BAV disease, which would be amenable to the more aggressive surgical strategy, still requires special future research efforts.

In conclusion, in the face of most recent *in vitro* and *in vivo* findings on BAV disease, we found it necessary to address the issue of phenotypes in BAV disease. We feel that a critical review of this clinical problem is crucial, because the different BAV phenotypes may be caused by unique pathogenetic mechanisms and may be amenable to different therapeutic approaches. Such observations are not simply theoretical in nature: they significantly affect our surgical approach to the proximal aorta in patients with this common clinical entity of BAV disease.

4. References

Arrington, C.; Sower, T.; Chuckwuk, N.; Stevens, J.; Leppert, M.; Yetman, A. & Bowles, N. (2008). Absence of TGFBR1 and TGFBR2 mutations in patients with bicuspid aortic valve and aortic dilatation. *American Journal of Cardiology*, Vol. 102, No. 5, (September 2008), pp. 629-631, ISSN 0002-9149

Bauer, M.; Gliech, V.; Siniawski, H. & Hetzer, R. (2006). Configuration of the ascending aorta in patients with bicuspid and tricuspid aortic valve disease undergoing aortic valve replacement with or without reduction aortoplasty. *Journal of Heart Valve Disease*, Vol. 15, No. 5, (September 2006), pp. 594-600, ISSN 0966-8519

Biner, S.; Rafique, A.; Ray, I.; Cuk, O.; Siegel, R. & Tolstrup, K. (2009). Aortopathy is prevalent in relatives of bicuspid aortic valve patients. *Journal of the American College of Cardiology*, Vol. 53, No. 24, (June 2009), pp. 2288-2295, ISSN 0735-1097

Conti, C.; Della Corte, A.; Votta, E.; Del Viscovo, L.; Bancone, C.; De Santo, L. & Redaelli, A. (2010). Biomechanical implications of the congenital bicuspid aortic valve: a finite element study of aortic root function from in vivo data. *Journal of Thoracic and Cardiovascular Surgery,* Vol. 140, No. 4, (October 2010), pp. 890-896, ISSN 0022-5223

Cotrufo, M.; Della Corte, A. (2009). The association of bicuspid aortic valve disease with asymmetric dilatation of the tubular ascending aorta: identification of a definite syndrome. *Journal of Cardiovascular Medicine,* Vol. 10, No. 4, (April 2009), pp. 291-297, ISSN 1558-2027

Cotrufo, M.; De Santo, L.; Esposito, S.; Renzulli, A.; Della Corte, A.; De Feo, M.; Marra, C. & Agozzino, L. (2001). Asymmetric medial degeneration of the intrapericardial aorta in aortic valve disease. *International Journal of Cardiology,* Vol.81, No.1, (November 2001), pp. 37-41, ISSN 0167-5273

Cotrufo, M.; Della Corte, A.; De Santo, L.; Quarto, C.; De Feo, M.; Romano, G.; Amarelli, C.; Scardone, M.; Di Meglio, F.; Guerra, G.; Scarano, M.; Vitale, S.; Castaldo, C. & Montagnani, S. (2005). Different patterns of extracellular matrix protein expression in the convexity and the concavity of the dilated aorta with bicuspid aortic valve: preliminary results. *Journal of Thoracic and Cardiovascular Surgery,* Vol. 130, No. 2, (August 2005), pp. 504-511, ISSN 0022-5223

Davies, R.; Kaple, R.; Mandapati, D.; Gallo, A.; Botta, D.; Elefteriades, J. & Coady, M. (2007). Natural history of ascending aortic aneurysms in the setting of an unreplaced bicuspid aortic valve. *Annals of Thoracic Surgery,* Vol. 83, No. 4, (April 2007), pp. 1338-1344, ISSN 0003-4975

Della Corte, A.; De Santo, L.; Montagnani, S.; Quarto, C.; Romano, G.; Amarelli, C.; Scardone, M.; De Feo, M.; Cotrufo, M. & Caianiello, G. (2006). Spatial patterns of matrix protein expression in dilated ascending aorta with aortic regurgitation: congenital bicuspid valve versus Marfan's syndrome. *Journal of Heart Valve Disease,* Vol. 15, No. 1, (January 2006), pp. 20-27, ISSN 0966-8519

Della Corte, A.; Bancone, C.; Quarto, C.; Dialetto, G.; Covino, F.; Scardone, M.; Caianiello, G. & Cotrufo, M. (2007). Predictors of ascending aortic dilatation with bicuspid aortic valve: a wide spectrum of disease expression. *European Journal of Cardiothoracic Surgery,* Vol. 31, No. 3, (March 2007), pp. 397-404, ISSN 1010-7940

Della Corte, A.; Quarto, C.; Bancone, C.; Castaldo, C.; Di Meglio, F.; Nurzynska, D.; De Santo, L.; De Feo, M.; Scardone, M.; Montagnani, S. & Cotrufo, M. (2008). Spatiotemporal patterns of smooth muscle sell changes in ascending aortic dilatation with bicuspid and tricuspid aortic valve stenosis: focus on cell-matrix signalling. *Journal of Thoracic and Cardiovascular Surgery,* Vol. 135, No. 1, (January 2008), pp. 8-18, ISSN 0022-5223

Della Corte, A. & Cotrufo, M. (2008). Bicuspid aortopathy or bicuspid aortopathies? The risk of generalizing. *Journal of Thoracic and Cardiovascular Surgery,* Vol. 136, No. 6, (December 2008) pp. 1604, ISSN 0022-5223

den Reijer, P.; Sallee 3rd, D.; van der Velden, P.; Zaaijer, E.; Parks, W.; Ramamurthy, S.; Robbie, T.; Donati, G.; Lamphier, C.; Beekman, R. & Brummer, M. (2010). Hemodynamic predictors of aortic dilatation in bicuspid aortic valve by velocity-encoded cardiovascular magnetic resonance. *Journal of Cardiovascular Magnetic Resonance,* Vol. 12, No. 1, (January 2010), pp. 4-17, ISSN 1097-6647.

Fazel, S.; Mallidi, H.; Lee, R.; Sheehan, M.; Liang, D.; Fleischmann, D.; Herfkens, R.; Mitchell, R. & Miller, DC. (2008). The aortopathy of bicuspid aortic valve disease has distinctive patterns and usually involves the transverse aortic arch. *Journal of Thoracic and Cardiovascular Surgery,* Vol. 135, No. 4, (April 2008), pp. 901-907, ISSN 0022-5223

Girdauskas, E.; Schulz, S.; Borger, M.; Mierzwa, M. & Kuntze, T (2011). Transforming growth factor-beta receptor type II mutation in a patient with bicuspid aortic valve disease and intraoperative aortic dissection. *Annals of Thoracic Surgery,* (in press), doi:10.1016/j.athoracsur.2010.12.060

Girdauskas, E.; Borger, M.; Secknus, M.; Girdauskas, G. & Kuntze, T. (2011). Is aortopathy in bicuspid aortic valve disease a congenital defect or a result of abnormal hemodynamics? A critical reappraisal of a one-sided argument. *European Journal of Cardiothoracic Surgery,* (February 2011), doi:10.1016/j.ejcts.2011.01.001

Guntheroth, W. (2008). A critical review of the ACC/AHA practice guidelines on bicuspid aortic valve with dilated ascending aorta. *American Journal of Cardiology,* Vol. 102, No. 1, (July 2008), pp. 107-110. ISSN 0002-9149

Itoh, A.; Fischbein, M.; Arata, K. & Miller, DC. (2010). „Peninsula-style" transverse aortic arch replacement in patients with bicuspid aortic valves. *Annals of Thoracic Surgery,* Vol. 90, No. 4, (October 2010), pp. 1369-1371, ISSN 0003-4975

Holmes, K.; Lehmann, C.; Dalal, D.; Nasir, K.; Dietz, H.; Ravekes, W.; Thompson, W. & Spevak, P. (2007). Progressive dilation of the ascending aorta in children with isolated bicuspid aortic valve. *American Journal of Cardiology,* Vol. 99, No. 7, (April 2007), pp. 978-983, ISSN 0002-9149

Hope, M.; Hope, T.; Meadows, A.; Ordovas, K.; Urbania, T.; Alley, M. & Higgins, C. (2010). Bicuspid aortic valve: four-dimensional MR evaluation of ascending aortic systolic flow pattern. *Radiology,* Vol.255, No.1, (April 2010), pp. 53-61, ISSN 0033-8419

Hope, M.; Hope, T.; Meadows, A.; Ordovas, K.; Urbania, T.; Alley, M. & Higgins, C. (2010). Bicuspid aortic valve: four-dimensional MR evaluation of ascending aortic systolic flow patterns. *Radiology,* Vol. 255, No. 1, (April 2010), pp. 53-61, ISSN 0033-8419

Lehoux, S.; Tronc, F. & Tedgui, A. (2002). Mechanisms of blood flow-induced vascular enlargement. *Biorheology,* Vol. 39, No. 3 4, (January 2002), pp. 319-324, ISSN 0006-355X

Loscalzo, M.; Goh, D.; Loeys, B.; Kent, K.; Spevak, P. & Dietz, H. (2007). Familial thoracic aortic dilation and bicommissural aortic valve: a prospective analysis of natural history and inheritance. *American Journal of Medical Genetics Part A,* Vol. 143A, No. 17, (September 2007), pp. 1960-1967, ISSN 1552-4825

Nistri, S.; Sorbo, M.; Marin, M.; Palisi, M.; Scognamiglio, R. & Thiene, G. (1999). Aortic root dilatation in young men with normally functioning bicuspid aortic valves. *Heart,* Vol. 82, No. 1, (July 1999), pp. 19-22, ISSN 1355-6037

Robicsek, F.; Thubrikar, M.; Cook, J. & Fowler, B. (2004). The congenitally bicuspid aortic valve: how does it function? Why does it fail? *Annals of Thoracic Surgery,* Vol. 77, No. 1, (January 2004), pp. 177-185, ISSN 0003-4975

Russo, C.; Cannata, A.; Lanfranconi, M.; Vitali, E.; Garatti, A. & Bonacina, E. (2007). Is aortic wall degeneration related to bicuspid aortic valve anatomy in patients with valvular disease? *Journal of Thoracic and Cardiovascular Surgery,* Vol. 136, No. 4, (October 2008), pp. 937-942, ISSN 0022-5223

Schaefer, B.; Lewin, M.; Stout, K.; Byers, P. & Otto, C. (2007). Usefulness of bicuspid aortic valve phenotype to predict elastic properties of the ascending aorta. *American Journal of Cardiology,* Vol. 99, No. 5, March 2007), pp. 686-690, ISSN 0002-9149

Schaefer, B.; Lewin, M.; Stout, K.; Gill, E.; Prueitt, A.; Byers, P. & Otto, C (2008). The bicuspid aortic valve: an integrated phenotypic classification of leaflet morphology and aortic root shape. *Heart,* Vol. 94, No. 12, (December 2008), pp. 1634-1638, ISSN 1355-6037

Sievers, H. & Schmidtke C (2007). A classification system for the bicuspid aortic valve from 304 surgical specimens. *Journal of Thoracic and Cardiovascular Surgery,* Vol. 133, No. 5, (May 2007), pp. 1226-1233, ISSN 0022-5223

Williams, DS. (2006). Bicuspid aortic valve. *Journal of Insurance Medicine,* Vol. 38, No. 1, pp. 72-74, ISSN 0743-6661

18

Surgical Treatment of Bicuspid Aortic Valve Disease

Ying-Fu Chen[1,3] and Shuo-Tsan Lee[2,3]
[1]*Division of Cardiovascular Surgery, Kaohsiung Medical University Hospital*
[2]*Division of Cardiology, Kaohsiung Medical University Hospital*
[3] *Graduate Institute of Medicine, Kaohsiung Medical University, Kaohsiung*
Taiwan

1. Introduction

Bicuspid aortic valve (BAV) disease is the most common congenital cardiac abnormality, occurring in 0.5% to 2% of the general population (Ward, 2000; Braverman et al., 2005), and in 0.9% as reported in autopsy studies (Roberts, 1970). It may be sporadic or familial and sporadically transmitted through families by an autosomal dominant pathway with a 4:1 male predominance (Cripe et al., 2004). The BAV may be associated with significant valvular dysfunction (Ward, 2000), will develop aortic stenosis and regurgitation, and will be at risk for infective endocarditis (Braverman et al., 2005; Sabet et al., 1999). The bicuspid valve includes different morphologic phenotypes (Sabet et al., 1999; Fernandes et al., 2004). It usually consists of two cusps unequal in size. The cusps are typically oriented right to left, and the larger cusp has a central raphe or ridge (Sievers & Schmidtke, 2007). Notably, pathologic examination of the raphe could not be demonstrated containing the valve tissue (Pomerance, 1972). A review of the echocardiograms of 1135 children with BAV revealed that the most common morphologic pattern is the fusion of the right and left cusps in 70% of all patients (Fernandes et al., 2004). Sievers & Schmidtke (2007) also reported that 71% of 304 BAV surgical specimens had right and left leaflet fusion. Raphal position was described between the right and left cusps in 86% of cases in surgical pathology study reported by Sabet et al (1999). Previously, much of the original focus centered on the abnormal bicuspid valve. Actually, BAV is not just only a disorder of valvulogenesis, but is also a coexistent genetic disorder of the aorta (Siu & Silversides, 2010). More recent studies have shown that structural abnormalities occur at the cellular level. The structural abnormalities of the thoracic aorta disclose a deficiency of fibrillin-1, increased activity of matrix metalloproteinases (MMPs), elastin fragmentation, and vascular smooth muscles cell (VSMC) apoptosis (Tadros et al., 2009). Genetic studies have reported that BAV is likely due to mutations in different genes with dissimilar patterns of inheritance (Cripe et al., 2004; Siu & Silversides, 2010). Typically, mutation in the *NOTCH1* gene leads to signaling abnormalities, which may be responsible for abnormal development of the aortic valve, and later to accelerated valvular calcium deposition (Garg et al., 2005; Mohamed et al., 2006).

In patients with BAV, the presence of BAV is an important risk factor for progressive dilatation of the aortic root and ascending aorta, even in BAV patients with normal valvular function (Nkomo et al., 2003; Gurvitz et al., 2004; Warren et al., 2006). Thus, because of its frequent association with aortic dilatation, BAV may predispose an individual to aortic dissection or rupture. Based on these findings, valve function as well as the diameter of aortoventricular annulus, sinuses of Valsalva, sinotublar junction, and ascending aorta should periodically checked (Tadros et al., 2009). In addition, the current American College of Cardiology (ACC)/American Heart Association (AHA) adult congenital heart disease guidelines suggest that echocardiographic screening for BAV in the first-degree relatives of BAV patients is necessary (Warnes et al., 2008).

2. Surgical treatment of valve pathology

Although the clinical presentation of BAV can vary from a benigh condition, often undetected throughout life, to severe valve disease in infancy (Fenoglio et al., 1977; Siu & Silversides, 2010), it is typically associated with aortic valve dysfunction in adulthood (Brown et al., 2007; Siu & Silversides, 2010). The common valve dysfunctions include stenosis, regurgitation, and endocarditis. Up to 85% of patients with BAV have aortic stenosis after the fifth decade of life (Sabet et al., 1999; Ashikhmina et al., 2010). In contrast, a pure aortic regurgitation (AR) is less common, develops in approximately 20% of patients with BAV, and usually manifests earlier in life than aortic stenosis (Sabet et al., 1999; Ashikhmina et al., 2010). These patients are typically treated with valvular surgery, often during the third and fourth decade of life (Sabet et al., 1999; Casselman et al., 1999; Ward, 2000; Badiu et al., 2011). Because the population of BAV patients is relatively young, in these young patients the choice of an appropriate heart valve substitute is difficult. The optimal substitute should be durable and have a minimal effect on quality of life and longevity (Schafers et al., 2007; Ashikhmina et al., 2010).

2.1 Balloon valvuloplasty

Percutaneous balloon valvuloplasty was first described in 1983 (Labobidi, 1983), and the effectiveness of this method, as well as the low incidence of restenosis shortly after the procedure, was first documented in children with congenital aortic stenosis (Labobidi et al., 1984) and then in a newborn with critical aortic stenosis (Labobidi & Weinhous, 1986). During childhood, valve replacement for the stenotic bicuspid valve is suboptimal because of the continuing growth of the child (Siu & Silversides, 2010). Therefore, in the current era, surgical valvotomy has been replaced by balloon valvuloplasty, which has become the procedure of choice in many centers for the treatment of critically ill infants with a severely stenotic aortic valve (Vida et al., 2005) because it has generally been reported to be a relatively low-risk procedure with reasonable short-term results (Mahle et al., 2010). At the University of Padova, (Padua, Italy), critical aortic stenosis in early infancy has been treated routinely with primary balloon valvuloplasty with a low early mortality (2.9%) and a low incidence of complications (2.9%) (Vida et al., 2005). Moreover, valvuloplasty is the interventional strategy of choice in children and in some young adults with BAV and aortic stenosis, because the aortic valve is usually not calcified at this stage and, therefore, the commissural adhesion can be successfully disrupted and the stenotic valve lesion relieved (Siu & Silversides, 2010). Nevertheless, incomplete relief of the valvar stenosis and significant AR are well-documented after percutaneous balloon valvuloplasty (Bacha et al., 2001). Mid-term results have shown a substantial incidence of restenosis, severe AR, and reintervention (Moore et al., 1996). Reich et al. (2004) demonstrated that a small aortic annulus and BAV were independent predictors of an unfavourable outcome. In such a

situation, patients with hypoplastic annuli and functional bicuspid valves may be primarily considered for surgery in order to prevent the risk of aortic regurgtation and the need for valve replacement (Reich et al., 2004).
Actually, any type of treatment for aortic stenosis in newborns and infants is palliative, and future aortic valve replacement is inevitable (Vida et al., 2005). Because the bioprosthetic valve has a high structural failure rate in young patients and mechanical valves have a risk of anticoagulant-related morbidity, the better option of aortic valve substitute in infants and children is the pulmonary autograft because of its potential for growth (Vida et al., 2005; Behery et al., 2009).

2.2 Aortic valve replacement

As outlined in the 2006 American College of Cardiology/American Heart Association Guidelines for the Management of Patients With Valvular Heart Disease (Bonow et al., 2006), aortic valve repair involves a lack of uniform applicability and lack of widespread experience with surgical techniques. Moreover, there are no clear indications on when repair should be performed and the regarding data demonstrating its safety and durability are limited (Rao et al., 2000; El Khoury et al., 2006; Aicher et al., 2007; Ashikhmina et al., 2010).
In adulthood, the major implication associated with BAV is a tendency toward premature degeneration of the aortic valve with premature presentation of calcific valvular stenosis (Braverman et al., 2005). If aortic valve repair is impossible because of the remarkable structural changes of the aortic valve, the definitive surgical treatment is aortic valve replacement (AVR) (Ali et al., 2010). AVR for aortic valve stenosis is the second most common reason for cardiac surgery in the industrialized countries, and BAV is the second most common cause of aortic valve disease requiring surgery (Etz et al., 2007).
In patients with congenital aortic valve disease such as BAV, Klieverik et al. (2008) reported that the durability of allografts for aortic valve replacement is better than that of bioprostheses, and that their hemodynamic profile is superior to that of mechanical prostheses and bioprostheses. However, the increasing reoperation risk within ten to twenty years remains a major concern. Wijesinghe et al. (2010) proved that transcatheter aortic valve implantation (TAVI) in selected high-risk patients with severe BAV stenosis can be successfully performed with acceptable early clinical outcomes, but that its long-term durability will require further evaluation. On the contrary, Zegdi et al. (2008a) proposed that the valvular opening shape tends to be elliptical rather than circular in patients with BAV; elliptical deployment of valved stents will inevitably create valve distortion that may impede their long-term durability. Thus, BAV stenosis has been considered a questionable indication or even a contraindication for endovascular valve implantation (Zegdi et al., 2008a; Zegdi et al., 2008b).

2.3 Ross procedure

Ross (1967) first described replacement of the diseased aortic valve by pulmonary autograft in 1967, and the full root technique with a pulmonary autograft was introduced in 1989 (Stelzer et al., 1989). The Ross operation is an acceptable alternative to conventional aortic valve replacement and has been shown to provide excellent hemodynamic results. The advantages of this therapeutic option are the use of a viable autologous valve and a low incidence of infection and thrombogenicity, avoidance of anticoagulant therapy, as well as its potential to grow in children (Hanke et al., 2007; Brown et al., 2010; Sievers et al., 2010; Ryan et al., 2011). Nevertheless, there is growing concern about autograft failure and surgical revisions because of the frequently concomitant aortic root and tubular ascending aorta pathology observed in many patients with BAV (Hanke et al., 2010), and the intrisic abnormalities in the wall of the pulmonary artery based on the common embryological origin of the aortic and pulmonary root, which may contribute to progressive neoaortic root dilatation and AR, or both, when the pulmonary root is placed in the systemic position (David et al., 2000; Siu & Silversides, 2010; Hanke et al., 2010).

Progressive dilatation of the pulmonary autograft with or without regurgitation of the autograft valve is a common indication of reoperation (David et al., 2000; Luciani et al., 2003; Takkenberg et al., 2006; Hanke et al., 2007; Ozaslan et al., 2009; Aljassim et al., 2011). In addition, factors contributing to a limited acceptance are the complexity of the operation and a dearth of long-term clinical information on the durability of the autograft in the aortic position and the durability of the pulmonary conduit substitute (Sievers et al., 2010). This concern has led many to reconsider the indication for the Ross operation in the adult population for whom other surgical options are available (Hanke et al., 2007; David, 2009). There are even some do not advocate the use of the Ross operation in patients with BAV disease (Siu & Silversides, 2010). Nevertheless, freedom from autograft or pulmonary conduit reoperation was 89% at 10-year follow-ups reported from the German-Dutch Registry (Sievers et al., 2010). They concluded that the autograft procedure is a valuable therapeutic option for treating aortic valve disease (including BAV) in children, adolescents, and young adults (Sievers et al., 2010). Recently, Ryan et al. (2011) reported that freedom from pulmonary autograft reoperation for aortic stenosis patients was 95% at 10 years. They concluded that the Ross procedure in adults provides excellent freedom from autograft failure in patients operated for aortic stenosis. Conversely, the freedom from autograft reoperation rate was 67% at 10 years in patients with AR preoperatively. Thus, the Ross operation provided suboptimal results in patients with aortic insufficiency (David et al., 2010; Ryan et al., 2011). Therefore, other therapeutic alternatives should be strongly considered in adults presenting primarily with aortic inssuffciency (Ryan et al., 2011).

Pulmonary autograft dilatation is common after the Ross procedure in adults, and this might be a cause of reoperation (David et al., 2000; Aljassim et al., 2011). Patients with BAV and dilated ascending aortas, or patients with dilated aortic root and primarily AR, have been considered the highest-risk groups for dilatation and neo-aortic valvular regurgitation (Tantengco et al., 1999; Simon-Kupilik et al., 2002; Kouchoukos et al., 2004; Brown et al., 2010). Perhaps the modified Ross procedure, as described by Ungerleider et al., in which the autograft is completely encased in a Dacron graft before implantation, may provide better results in patients with preoperative ascending aortic and sinus dilation. A long-term follow-up for successful valve function will be needed for this technique to be recommended for wider use (Ungerleider et al., 2010).

In summary, although the early outcomes continue to be excellent, follow-ups after more than 10 years show continued deterioration of the autografts and a need for reoperation in a substantial percentage of patients, particularly those in whom the root replacement technique was used. Thus, some investigators suggested that the Ross procedure should not routinely be used for aortic valve replacement in adults (Kouchoukos, 2011).

2.4 Repair of regurgitant valve

Clinically, up to 15% to 20% of patients with BAV are reported to have had significant AR as young or middle-aged adults (Roberts, 1970; Olson et al., 1984; Ward, 2000). Although chronic AR is well tolerated for a long time, progressive left ventricular dilatation is a sign with ominous results if timely intervention is not undertaken (Pretre et al., 2006). This makes the choice of valve substitutes difficult because of the limitations of current prostheses. Mechanical valves have an excellent freedom from reoperation, but the cumulative risk of thromboembolic complications and anticoagulation-related hemorrhage may be substantial due to the long exposure time (Khan, 2002; Salem et al., 2004). The Ross procedure is ideal for young patients with BAV stenosis because of its low operative mortality, excellent hemodynamic performance, low prevalence of infection, avoidance of anticoagulant therapy, and potential to grow in children (El Behery et al., 2009; Takkenberg et al., 2009). However, the presence of preoperative AR and aortic root dilatation are important independent determinants of reoperation for pulmonary autograft failure (Elkins et al., 2008; de Kerchove et al., 2009; Ryan et al., 2011). For these reasons, repairing the BAV is an attractive therapeutic option (Ashikhmina et al., 2010; Boodhwani et al., 2011; Ryan et al., 2011).

Reconstruction of the regurgitant bicuspid valve was proposed as early as 1991 by Cosgrove et al. (1991). Subsequently, others have been able to reproduce reconstructive surgery for regurgitant BAV with good results (Aicher et al., 2004); although some others who used the Cosgrove technique proposed that the intraoperative results were rarely predictable and that there was a high reoperation rate in the early phase (Moidl et al., 1995).

Cusp prolapse may be an isolated cause of AR or may exist in conjunction with dilatation of the proximal aorta. Prolapse can be corrected by central plication, triangular resection, or pericardial patch implantation (Aicher et al., 2007b). In the case of limited cusp prolapse, Aicher et al. (2007b) used plication stitches in the central portion of the free edge of the cusp, which were possibly first used by Spencer et al. (1962). The concept of paracommissural plication has been used in AR with ventricular septal defects (Starr et al., 1960; Garamella et al., 1960). Aicher et al. (2007b) showed that central plication had better valve stability with freedom from recurrent AR and freedom from reoperation at 10 years postoperatively compared with the paracommissural approach. In the presence of a more extensive prolapse, a triangular resection was adopted to avoid excessive bulging of plicated cusp tissue (Aicher et al., 2007b). The reason for their low failure rate may be that they frequently corrected prolapse of both cusps in bicuspid aortic valves. On the other hand, using pericardial patch augmentation to close congenital fenestrations that had led to increase coaptation surface provides reliable early and midterm competence of reconstructed bicuspid aortic valves (Aicher et al., 2007b; Doss et al., 2008).

The systemic segmental approach suggested by Pettersson et al. (2008) is based on echocardiographic evaluation. Their findings emphasized that restrictive cusp motion, due to fibrosis or calcification, is an important predictor for recurrent AR following valve repair. On the contrary, redundant or sufficient cusp tissue offers a greater potential for reparability. Several studies have suggested risk factors for failure of BAV repair. Casselman et al. (1999) described left ventricular dysfunction as a predictor of immediate, persistant regurgitation after valve repair. Nash et al. (2005) reported that the paramenters included an eccentric jet of AR, absence of cuspal or commissural thickening, and lack of cusp calcification associated with an increased likelihood of successful valve repair. De Kerchove et al. (2008) suggested that methods of repair of the prolapsed cusp and increased left ventricular end-diastolic diameter were predictors of BAV repair failure. Recently, the size of the aortoventricular junction was also shown to be an independent risk factor for recurrence of regurgitation after repair (Aicher et al., 2011). One should be hesitant to repair a BAV if the aortoventricular diameter is $\geq$ 29mm, if commissural orientation is $< 160°$, and if a pericardial patch is required for partial cusp replacement (Aicher et al., 2011).

In summary, bicuspid aortic valve repair is a viable alternative to replacement with a bioprosthesis because durability and safety are similar between both surgical management methods for AR. Nevertheless, after initial repair, approximately half of the patients require aortic valve replacement within 10 years (Ashikhmina et al., 2010).

3. Surgical treatment of bicuspid aortic valve with aortopathy

Studies on children (Beroukhim et al., 2006; Warren et al., 2006; Holmes et al., 2007) and adults (Yasuda et al., 2003; Davies et al., 2007; Tadros et al., 2009) have reported significantly faster aortic dilatation in the significantly younger with BAV versus trileaflet aortic valve (Figure). BAV is associated with ascending aortic dilatation and enlargement of the aortic root annulus in as many as half of all individuals (Nkomo et al., 2003; Park et al., 2011). Therefore, the size and shape of the ascending aorta should be serially followed. Measurements of the aortic root dimensions should be performed at the level of the ventriculoaortic diameter, sinuses of Valsalva, sinotubular junction, and proximal ascending aorta (Braverman et al., 2005). Surgery to repair the aortic root or replace the ascending aorta has been recommended for those patients with dilated aortic roots or ascending aortas, with possible early prophylactic surgical intervention to prevent dissection or rupture (Bonow et al., 2008; Tadros et al., 2009).

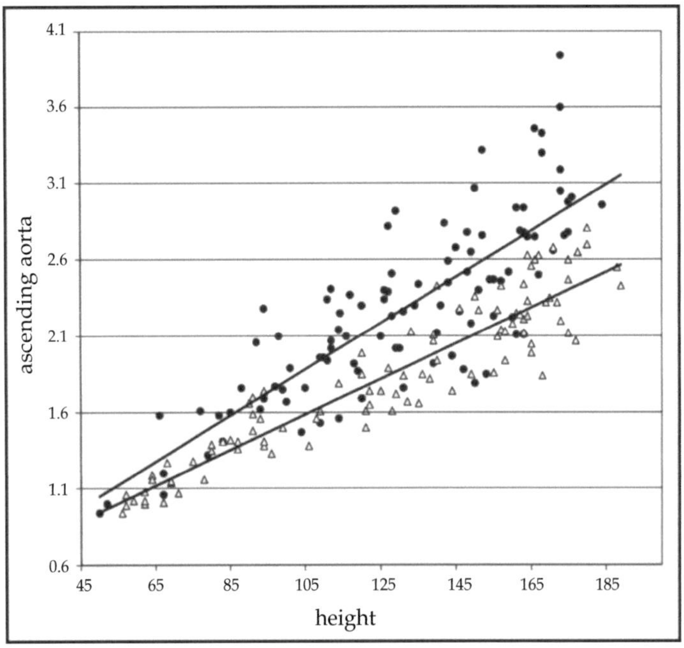

Reprinted from Beroukhim et al. (2006), with permission from Elsevier. Copright 2006.

Fig. 1. Measurements of the ascending aorta in centimeters for patients with BAVs (n = 101) and controls (n = 97). The upper slope *(circles)* represents the BAV group, and the lower slope *(triangles)* represents the control group. Regression equations are in the same order (y = 0.0151x = 0.2926; y = 0.0117x + 0.362). Measurements and height are expressed in centimeters

3.1 Valve sparing aortic root replacement

Valve-sparing aortic root replacements are becoming more popular in view of the potential thromboembolic, and infection complications after composite graft replacement (Cozijnsen et al., 2011). Currently, there are two different techniques of valve-sparing root replacement. In the remodeling technique of the aortic root described by Sarsam and Yacoub (1993), the graft is sewn to the remaining aortic wall around the commissures. In the reimplantation technique proposed by David and Feindel (1992), the graft is fixed at the subannular level, and the valve and commissures are reimplanted inside the graft. Both procedures provide an alternative to composite root replacement with excellent short- and medium-term results, but the long-term durability is not yet established (Cozijnsen et al., 2011). Of note, the main limitation of valve-sparing procedures compared with aortic root replacement with a composite graft remains the predominant risk for reoperation on the bicuspid aortic valve due to recurrent regurgitation (Zehr et al., 2004; Badiu et al., 2010). Cattaneo et al. (2004) reported that late results with valve-sparing procedure in children have been compromised by late root dilatation. Kallenbach et al. (2002) reported that some of their patients subsequently required valve replacement after valve-sparing operations because of subsequent increases in AR. On the contrary, Badiu et al. (2010) said that root replacement with aortic valve-sparing should be offered even in the presence of a BAV or severe AR. Aicher et al. (2007a) reported that remodeling of the aortic root can be treated in patients with dilatation of the aortic root and concomitant AR whenever the aortoventricular junction was not dilated. Freedom from reoperation was 96% at 5 and 10 years, and freedom from valve replacement was 98% at 5 and 10 years. Thus, they concluded that root remodeling leads to durable restoration of bicuspid valve function and that the risk of reoperation is low. Therefore, root remodeling is a good option in patients with aortic dilatation and AR undergoing valve-sparing aortic replacement (Aicher et al., 2007a).
Cusp pathology is frequently encountered in patients with supracoronary ascending aortic aneurysm and AR. Severe AR is not a contraindication to valve-sparing surgery, but careful identification and repair of cusp pathology, in addition to sinotubular junction reduction, is critical for durable, long-term outcome (Boodhwani et al., 2011). There is no actual recommendation in the ACC/AHA guidelines for valve-sparing aortic root replacement (Bonow et al., 2006). The guidelines indicate that this may be possible in selected patients for valve-sparing procedures at experienced centers when there is no AR or deformed or calcified aortic valves (Bonow, 2008). Despite reports of good mid-term results with valve-sparing operations (Doss et al., 2010; De Paulis et al., 2010), some experts believe that leaving behind the abnormal BAV is ill-advised. Therefore, the optimal surgical approach for patients with BAV remains to be defined (Siu & Silverslides, 2010).

3.2 Ascending aorta replacement

It is now widely accepted that an inherent aortopathy exists regardless of whether the valve has any functional abnormalities. Ascending aortic dilatation occurs more frequently and at a younger age in patients with a BAV than in patients with a tricuspid aortic valve (Hahn et al., 1992; Nkomo et al., 2003), and, according to Yasuda et al. (2003), the aorta continues to dilate, even after valve replacement. Because of this, reoperation for aortic aneurysm as well as late aortic dissection and sudden rupture are significantly higher in this group of patients (Russo et al., 2002; Borger et al., 2004). Although the proximal ascending aorta is thought to be the most commonly affected segment (Nkomo et al., 2003; Alegret et al., 2003; Westhoff-Bleck et al., 2005; Tadros et al., 2009; Biner et al., 2009), recent computed tomographic angiography or magnetic resonance angiography and echocardiography studies of the thoracic aorta morphology in patients with BAV show more diffuse and distinct patterns of aortopathy extending from the aortic root to the proximal aortic arch (Westhoff-Bleck et al., 2005; Fazel et al., 2008; Nazer et al., 2010).

The two main theories explaining the phenomenon of aortopathy in patients with BAV are: (1) the genetic theory, and (2) the hemodynamic theory. Both genetic and hemodynamic causes of aortic pathology associated BAV have been postulated, and there is still a great deal of controversy about the pathogenesis of the dilatation of the ascending aorta. Given the marked heterogeneity of BAV disease, further studies are required in order to more accurately determine which theory is the correct one for explaining BAV-derived aortopathy (Bonow et al., 2008; Tadros et al., 2009; Girdauskas et al., 2011).

Looking at the time of rupture or dissection on a lifetime basis, it can be seen that there are sharp hinge points when the ascending aorta reaches 6 cm in diameter (i.e., the patient has incurred a 34% risk of rupture or dissection) (Elefteriades & Farkas, 2010). The mortality rate for elective surgical correction of ascending aortic aneurysm in an experienced center is 2.5% to 5.0% (Elefteriades, 2002; Isselbacher, 2005; Tadros et al., 2009). Ascending aortic aneurysms with an annual risk of rupture or dissection higher than the combined risks of perioperative mortality should be repaired electively (Tadros et al., 2009). These data permit evidence-based criteria for surgical intervention. Because rupture or dissection occurs at 6 cm or more, most adverse events can be prevented by operating at a criterion of less than 6 cm (Elefteriades, 2010). Therefore, for idiopathic ascending aortic aneurysms, surgical intervention at up to 5.5 cm has been recommended on the basis. In contrast, to accommodate differences in body size for optimal operative decision making, Elefteriades (2002) proposed using the aortic size indexed to body mass, rather than using absolute aortic dimensions to predict risk. In other words, adults with small body size should undergo earlier intervention because a higher ratio of aortic size to body size is a predictor of increased risk (Svensson & Khitin, 2002; Svensson et al., 2003; Davies et al., 2006; Tadros et al., 2009). The risk of rupture, dissection, or death is high (approximately 20% per year) when the aortic size index is above 4.25 cm/m^2 (Davies et al., 2006). However, an aorta less than 5 cm in diameter does not guarantee freedom form aortic complications. Autopsies and clinical studies have shown that aortic dissection certainly occurs in near-normal-sized aortas that do not fall within current guidelines for elective aneurysm surgery (Neri et al., 2005; Pape et al., 2007; Bajona et al., 2010).

Between 2006 and 2008, 3 guidelines that focused on advice for patients with a dilating ascending aorta in combination with BAV or AR were published: (1) the 2006 ACC/AHA guidelines for the management of valvular heart disease (Bonow et al., 2006); (2) the 2007 European Society of Cardiology (ESC) guidelines on the management of valvular heart disease (Vahanian et al., 2007); and (3) the 2008 ACC/AHA guidelines for managing adults with congenital heart disease (Warnes et al., 2008). All give practically the same recommendations as the following guidelines.

Management Guidelines for Patients with Bicuspid Aortic Valve with Dilated Ascending Aorta proposed by the 2008 ACC/AHA guidelines (Bonow et al., 2008).

Class I

1. Patients with known bicuspid aortic valves should undergo an initial transthoracic echocardiogram to assess the diameters of the aortic root and ascending aorta. (Level of Evidence: B)

2. Cardiac magnetic resonance imaging or cardiac computed tomography is indicated in patients with bicuspid aortic valves when morphology of the aortic root or ascending aorta cannot be assessed accurately by echocardiography. (Level of Evidence: C)
3. Patients with bicuspid aortic valves and dilatation of the aortic root or ascending aorta (diameter greater than 4.0 cm*) should undergo serial evaluation of aortic root/ascending aorta size and morphology by echocardiography, cardiac magnetic resonance, or computed tomography on a yearly basis. (Level of Evidence: C)
4. Surgery to repair the aortic root or replace the ascending aorta is indicated in patients with bicuspid aortic valves if the diameter of the aortic root or ascending aorta is greater than 5.0 cm* or if the rate of increase in diameter is 0.5 cm per year or more. (Level of evidence: C)
5. In patients with bicuspid valves undergoing AVR because of severe AS or AR repair of the aortic root or replacement of the ascending aorta is indicated if the diameter of the aortic root or ascending aorta is greater than 4.5 cm*. (Level of evidence: C)

Class IIa

6. It is reasonable to give beta-adrenergic blocking agents to patients with bicuspid valves and dilated aortic roots (diameter greater than 4.0 cm*) who are not candidates for surgical correction and who do not have moderate to severe AR. (Level of Evidence: C)
7. Cardiac magnetic resonance imaging or cardiac computed tomography is reasonable in patients with bicuspid aortic valves when aortic root dilatation is detected by echocardiography to further quantify severity of dilatation and involvement of the ascending aorta. (Level of Evidence: B).

The recent 2010 ACC Foundation/AHA guidelines (Hiratzka et al., 2010) have provided adjusted indications for prophylactic surgery of asymptomatic patients with ascending aortic anneurysm.

Class I

Patients with Marfan syndrome or other genetically mediated disorders (vascular Ehlers-Danlos syndrome, Turner syndrome, bicuspid aortic valve, or familial thoracic aortic aneurysm and dissection) should undergo elective operation at smaller diameters (4.0 to 5.0 cm depending on the condition) to avoid acute dissection or rupture. (Level of Evidence: C)

Class IIa

Elective aortic replacement is reasonable for patients with Marfan syndrome, other genetic diseases, or bicuspid aortic valves, when the ratio of maximal ascending or aortic root area (πr^2) in cm^2 divided by the patient's height in meters exceeds 10. (Level of Evidence: C)

More recently, Svensson et al. (2011) proposed that an aortic size larger than 4.5 cm or aortic cross-sectional area/height ratio greater than 8 to 10 should be considered triggers for concurrent aortic repair, because there is no added risk, and late survival is better.

3.3 Thoracic endovascular aneurysm repair (TEVAR)

TEVAR is a minimally invasive method for managing descending aortic aneurysms in the acute and chronic settings (Dake et al., 1994; Dake et al., 1999) and is becoming more frequently used (Gopaldas et al., 2010; Coady et al., 2010). TEVAR has been suggested as an alternative, although controversial, approach for the elderly with comorbidities because of the high risk of open repair (Tadros et al., 2009). Nevertheless, TEVAR is not currently a definitive approach for managing ascending aortic dilatation with BAV because the contour of the ascending aorta is complex and has inadequate landing zones to anchor the stent grafts, especially when dilatation involves the aortic annulus and extends into the arch (Tadros et al., 2009). Whether future developments in these techniques may render them more widely applicable as therapy for ascending aortic aortopathy is still unknown (Atkins et al., 2006; Vallely et al., 2008). On the other hand, the data are limited on TEVAR in patients with connective tissue disease, as well as on continued aortic expansion and higher reintervention rates (Geisbusch et al., 2008). Furthermore, patients with BAV aortopathy typically need intervention at a younger age, and currently TEVAR has not been shown to provide as durable long-term results as does open repair (Tadros et al., 2009).

4. Conclusion

BAV is the most common form of congenital heart defect. Although BAV can be found in isolation because of a disorder of valvulogenesis, it is also represented as coexistent aspects of a genetic disorder of aortopathy, and is most frequently associated with dilatation of the proximal ascending aorta. With or without intervention, patients with BAV require continued surveillance. Because BAV is a disease of both valvular pathology and aortopathy, surgical decision making is more complicated than previously believed. There are several surgical options available to patients with BAV. New surgical techniques have been developed, especially for valve repair and transcatheter aortic valve implantation. The surgical intervention option should be individualized to each patient, depending on the surgical experience and skill of the surgeon. If aortic valve repair for valvular regurgitation or an aortic valve sparing procedure is to be considered, patients should be referred to experienced centers where there is both interest and experience with surgical options available for these patients. Compared with trileaflet aortic valve patients, BAV disease patients have a connective tissue disorder leading to a higher prevalence and faster yearly growth rate of the ascending aorta, which increases the risk of dissection or rupture at a younger age. Thus, ascending aortic dilatation associated with BAV warrants frequent monitoring, with possible early prophylactic intervention to prevent dissection or rupture.

5. References

Aicher D, Langer F, Kissinger A, Lausberg H, Fries R, & Schafers HJ (2004). Valve-sparing aortic root replacement in bicuspid aortic valve: a reasonable option. *J Thorac Cardiovasc Surg*, Vol 128, No. 5,(November 2004),pp. 662-668, ISSN 0022-5223.

Aicher D, Langer F, Lausberg H, Bierbach B, & Schafers HJ (2007a). Aortic root remodeling: ten-year experience with 274 patients. *J Thorac Cardiovasc Surg*, Vol 134, No. 4,(October 2007), pp. 909-915, ISSN 0022-5223.

Aicher D, Langer F, Adam O, Tscholl D, Lausberg H, & Schafers HJ (2007b). Cusp repair in aortic valve reconstruction: does the technique affect stability? *J Thorac Cardiovasc Surg*, Vol 134, No. 6,(December 2007), pp. 1533-1538, ISSN 0022-5223.

Aicher D, Kunihara T, Issa OA, Brittner B, Graber S, & Schafers HJ (2011). Valve configuration determines long-term results after repair of the bicuspid aortic valve. *Circulation*, Vol 123, No. 2, (January 2011),pp. 178-185, ISSN 1524-4539.

Alegret JM, Duran I, Parazon O, Vernis JM, Ameijide A, Rabassa A, & Masana L (2003). Prevalence of and predictors of bicuspid aortic valves in patients with dilated aortic roots. *Am J Cardiol*, Vol 91, No. 5, (March 2003), pp. 619-622, ISSN 0002-9149.

Ali A, Patel A, Ali ZA, Abu-Omar Y, Freed D, Sheikh AY, Athanasiou T, & Pepper J (2010). Stentless aortic valve replacement in patients with bicuspid aortic valve disease: clinical outcome and aortic diameter changes during follow-up. *Eur J Cardiothorac Surg*, Vol 38, No. 2, (August 2010), pp. 134-140, ISSN 1010-7940.

Aljassim O, Svensson G, Perrotta S, Jeppsson A, & Bech-Hanssen O (2011). Dilatation of the pulmonary autograft and native aorta after the Ross procedure: a comprehensive echocardiographic study. *J Thorac Cardiovasc Surg*, (In press), ISSN 0022-5223.

Ashikhmina E, Sundt TM III, Dearani JA, Connolly HM, Li Z, & Schaff HV (2010). Repair of the bicuspid aortic valve: a viable alternative to replacement with a bioprosthesis. *J Thorac Cardiovasc Surg*, Vol 139, No. 6, (June 2010), pp. 1395-1401, ISSN 0022-5223.

Atkins MD Jr, Black JH 3rd, & Cambria RP (2006). Aortic dissection: perspectives in the era of stent-graft repair. *J Vasc Surg*, Vol 43, No. Suppl A, (February 2006), pp. 30A-43A, ISSN 1097-6809.

Bacha EA, Satou GM, Moran AM, Zuraakowski D, Marx GR, Keane JF, & Jonas RA (2001). Valve-sparing operation for balloon-induced aortic regurgitation in congenital aortic stenosis. *J Thorac Cardiovasc Surg*, Vol 122, No. 1, (July 2001), pp. 162-168, ISSN 0022-5223.

Badiu CC, Eichinger W, Bleiziffer S, Hermes G, Hettich I, Krane M, Bauernschmitt R, & Lange R (2010). Should root replacement with aortic valve-sparing be offered to patients with bicuspid valves or severe aortic regurgitation? *Eur J Cardiothorac Surg*, Vol 38, No 5, (November 2010), pp. 515-522, ISSN 1010-7940.

Badiu CC, Bleiziffer S, Erchinger WB, Zaimova I, Hutter A, Mazzitelli D, Voss B, & Lange R (2011). Are bicuspid aortic valves a limitation for aortic valve repair? *Eur J Cardiothorac Surg* (In Press), ISSN 1010-7940.

Bajona P, & Feindel CM (2010). Bicuspid-aortic valve surgery: repair or repair or replace? *Curr Opin Cardiol*, Vol 25, No. 2, (March 2010). pp. 119-123, ISSN 0268-4705.

Behery SE, Rubay J, Sluysmans T, Absil B, & Oaert C (2009). Midterm results of the Ross procedure in a pediatric population: bicuspid aortic valve is not a contraindication. *Pediatr Cardiol*, Vol 30, No. 3, (April 2009), pp. 219-224, ISSN 0172-0643.

Berouhim RS, Kruzick TL, Taylor AL, Gao D, & Yetman AT (2006). Progression of aortic dilation in children with a functionally normal bicuspid aortic valve. Am j Cardiol, Vol 98, No. 6, (September 2006),pp. 828-830, ISSN 0002-9149.

Biner S, Rafique AM, Ray I, Cuk O, Siegel RJ, & Tolstrup K (2009). Aortopathy is prevalent in relative of bicuspid aortic valve patients. *J Am Coll Cardiol*, Vol 53, No. 24, (June 2009), pp. 2288-2295, ISSN 0735-1097.

Bonow RO, Carabello BA, Chatterjee K, de Leon AC Jr, Faxon DP, Freed MD, Gaasch WH, Lytle BW, Nishimura RA, O'Gara PT, O'Rourke RA, Otto CM, Shah PM, Shanewise JS, Smith SC Jr, Jacobs AK, Adams CD, Anderson JL, Antman EM, Fuster V, Halperin Jl, Hiratzka LF, Hunt SA, Page RL, & Riegl B (2006). ACC/AHA 2006 guidelines for the management of patients with valvular Heart disease: a report of the American College of Cardiology/American Heart Association Task Force on Practice Guidelines (Writing Committee to Revise the 1998 Guidelines for the Management of Patients with Valvular Heart Disease) developed in collaboration with the Society of Cardiovascular Anesthesiologists endorsed by the Society for Cardiovascular Angiography and Interventions and the Society of Thoracic Surgeons. J Am Coll Cardiol, Vol 48, No. 3, (August 2006), pp. e1-e148, ISSN 0735-1097

Bonow RO (2008). Bicuspid aortic valves and dilated aortas: a critical review of the critical review of the ACC/AHA practice guidelines recommendations. *Am J Cardiol,* Vol 107, No. 1, (July 2008), pp. 111-114, ISSN 0002-9149.

Bonow RO, Carabello BA, Chatterjee K, de Leon AC Jr, Faxon DP, Freed MD, Gaasch WH, Lytle BW, Nishimura RA, O'Gara PT, O'Rourke RA, Otto CM, Shah PM, & Shanewise JS (2008). 2008 Focused Update Incorporated Into the ACC/AHA 2006 Guidelines for the Management of Patients With Valvular Heart Disease. A Report of the American College of Cardiology/American Heart Association Task Force on Practice Guideline (Writing Committee to Revise the 1998 Guidelines for the Management of Patients with Valvular Heart Disease). *Circulation,* Vol 118, No. 15, (October 2008), pp. e523-e661, ISSN 1524-4539.

Boodhwani M, de Kerchove L, Glineur D, Rubay J, Vanoverschelde JL, Van Dyck M, Noirhomme P, & El Khoury G (2011). Aortic valve repair with ascending aortic aneurysms: associated lesions and adjunctive techniques. *Eur J Cardiothorac Surg* (In press), ISSN 1010-7940.

Borger MA, Preston M, Ivanov J, Fedak PW, Davierwala P, Armstrong S, & David TE (2004). Should the ascending aorta be replaced more frequently in patients with bicuspid aortic valve disease? *J Thorac Cardiovasc Surg,* Vol 128, No. 5, (November 2004), pp. 677-683, ISSN 0022-5223.

Braverman AC, Guven H, Beardslee MA, Makan M, Kates AM, & Moon MR (2005). The bicuspid aortic valve. *Curr Probl Cardiol,* Vol 30, No. 9, (September 2005), pp. 470-522, ISSN 0146-2806.

Brown JW, Ruzmetov M, Rodefeld MD, Mahomed Y, & Turrentine MW. (2007). Incidence of and risk factors for pulmonary autograft dilation after Ross aortic valve replacement. *Ann Thorac Surg,* Vol.83, No. 5, (May 2007), pp. 1781-1817, ISSN 0003-4975.

Brown JW, Ruzmetov M, Shahriari AP, Rodefeld MD, Mahomed Y, & Turrentine MW (2010). Modification of the Ross aortic valve replacement to prevent autograft dilatation. *Eur J Cardiothorac Surg,* Vol 37, No. 5, (May 2010),pp. 1002-1007, ISSN 1010-7940.

Casselman FP, Gillinov AM, Akhrass R, Kasirajan V, Blackstone AH, & Cosgrove DM (1999). Intermediate-term durability of bicuspid aortic valve repair for prolapsing leaflet. *Eur J Cardiothorac Surg.* Vol 15, No. 3, (March 1999), pp. 302-308, ISSN 1010-7940.

Cattaneo SM, Bethea BT, Alejo DE, Spevak PJ, Clauss SB, Dietz HC, Gott VL, & Cameron DE (2004). Surgery for aortic root aneurysms in children: a 21-year experiencec in 50 pateints. *Ann Thorac Surg,* Vol. 77, No. 1, (January 2004), pp. 168-176, ISSN 0003-4975.

Coady MA, Ikonomidis JS, Cheung AT, Matsumoto AH, Dake MD, Chaikof EL, Cambria RP, Mora-Mangano CT, Sundt TM, Sellke FW, & on behalf of the American Heart Association Council on Cardiovascular Surgery and Anesthesia and Council on Peripheral Vascular Disease (2010). Surgical Management of Descending Thoracic

Aortic Disease: Open and Endovascular Approaches. A Scientific Statement From the American Heart Association. *Circulation*, Vol 121, No. 25, (January 2010), pp. 2780-2804, ISSN 1524-4539.

Cosgrove DM, Rosenkranz ER, Hendren WG, Bartlett JC, & Stewart WJ (1991). Valvuloplasty for aortic insufficiency. *J Thorac Cardiovasc Surg*, Vol 102, No. 4, (October, 1999), pp. 571-576, ISSN 0022-5223.

Cozijnsen L, Braam RL, Waalewijn RA, Schepens MAAM, Loeys BL, van Oosterhout MFM, Barge-Schaapveld DQCM, & Mulder BJM (2011). What is new in dilatation of the ascending aorta? Review of current literature and practical advice for the cardiologist. *Circulation*, Vol 123, No. 8, (March 2011), pp. 924-928, ISSN 1524-4539.

Cripe L, Andelfinger G, Martin LJ, Shooner K, & Benson DW (2004). Bicuspid aortic valve is heritable. *J Am Coll Cardiol*, Vol 44, No. 1, (July 2004), pp. 138-143, ISSN 0735-1097.

Dake MD, Miller DC, Semba CP, Mitchell RS, Walker PJ, & Liddell RP (1994). Transluminal placement of endovascular stent-grafts for the treatment of descending thoracic aortic aneurysms. *N Engl J Med*, Vol 331, No. 26, (December 1994), pp. 1729-1734, ISSN 1533-4406.

Dake D, Kato N, Mitchell RS, Semba CP, Razavi MK, Shimono T, Hirano T, Takeda K, Yada I, & Miller DC (1999). Endovascular stent-graft placement for the treatment of acute aortic dissection. *N Engl J Med*, Vol 340, No. 20, (May 1999), pp. 1546-1552, ISSN 1533-4406.

David TE, & Feindel CM (1992). An aortic valve-sparing operation for patients with aortic incompetence and aneurysm of the ascending aorta. *J Thorac Cardiovasc Surg*, Vol 103, No. 4, (April 1992), pp. 617-621, ISSN 0022-5223.

David TE, Omran A, Ivanov J, Armstrong S, de Sa MP, Sonnenberg B, & Webb G, (2000). Dilatation of the pulmonary autograft after the Ross procedure. *J Thorac Cardiovasc Surg*, Vol 119, No. 2, (February 2000), pp. 210-220, ISSN 0022-5223.

David TE, (2009). Ross procedure at the crossroads. *Circulation*, Vol 119, No. 2, (January 2009), pp. 207-209, ISSN 1524-4539.

David TE, Woo A, Armstrong S, & Maganti M (2010). When is the Ross operation a good option to treat aortic valve disease? *J Thorac Cardiovasc Surg*, Vol 139, No. 1, (January 2010), pp. 68-75, ISSN 0022-5223.

Davies RR, Gallo A, Coady MA, Tellides G, Botta DM, Tellides G, Botta DM, Burke B, Coe MP, Kopf GS, & Elefteriades JA (2006). Novel Measurement of relative aortic size predicts rupture of thoracic aortic aneurysms. *Ann Thorac Surg*, Vol 81, No. 1, (January 2006), pp. 169-177, ISSN 0003-4975.

Davies RR, Kaple RK, Mandapati D, Gallo A, Botha DM Jr, Elefteriades JA, & Coady MA (2007). Natural history of ascending aortic aneurysms in the setting of an unreplaced bicuspid aortic valve. *Ann Thorac Surg*, Vol 83, No. 4, (April 2007), pp. 1338-1344, ISSN 0003-4975.

De Kerchove L, Glineur D, Poncelet A, Boodhwani M, Rubay J, Dhoore W, Noirhomme P, & El Khoury G (2008). Repair of aortic leaflet prolapse: a ten-year experience. *Eur J Cardiothorac Surg*, Vol 34, No. 4, (October 2008), pp. 785-791, ISSN 1010-7940.

De Kerchove L, Rubay J, Pasquet A, Poncelet A, Ovaert C, Pirotte M, Buche M, D'Hoore W, Noirhomme P, & El Khoury G(2009). Ross operation in the adult: long-term outcomes after root replacement and inclusion techniques. *Ann Thorac Surg*, Vol 87, No. 1, (January 2009), pp. 95-102, ISSN 0003-4975.

De Paulis R, Scaffa R, Nardella S, Maselli D, Weltert L, Bertoldo F, Pacini D, Settepani F, Tarelli G, Gallotti R, Di Bartolomeo R, & Chiariello L (2010). Use of the Valsalva graft and long-term follow-up. *J Thorac Cardiovasc Surg,* Vol 140, No. 6S, (December 2010), pp. S23-S27, ISSN 0022-5223.

Doss M, Sirat S, Risteski P, Martens S, & Moritz A (2008). Pericardial patch augmentation for repair incompetent bicuspid aortic valves at midterm. *Eur J Cardiothorac Surg,* Vol 33, No. 5, (May 2008), pp. 881-884, ISSN 1010-7940.

Doss M, Risteski P, Sirat S, Bakhtiary F, Martens S, & Moritz A (2010). Aortic root stability in bicuspid aortic valve disease: patch augmentation plus reduction aortoplasty versus modified David type repair. *Eur J Cardiothorac Surg,* Vol 38, No. 5, (November 2010), pp. 523-527, ISSN 1010-7940.

El Khoury G, Vanoverschelde JL, Glineur D, Pierard F, Verhelst RR, Rubay J, Funken JC, Watremez C, Astarci P, Lacroix V, Poncelet A, & Noirhomme P (2006). Repair of bicuspid aortic valves in patients with aortic regurgitation. *Circulation,* Vol 114, No. Suppl I, (July 2006), pp. I 610-I 616, ISSN 1524-4539.

EL Behery, Rubay J, Sluysmans T, Absil B, & Ovaert C (2009). Midterm results of the Ross Procedure in a pediatric population: bicuspid aortic valve is not a contraindication. *Pediatr Cardiol,* Vol 30, No. 3, (April 2009), pp. 219-224, ISSN 0172-0643.

Elefteriades JA (2002). Natural history of thoracic aortic aneurysms: indications for surgery, and surgical versus nonsurgical risks. *Ann Thorac Surg,* Vol 74, No. 5, (November 2002), pp. S1877-S1880.

Elefteriades JA, & Farkas E (2010). Thoracic aortic aneurysm: clinically pertinent cortroversies and uncertainties. *J Am Coll Cardiol,* Vol 55, No. 9, (March 2010), pp. 841-857, ISSN 0735-1097.

Elkins RC, Thompson DM, Lane MM, Elkin CC, & Peyton MD (2008). Ross operation: 16-year experience. *J Thorac Cardiovasc Surg,* Vol 136, No. 3, (September 2008), pp. 623-630, ISSN 0022-5223.

Etz C, Homann TM, Silovitz D, Spielvogel D, Bodian CA, Luehr M, DiLuozzo G, Plestis KA, & Griepp RB (2007). Long-term survival after the Bentall procedure in 206 patients with bicuspid aortic valve. *Ann Thorac Surg,* Vol 84, No. 4, (October 2007), pp. 1186-1194, ISSN 0003-4975.

Fazel SS, Mallidi HR, Lee RS, Sheehan MP, Liang D, Fleischman D, Herfkens R, Mitchell RS, & Miller DC (2008). The aortopathy of bicuspid aortic valve disease has distinctive patterns and usually involves the transverse aortic arch. *J Thorac Cardiovasc Surg,* Vol 135, No. 4, (April 2008), pp. 901-907, ISSN 0022-5223.

Fenoglio JJ Jr, McAllister HA Jr, DeCastro CM, Davia JE, & Cheitlin MD (1977). Congenital bicuspid aortic valve after age 20. *Am J Cardiol.* Vol.39, No. 2, (February 1977), pp. 164-169, ISSN 0002-9149.

Fernandes SM, Sanders SP, Khairy P, Jenkins KJ, Gauvreau K, Lang P, Simonds H, & Colan SD (2004). Morphology of bicuspid aortic valve in children and adolescents. *J Am Coll Cardiol,* Vol 44, No. 8, (October 2004), pp. 1648-1651, ISSN 0735-1097.

Garamella JJ, Cruz AB Jr, Heupel WH, Dahl JC, Jensen NK, & Berman R (1960). Ventricular septal defect with aortic insufficiency. Successful surgical correction of both defects by the transaortic approach. *Am J Cardiol,* Vol 5, No. 2, (February 1960), pp. 266-272. ISSN 0002-9149.

Garg V, Muth AN, Ransom JF, Schluterman MK, Barnes R, King IN, Grossfeld PD, & Srivastava D (2005). Mutations in NOTCH1 cause aortic valve disease. *Nature*, Vol 437, No. 7056, (September 2005),pp. 270-274, ISSN 0028-0836.

Geisbusch P, Kotelis D, von Tengg-Kobligk H, Hyhlik-Durr A, Allenberg JR, & Bockler D (2008). Thoracic aortic endografting in patients with connective tissue diseases. *J Endovasc Ther*, Vol 15, No. 2, (April 2008), ISSN 1526-6028.

Girdauskas E, Borger MA, Secknus MA, Girdauskas G, & Kuntze T (2011). Is aortopathy in bicuspid aortic valve disease a congenital defect or a result of abnormal hemodynamics? A critical reappraisal of a one-sided argument. *Eur J Cardiothorac Surg*, Vol 39, No. 6, (January 2011), pp. 809-814. ISSN 1010-7940.

Gopaldas RR, Huh J, Dao TK, LeMaire SA, Chu D, Bakaeen FG, & Coselli JS (2010). Superior nationwide outcomes of endovascular versus open repair for isolated descending thoracic aortic aneurysm in 11669 patients *J Thorac Cardiovasc Surg*, Vol 140, No. 5, (November 2010), pp. 1001-1010, ISSN 0022-5223.

Gurvitz M, Chang RK, Drant S, & Allada V (2004). Frequency of aortic root dilation in children with a bicuspid aortic valve. *Am J Cardiol*, Vol 94, No. 10, (November 2004), pp. 1337-1340, ISSN 0002-9149.

Hahn RT, Roman MJ, Mogtader AH, & Devereux RB (1992). Association of aortic dilation with regurgitant, stenotic and functionally normal bicuspid aortic valves. *J Am Coll Cardiol*, Vol 19, No. 2, (February 1992), pp. 283-288, ISSN 0735-1097.

Hanke T, Stierle U, Boehm JO, Botha CA, Bechtel JFM, Erasmi A, Misfeld M, Hemmer W, Rein JG, Robinson DR, Lange R, Horer J, Moritz A, Ozaslan F, Wahlers T, Franke UFW, Hetzer R, Hubler M, Ziemer G, Graf B, Ross DM, Sievers HH, & on behalf of the German Ross Registry (2007). Autograft regurgitation and aortic root dimensions after the Ross procedure: the German Ross Registry Experience. *Circulation,* Vol 116, No. 11 Suppl I, (September 2007), pp. I 251-I 258, ISSN 1524-4539.

Hanke T, Charitos EI, Stierle U, Robinson DR, Hemmer W, Moritz A, Lange R, Sievers HH, & on behalf of the German Ross Registry (2010). The Ross operation - a feasible and safe option in the setting of a bicuspid aortic valve? *Eur J Cardiothorac Surg*, Vol 38, No. 3, (September 2010), pp. 333-339, ISSN 1010-7940.

Hiratzka LF, Bakris GL, Beckman JA, Bersin RM, Carr VF, Casey Jr DE, Eagle KA, Hermann LK, Isselbacher EM, Kazerooni EA, Kouchoukos NT, Lytle BW, Milewicz DM, Beich DL, Sen S, Shinn JA, Svensson LG, & Williams DM (2010). 2010 ACCF/AHA/AATS/ACR/ASA/SCAI/SIR/STS/SVM Guidelines for the Diagnosis and Management of Patients with Thoracic Aortic Disease. *J Am Coll Cardiol*, Vol 55, No. 14, (April 2010), pp. e27-e129, ISSN 0735-1097.

Holmes KW, Lehmann CU, Dalal D, Nasir K, Dietz HC, Ravekes WJ, Thompson WR, & Spevak PJ (2007). Progression dilation of the ascending aorta in children with isolated bicuspid aortic valve. *Am J Cardiol*, Vol 99, No. 7, (April 2007), pp. 978-983, ISSN 0002-9149.

Isselbacher EM (2005). Thorcic and abdominal aortic aneurysms. *Circulation*, Vol 111, No. 6, (February 2005), pp. 816-828, ISSN 1524-4539.

Kallenbach K, Hagl C, Walles T, Leyh RG, Pethid K, Haverich K, & Harringer W (2002). Results of a valve-sparing aortic root reconstruction in 158 consecutive patients. *Ann Thorac Surg*, Vol. 74, No. 6, (December 2002), pp. 2026-2032, ISSN 0003-4975.

Khan S (2002). Long-term outcomes with mechanical and tissue valves. *J Heart Valve Dis*, Vol 11, No. Supple I, (January 2002), pp. I8- I14, ISSN 0966-8519.

Klieverik LMA, Bekkers JA, Roos JW, Eijkemans MJC, Raap GB, Bogers JJC, & Takkenberg JJM (2008). Autograft or allograft aortic valve replacement in young adult patients with congenital aortic valve disease. *Eur Heart J*, Vol 29, No. 11, (June 2008), pp. 1446-1453, ISSN 0195-668X.

Kouchoukos NT, Masetti P, Nickerson NJ, Castner CF, Shannon WD, & Davila-Roman VG (2004). The Ross procedure: long-term clinical and echocardiographic follow-up. *Ann Thorac Surg*, Vol 78, No. 3, (September 2004), pp. 773-781, ISSN 0003-4975.

Kouchoukos NT (2011). Should we still do the Ross operation in adult? *Curr Opin Cardiol*, Vol 26, No. 2, (March 2011), pp. 94-98, ISSN 0268-4705.

Labobidi Z (1983). Aortic balloon valvuloplasty. *Am Heart J*, Vol 106, No. 4, (October 1983), pp. 751-752, ISSN 0002-8703.

Labobidi Z, Wu JR, & Walls JT (1984). Percutaneous balloon aortic valvuloplasty: results in 23 patients. *Am J Caradiol*, Vol 53, No. 1, (January 1984), pp. 194-197, ISSN 0002-9149.

Labobidi Z, & Weinhous L (1986). Successful balloon valvuloplasty for neonatal critical aortic stenosis. *Am Heart J*. Vol 112, No. 5, (January 1986), pp. 913-916, ISSN 0002-8703.

Luciani GB, Casali G, Favaro A, Prioli MA, Barozzi L, Santini F, & Mazzucco A (2003). Fate of the aortic root late after the Ross operation. *Circulation*, Vol 108, No. Suppl II, (September 2003), pp. II61-II67, ISSN 1524-4539.

Mahle WT, Sutherlard JL, & Frias PA (2010). Outcome of isolated bicuspid aortic valve in childhood. *J Pediatr*, Vol 157, No. 3, (September 2010), pp. 445-449, ISSN 0022-3476.

Mohamed SA, Aherrahrou Z, Liptau H, Erasmi AW, Hagemann C, Wrobel S, Borzym K, Schunkert H, Sievers HH, & Erdmann J (2006). Novel missense mutations (p.T596M and p.P1797H) in NOTCH1 in patients with bicuspid aortic valve. *Biochem Biophys Res Commun*, Vol 345, No. 4, (July 2006), pp. 1460-1465, ISSN 0006-291X.

Moidl R, Moritz A, Simon P, Kupilik N, Wolner E, & Mohl W (1995). Echocardiographic results after repair of incompetent bicuspid aortic valves. *Ann Thorac Sirg*, Vol 60, No. 3, (September 1995), pp. 669-672. ISSN 0003-4975.

Moore P, Egilo E, Mowrey H, Perry SB, Lock JE, & Keane JF (1996). Midterm results of balloon dilation of congenital aortic stenosis: predictors of success. J *Am Coll Cardiol*, Vol 27, No. 5, (April 1996), pp. 1257-1263, ISSN 0735-1097.

Nash PJ, Vitvitsky E, Li J, Cosgrove DM 3rd, Pettersson G, & Grimm RA (2005). Feasibility of valve repair for regurgitant biscupid aortic valves: an ecchocardiographic study. *Ann Thorac Surg*, Vol 79, No. 5, (May 2005), pp. 1473-1479, ISSN 0003-4975.

Nazer RI, Elhenawy AM, Fazel SS, Garrido-Olivares LE, Armstrong S, & David TE (2010). The influence of operative techniques on the outcomes of bicuspid aortic valve disease and aortic dilatation. *Ann Thorac Surg*, Vol 89, No. 6, (June 2010), pp. 1918-1924, ISSN 0003-4975

Neri E, Barabesi L, Buklas D, Vricella LA, Benvenuti A, Tucci E, Sassi C, & Massetti M (2005). Limited role of aortic size in the genesis of acute type A aortic dissection. *Eur J Cardiothorac Surg*, Vol 28, No. 6, (December 2005), pp. 857-863, ISSN 1010-7940.

Nkomo VT, Enriquez-Sarano M, Ammash NM, Melton LJ 3rd, Bailey KR, Desjardins V, Horn RA, & Tajik (2003). Bicuspid aortic valve associated with aortic dilatation: a community-based study. *Arterioscler Thromb Vasc Biol,* Vol 23, No. 4, (February 2003), pp. 351-356, ISSN 1524-4636.

Olson LJ, Subramanian R, & Edwards WD (1984). Surgical pathology of pure aortic insufficiency: a study of 225 cases. *Mayo Clin Proc,* Vol 59, No. 12,(December 1984), pp. 835-841, ISSN 0025-6196.

Ozaslan F, Wittlinger T, Monsefi N, Bouhmidi T, Theres S, Doss M, Wimmer-Greinecker G, & Moritz A (2009). Long-term follow-up of supra-annular pulmonary autograft aortic root replacement in patients with bicuspid aortic valve. *Eur J Cardiothorac Surg,* Vol 34, No. 3, (September 2009), pp. 583-588, ISSN 1010-7940.

Pape LA, Tsai TT, Isselbacher EM, Oh JK, O'Gara PT, Evangelista A, Fattori R, Meinhardt G, Trimarchi S, Bossone E, Suzuki T, Cooper JV, Froehlich JB, Nienaber CA, & Eagle KA (2007). Aortic diameter ≥ 5.5 cm is not a good predictor of type A aortic dissection: observations from the International Registry of Acute Aortic Dissection (IRAD). *Circulation,* Vol 116, No. 10, (September 2007), pp. 1120-1127, ISSN 0009-7322.

Park CB, Greason KL, Suri RM, Michelena HI, Schaff HV, & Sundt TM 3rd (2011). Fate of nonreplaced sinuses of Valsalva in bicuspid aortic valve disease. *J Thorac Cardiovasc Surg,* Vol 142, No.2, (August 2011), pp.278-284, ISSN 0022-5223.

Pettersson GB, Crucean AC, Savage R, Halley CM, Grimm RA, Svensson LG, Naficy S, Gillinov AM, Feng J, & Blackstone EH (2008). Toward predictable repair of regurgitant aortic valves. A systemic morphology-directed approach to bicommissural repair. *J Am Coll Cardiol,* Vol 52, No. 1, (July 2008), pp. 40-49, ISSN 0735-1097.

Pomerance A (1972). Pathogenesis of aortic stenosis and its relation to age. *Br Heart J,* Vol 34, No. 6, (June 1972), pp. 569-574, ISSN 0007-0769.

Pretre R, Kadner A, Dave H, Bettex D, & Genoni M (2006). Tricuspidisation of the aortic valve with creation of a crown-like annulus is able to restore a normal valve function in bicuspid aortic valves. *Eur J Cardiothorac Surg,* Vol 29, No. 6, (June 2006),pp. 1001-1007, ISSN 1010-7940.

Rao V, van Arsdell GS, David TE, Azakie A, & William WG (2000). Aortic valve repair for adult congenital heart disease: a 22-year experience. *Circulation,* Vol 102 (Suppl 3), No 19, (November 2000), pp.III40-III43, ISSN 1524-4539.

Reich O, Tax P, Marek J, Gilik J, Tomek V, Chaloupecky V, Bartakova H, & Skovranek J (2004). Long term results of percutaneous balloon valvoplasty of congenital aortic stenosis: independent predictors of outcome. *Heart,* Vol 90, No. 1, (January 2004), pp. 70-76, ISSN 1355-6037.

Roberts WC (1970). The congenitally bicuspid aortic valve: a study of 85 autopsy cases. *Am J Cardiol,* Vol 26, No. 1, (July 1970), pp. 72-83, ISSN 0002-9149.

Ross DN (1967). Replacement of aortic and mitral valves with a pulmonary autograft. *Lancet,* Vol 2, No. 7523, (November 1967), pp. 956-958, ISSN 0140-6736.

Russo CF, Mazzetti S, Garatti A, Ribera E, Milazzo A, Bruschi G, Lanfranconi M, Colombo T, & Vitali E (2002). Aortic complications after bicuspid aortic valve replacement: Long-term results. *Ann Thorac Surg,* Vol 74, No. 5, (November 2002),pp. S1773-S1776, ISSN 0003-4975.

Ryan WH, Prince SL, Culica D, & Herbert MA (2011). The Ross procedure performed for aortic insufficiency is associated with increased autograft reoperation. *Ann Thorac Surg*, Vol 91, No. 1, (January 2011), pp. 64-70, ISSN 0003-4975.

Sabet HY, Edwards WD, Tazelaar HD, & Daly RC (1999). Congenitally bicuspid aortic valves: a surgical pathology study of 542 cases (1991 through 1996) and a literature review of 2715 additional cases. *Mayo Clin Proc*, Vol 74, No. 1, (January 1999), pp. 14-26, ISSN 0025-6196.

Salem DN, Stein PD, Al-Ahmad A, Bussey HI, Horstkotte D, Miller N, & Pauker SG (2004). Antithrombotic therapy in valvular heart disease - native and prosthetic; Seventh ACCP Conference on Antithrombotic and Thrombolytic Therapy. *Chest*, Vol 126, No. 3 Suppl, (September 2004), pp. S457-S482, ISSN 0012-3692.

Sarsam MA, & Yacoub M (1993). Remodeling of the aortic valve annulus. *J Thorac Cardiovasc Surg*, Vol 105, No. 3, (March 1993), pp. 435-438, ISSN 0022-5223.

Schafers HJ, Aicher D, Langer F, & Lausberg HF (2007). Preservation of the bicuspid aortic valve. *Ann Thorac Surg*, Vol 83, No. 2, (February 2007), pp. S740-S745, ISSN 0003-4975.

Sievers HH, & Schmidtke C (2007). A classification system for the bicuspid aortic valve from 304 surgical specimens. *J Thorac Cardiovasc Surg*, Vol 133, No. 5, (May 2007), pp. 1226-1233, ISSN 0022-5223.

Sievers HH, Stierle U, Charitos EI, Hanke T, Misfeld M, Bechtel M, Gorski A, Franke UFW, Graf B, Robinson DR, Bogers AJJC, Dodge-Khatami A, Boehm JO, Rein JG, Botha CA, Lange R, Hoerer J, Moritz A, Wahlers T, Breuer M, Ferrari-Kuehne K, Hetzer R, Huebler M, Ziemer G, Takkenberg JJM, Hemmer W, & on behalf of the German-Dutch Ross Registry (2010). Major adverse cardiac and cerebrovascular events after the Ross procedure. A report from the German-Dutch Ross Registry. *Circulation*, Vol 122, No. 11 Suppl, (September 2010), pp. S216-S223, ISSN 1524-4539.

Simon-Kupilik N, Bialy J, Moidl R, Kasimir MT, Mittlbock M, Seebacher G, Wolner E, & Simon P (2002). Dilatation of the autograft root after the Ross operation. Eur J Cardiothorac Surg, Vol 21, No. 3, (March 2002), pp. 470-473, ISSN 1010-7940.

Siu SC, & Silversides CK (2010). Bricuspid aortic valve disease. *J Am Coll Cardiol*, Vol 55, No. 25, (January 2010), pp. 2789-2800, ISSN 0735-1097.

Spencer FC, Bahnson HT, & Neill CA (1962). The treatment of aortic regurgitation associated with a ventricular septal defect. *J Thorac Cardiovasc Surg*, Vol 43, No. 2, (Febrauary 1962), pp. 222-233, ISSN 0022-5223.

Starr A, Menasche V, & Dotter C (1960). Surgical correction of aortic insufficiency associated with ventricular septal defect. *Surg Gynecl Obstet*, Vol 111, No. 1, (July 1960),pp. 71-76, ISSN 1072-7515.

Stelzer P, Jones DJ, & Elkins RC (1989). Aortic root replacement with pulmonary autograft. *Circulation*, Vol 80, No. 5 Suppl III, (November 1989), pp. III 209-III 213, ISSN 1524-4539.

Svensson LG, & Khitin L (2002). Aortic cross-sectional area/height ratio timing od aortic surgery in asymptomatic patients with Marfan syndrome. *J Thorac Cardiovasc Surg*, Vol 123, No. 2,(February 2002), pp. 360-361, ISSN 0022-5223.

Svensson LG, Kim K-H, Lytle BW, & Cosgrove DM (2003). Relationship of aortic cross-sectional area to height ratio and the risk of aortic dissection in patients with bicuspid aortic valves. *J Thorac Cardiovasc Surg*, Vol 126, No. 3, (September 2003), pp. 892-893, ISSN 0022-5223.

Svensson LG, Kim KH, Blackstone EH, Rajeswaran J, Gillinov AM, Mihaljevic T,griffin BP, Grimm R, Stewart WJ, Hammer DF, & Lytle BW (2011). Bicuspid aortic valve surgery with proactive ascending aorta repair. *J Thorac Cardiovasc Surg* Vol 142, No.3, (September 2011), pp.622-629, ISSN 0022-5223.

Tadros TM, Klein MD, & Shapira OM (2009). Ascending aortic dilatation associated with bicuspid aortic valve: pathophysiology, molecular biology, and clinical implication. *Circulation*, Vol 119, No. 6, (February 2009), pp. 880-890, ISSN 1524-4539.

Takkenberg JJ, van Herwerden LA, Galema TW, Bekkers JA, Kleyburg-Linkers VE, Eijkemans MJC, & Bogers AJ (2006). Serial echocardiographic assessment of autograft regurgitation and root dimensions after the modified Ross procedure. *J Heart Valve Dis*, Vol 15, No. 1, (January 2006),pp. 100-107, ISSN 0966-8519.

Takkenberg JJ, Klieverik LM, Schoof PH, van Suylen RJ, van Herwerden LA, Zondervan PE, Ross-Hesselink JW, Eijkemans MJ, Yacoub MH, & Bogers AJ (2009). The Ross procedure: a systemic review and meta-analysis. *Circulation*, Vol 119, No. 2, (January 2009),pp. 222-228, ISSN 1524-4539.

Tantengco MV, Humes RA, Clapp SK, Lobdell KW, Walters HL 3rd, Hakimi M, & Epstein ML (1999). Aortic root dilation after the Ross procedure. *Am J Cardiol*, Vol 83, No. 6, (March 1999), pp. 915-920, ISSN 0002-9149.

Urgerleider RM, Ootaki Y, Shen I, & Welke KF (2010). Modified Ross procedure to prevent autograft dilatation. *Ann Thorac Surg*, Vol 90, No. 3, (September 2010), pp. 1035-1037, ISSN 0003-4975.

Vahanian A, Baumgartner, Baumgartner H, Bax J, Butchart E, Dion R, Filipattos G, Flachskampf F, Hall R, Iung B, Kasprzak J, Nataf P, Tirnos P, Toracca L, & Wenink A (2007). Guidelines on the management of valvular heart disease. *Eur Heart J*, Vol 28, No. 2, (January 2007), pp. 230-268, ISSN 0915-668X.

Vallely MP, Semsarian C, & Bannon PG (2008). Management of the ascending aorta in patients with bicuspid aortic valve disease. *Heart Lung Circ*, Vol 17, No. 5, (October 2008), pp. 357-363, ISSN 1444-2892.

Vida VL, Bottio T, Milanesi O, Reffo E, Biffanti R, Bonato R, & Stellin G (2005). Critical aortic stenosis in early infancy: surgical treatment for residual lesions after balloon dilation. *Ann Thorac Surg*. Vol 79, No. 1, (January 2005), pp. 47-51, ISSN 0003-4975.

Ward C (2000). Clinical significance of the bicuspid aortic valve. *Heart*, Vol 83, No. 1, (January 2000),pp. 81-85, ISSN 1355-6037.

Warnes CA, Williams RG, Bashore TM, Child JS, Connolly HM, Dearani JA, del Nido P, Fasules JW, Graham TP Jr, Hijazi ZM, Hunt SA, King ME, Landzberg MJ, Miner PD, Radford MJ, Walsh EP, Webb GD, Smith SC Jr, Jacobs AK, Adams CD, Anderson JL, Antman EM, Buller CE, Creager MA, Ettinger SM, Halperin JL, Hunt SA, Krumholz HM, Kushner FG, Lytle BW, Nishimura RA, Page RL, Riegel B, Tarkington LG, Yancy CW; American College of Cardiology; American Heart Association Task Force on Practice Guidelines (Writing Committee to Develop Guidelines on the Management of Adults With Congenital Heart Disease); American Society of Echocardiography; Heart Rhythm Society; International Society for Adult Congenital Heart Disease; Society for Cardiovascular Angiography and Interventions; & Society of Thoracic Surgeons.(2008). ACC/AHA 2008 guidelines for the management of adults with congenital heart disease: a report of the American College of Cardiology/American Heart Association Task

Force on Practice Guidelines (Writing Committee to Develop Guidelines on the Management of Adults with Congenital Heart Disease) developed in collaboration With the American Society of Echocardiography, Heart Rhythm Society, International Society for Adult Congenital Heart Disease, Society for Cardiovascular Angiography and Interventions, and Society of Thoracic Surgeons. *J Am Coll Cardiol*, Vol. 52, No. 23, (December 2008), pp. e1-e121, ISSN 0735-1097.

Warren AE, Boyd ML, O'Connell C, & Dodds L (2006). Dilatation of the ascending aorta in paediatric patients with bicuspid aortic valve: frequency, rate of progression and risk factors. *Heart*, Vol 92, No. 10, (October 2006), pp. 1496-1500, ISSN 1355-6037.

Westhoff-Bleck M, Meyer GP, Lotz J, Tutarel O, Weiss T, Rafflenbeul W, Drexler H, & Schroder E (2005). Dilatation of the entire thoracic aorta in patients with bicuspid aortic valve: a magnetic resonance angiography study. *Vasa*, Vol 34, No. 3, (August 2005),pp. 181-185, ISSN 0000-0000.

Wijesinghe N, Ye J, Rodes-Cabau J, Cheung A, Velianou JL, Natarajan MK, Dumont E, Nietlispach F, Gurvitch R, Wood DA, Tay E, & Webb JG (2010). Transcatheter aortic valve implantation in patients with bicuspid aortic valve stenosis. *J Am Coll Cardiol Intv*, Vol 3, No. 11, (March 2010), pp. 1122-1125, ISSN 1936-8798.

Yasuda H, Nakatani S, Stugaard M, Tsujita-Kuroda Y, Bando K, Kobayashi J, Yamagishi M, Kitakaze M, Kitamura S, & Miyatake K (2003). Failure to prevent progressive dilation of ascending aorta by aortic valve replacement in patients with bicuspid aortic valve: comparison with tricuspid aortic valve. *Circulation*, Vol 108, No. Suppl II, (September 2003), pp.II291-II294, ISSN 1524-4539.

Zegdi R, Khabbaz Z, Ciobotaru V, Noghin M, Deloche A, & Fabiani JN (2008a). Calcific bicuspid aortic stenosis: a questionable indication for endovascular valve implantation? *Ann Throac Surg*, Vol 85, No. 1, (January 2008),pp. 342, ISSN 0003-4975.

Zegdi R, Ciobotaru V, Noghin M, Sleilaty G, Lafont A, Latremouille C, & Fabiani JN (2008b). Is it reasonable to treat all calcified stenotic aortic valves with a valved stent? *J Am Coll Cardiol*, Vol 51, No. 5, (February 2008),pp. 579-584, ISSN 0735-1097.

Zehr KJ, Orszulak TA, Mullany CJ, Matloobi A, Daly RC, Dearani JA, Sundt 3rd TM, Puga FJ, Danielson GK, & Schaff RV (2004). Surgery for aneurysms of the aortic root: a 30-year experience. *Circulation*, Vol 110, No. 11, (September 2004), pp. 1364-1371, ISSN 1524-4539.